Principles and Practice of Child Neurology in Infancy

Edited by Colin Kennedy

Professor of Neurology and Paediatrics, Clinical Neurosciences,
University of Southampton, and Honorary Consultant
Paediatric Neurologist, Southampton University Hospital NHS
Foundation Trust, Southampton, United Kingdom

2012
Mac Keith Press

© 2012 Mac Keith Press

Editor: Hilary M. Hart
Managing Director: Ann-Marie Halligan
Production Manager: Udoka Ohuonu
Project Manager: Mirjana Misina

First published in this edition in 2012 by Mac Keith Press
6 Market Road, London N7 9PW, UK

British Library Cataloguing-in-Publication data
A catalogue record for this book is available from the British Library

ISBN: 978-1-908316-35-6

Printed by Latimer Trend & Company, Plymouth, UK
Mac Keith Press is supported by Scope

Contents

Contents

Authors' appointments

Ulrika Ådén, Associate Professor, Department of Women's and Children's Health, Karolinska Institutet, Stockholm, Sweden

Ilona Autti-Rämö, Pediatric Neurologist, Chief of Health Research, The Social Insurance Institution, Helsinki, Finland

Peter Baxter, Consultant Paediatric Neurologist, Sheffield Childrens Hospital; Honorary Senior Lecturer, University of Sheffield, Sheffield, UK

Vittorio Belmonti, Child Neuropsychiatrist and PhD Student, Department of Developmental Neuroscience, Stella Maris Scientific Institute and University of Pisa, Pisa, Italy

Gian Paolo Chiaffoni, Head, Department of Pediatrics, Conegliano and Vittorio Veneto Hospitals, Conegliano, Italy and WHO-Europe Temporary Advisor for Perinatal Care

Richard Chin, Director of the Muir Maxwell Epilepsy Centre and Clinical Senior Lecturer in Paediatric Neurosciences, Child Life and Health, University of Edinburgh, Scotland, and Consultant Paediatric Neurologist, Royal Hospital for Sick Children, Edinburgh, Scotland, UK

Imti Choonara, Professor of Child Health, Academic Division of Child Health (University of Nottingham), The Medical School, Derbyshire Children's Hospital, Derby, UK

Giovanni Cioni, University Professor and Head, Department of Developmental Neuroscience, Stella Maris Scientific Institute and University of Pisa, Pisa, Italy

J. Helen Cross, The Prince of Wales's Chair of Childhood Epilepsy; UCL-Institute of Child Health, Great Ormond Street Hospital for Children, London and Young Epilepsy, Lingfield, UK

Leena Haataja, Professor, Deptartment of Pediatric Neurology, Turku University Hospital, Turku, Finland

Hans Hartmann, Consultant Neuropaediatrician, Department of Pediatric Kidney, Liver and Metabolic Diseases, Hannover Medical School, Hannover, Germany

Florian Heinen Professor of Paediatrics and Head of Department, Paediatric Neurology and Developmental Medicine, University of Munich, Hauner Children's Hospital, Center for International Health (CIH), LMU, Munich, Germany

Varsine Jaladyan, Child Neurology, "Arabkir" Joint Medical Centre & Institute of Child and Adolescent Health, Yerevan, Armenia

Colin Kennedy, Professor of Neurology and Paediatrics, Clinical Neurosciences, University of Southampton, and Honorary Consultant Paediatric Neurologist, University Hospital Southampton NHS Foundation Trust, Southampton, UK

Rachel Kneen, Consultant Paediatric Neurologist, Department of Neurology, Littlewood's Neuroscience Unit, Alder Hey Children's NHS Foundation Trust and Institute of Infection and Global Health, University of Liverpool, Liverpool, UK

Fenella Kirkham, Consultant Paediatric Neurologist, Department of Child Health, University Hospitals Southampton NHS Foundation Trust, Southampton and Professor of Paediatric Neurology, Neurosciences Unit, University College London Institute of Child Health, London, UK

Andrew L. Lux, Consultant in Paediatric Neurology, Bristol Royal Hospital for Children, Bristol Education Centre, Bristol, UK

Vlatka Mejaski-Bosnjak, Professor of Child Neurology, Head of Department of Neuropediatrics, Children's Hospital Zagreb, School of Medicine, University of Zagreb, Zagreb, Croatia

Tuuli Metsvaht, Associate Professor, University of Tartu, Department of Paediatrics; Head of Paediatric Intensive Care Unit, Tartu University Hospital, Department of Anaesthesiology and Intensive Care, Tartu, Estonia

Mary Morgan, Consultant Paediatric Haematologist, Department of Paediatric Haematology/Oncology, University Hospital Southampton NHS Foundation Trust, Southampton, UK

Alla Nechay, Paediatric Neurologist, Neurology Department, Paediatric Hospital of Kiev, Bogatyrska, Kiev, Ukraine.

Charles Newton, Cheryl and Reece Scott Professor of Psychiatry, University of Oxford, Oxford, UK

Richard W. Newton, Consultant Paediatric Neurologist, Royal Manchester Children's Hospital, Manchester, UK

Barbara Plecko, Professor of Paediatric Neurology, University of Zurich, Zurich,Switzerland

Audrone Prasauskiene, Child Neurologist, Director of the Children's Rehabilitation Hospital (Lithuanian University of Health); Lecturer, Department of Rehabilitation, Lithuanian University of Health Sciences, Kaunas, Lithuania

Dainius Puras, Head and Associate Professor, Centre of Child Psychiatry and Social Paediatrics, Clinic of Psychiatry, Vilnius University, Lithuania

Boika Rechel, Clinical Lecturer in Public Health, Honorary Consultant in Public Health Medicine, Norwich Medical School, University of East Anglia, Norwich, UK

Maryze Schoneveld van der Linde, Cultural Anthopologist and Consultant, Patient Centered Solutions, Varsseveld, The Netherlands

Bernhard Schmitt, Professor of Paediatrics and Paediatric Neurology, Division of Clinical Neurophysiology/Epilepsy, University Children's Hospital, Zurich

Thomas Sejersen, Senior Consultant, Neuropaediatric Unit, Astrid Lindgrens Barnsjukhus, Karolinska University Hospital, Stockholm, Sweden

John B.P. Stephenson, Honorary Professor of Paediatric Neurology, University of Glasgow and Retired Consultant Paediatric Neurologist, Fraser of Allander Neurosciences Unit, Royal Hospital for Sick Children, Glasgow, Scotland, UK

Inga Talvik, Associate Professor, University of Tartu; Department of Paediatrics, Tartu University Hospital, Children's Clinic, Head of Child Neurology Unit, Tartu, Estonia

Tiina Talvik, Professor Emerita, Senior Consultant in Paediatric Neurology, Department of Paediatrics, University of Tartu, Tartu University Hospital, Children's Clinic, Tartu, Estonia

Meral Topcu, Professor of Paediatrics and Paediatric Neurologist, Hacettepe Children's Hospital, Department of Child Neurology, Ankara, Turkey

Daniele Trevisanuto, Consultant Neonatologist, Neonatal Intensive Care Unit, Pediatric Department, University of Padua, Azienda Ospedaliera di Padova, Padua, Italy.

Brigitte Vollmer, Senior Lecturer in Paediatric and Neonatal Neurology; Hon. Consultant Paediatric Neurologist, University Hospital Southampton NHS Foundation Trust, Southampton, UK

Valerie Walker, Honorary Consultant Chemical Pathologist, Southampton University Hospitals NHS Trust, Southampton, UK

Jane Williams, Consultant Community Paediatrician, Nottingham University Hospitals NHS Trust, Nottingham, United Kingdom

Dilek Yalnizoglu, Professor of Pediatrics and Pediatric Neurologist, Hacettepe Children's Hospital, Department of Child Neurology, Ankara, Turkey

Foreword

The publication of a handbook on neurological disorders in infancy is an important contribution to health professional practice. The first 1000 days – 9 months of gestation followed by the first two years of life – are critical to the healthy development of a child and it is in this period that the foundations of neurological function are established. The first year is frequently the period of first presentation of neurological disorders and having a handbook focused on the this period is of particular value.

One of the challenges that the book highlights is the wide variation in clinicians' understanding of development, their recognition of the importance of prevention and promotion practices that support healthy development, and the challenges of diagnosis and management of common neurological conditions during this period. In order to address these concerns the book is structured to first provide this background information in a number of chapters that cover basic definitions, the importance of teamwork and the role of families in supporting development, prevention and promotion strategies and developmental assessment.

The first section covers the key diagnostic resources that are required in this age group, some or all of which may be available to clinicians in their assessment of infants with an apparent neurological disorder.

The chapter on evidence-based medicine is an important reminder that practising evidence-based medicine helps ensure that as clinicians, the concept foremost in our minds is to do no harm.

Therapeutics for infants can be challenging and an area of potential risk given that some physicians treating infants may not be specifically trained in their care and therapeutic windows can be narrow. This chapter combined with the specific clinical chapters will be a useful support to clinicians with limited experience with this age group. Reference to the World Health Organization information on essential medicines for children will be supportive to those clinicians working in resource-limited regions of the world.

The second section of the handbook has chapters focused on the major disorders that present in infancy, including febrile and non-febrile encephalopathies, the range of presentations that occur with seizures, macro- and microcephaly, and neuromotor disorders including the 'floppy infant', cerebral palsy and other movement disorders. The section concludes with a most important chapter on progressive loss of skills.

The Chapters in the handbook are structured in a way that allows the reader to easily identify areas of interest while skipping over those chapters where the content is familiar to them.

International authorities in child development and child neurology have contributed to this important handbook with the able editorial support of Professor Colin Kennedy. The content will be an accessible and valuable resource to clinicians globally, from resource poor to resource rich environments and to clinicians whose focus is exclusively the care of young children to those clinicians, often in resource poor countries, who are charged with the care of individuals across the age span. Infancy can be a daunting period of diagnostic and therapeutic challenge and this handbook will bring much needed support to those charged with the care of infants, no matter what their individual level of experience may be. Effective management of neurological disorders during this period can have a long-term impact on the health and further development of these infants and this handbook makes an important contribution to the knowledge clinicians need in order to be most effective.

Robert W Armstrong, MD PhD FRCPC
Professor and Foundation Dean
Aga Khan University, Kenya

Preface

The spark that eventually led to this book was the publication of a systematic observational assessment of paediatric hospital care in parts of Eastern Europe and Central Asia by the World Health Organization (WHO).[1] The study identified over-investigation, over-diagnosis and over-treatment of neurological disease, especially in infancy. Discrepancies between local and international diagnostic classification systems were a major contributory cause of these problems. At around the time of that publication, senior clinicians from the region were seeking to strengthen links with the relevant Western European specialty groups. A dialogue with the European Office of WHO ensued and a plan to provide guidance for neurological management was included within a 2009–2011 grant from the European Commission to WHO to improve maternal and child health in the Republic of Kazakhstan.

The present book provides not only clinical guidance but also defines normality and abnormality in the field of child neurology and neurodevelopment and sets out principles of prevention and management of neurological disease in infancy. The final result is a volume outlining the management of suspected neurological and neurodevelopmental disorders that is applicable in all parts of the globe.

The book is in two parts. The first part sets out the principles of working with families, of clinical assessment and of the use of investigations, treatments and evidence-based medicine. The second part provides detailed guidance on the practice of child neurology as it applies to infancy. This symptom-based, rather than disease-based,

[1]Duke T Keshishiyan E, Aigul Kuttumuratova A et al. Quality of hospital care for children in Kazakhstan, Republic of Moldova, and Russia: systematic observational assessment. *The Lancet* 2006, 367: 919–25.

approach should make the content accessible to all, whatever their background knowledge of disease classification.

This book is the result of the work of an international working group, drawn from the European Paediatric Neurology Society and the European Academy of Childhood Disability and chaired by myself, and a Kazakh working group, chaired by Dr Altynshash Jaxybayeva. There have been two striking features of this project. The first is that the contributors displayed their enthusiasm to share their expert knowledge. The second feature has been the engagement of clinical colleagues on the working group in the Republic of Kazakhstan. Their willingness to change and desire to modernise is apparent not only from their attitude to the content of this book but also in their commitment to undergraduate and postgraduate medical training based on knowledge of internationally accepted principles and practice in the care of children with neurological problems.

The book is an up-to-date summary of current clinical practice that will be useful in both resource-rich and resource-poor health systems to those practising as specialists in paediatric neurology and disability, to any paediatrician dealing with epilepsy and other neurological disorders and to other health professionals in the multidisciplinary team.

Colin Kennedy
Southampton, September 2012

Acknowledgements

This book would not have been possible without Alberta Bacci, Vivian Barnekow, Aigul Kuttumuratova, and Olga Pettersson at the WHO European Office; Abuova Gaukar and others at the WHO Kazakhstan Country Office; my fellow members of the international working group; Dr Altynshash Jaxybayeva and others on the Kazakh working group; the executive boards of the European Paediatric Neurology Society and the European Academy of Childhood Disability; my fellow authors; and Caroline Black, Ann-Marie Halligan, Hilary Hart, Mirjana Misina, Udoka Ohuonu and James Dufficy at Mac Keith Press. I would also particularly like to thank Drs Gian Paolo Ciaffoni, Leena Haataja, Richard Newton, Thomas Sejerson, and Jane Williams: this group of co-authors also acted as sub-editors to support me by providing their individual perspectives to help shape the book and their independent reviews of individual chapters.

Many thanks to you all for the team effort that made this book possible.

This book was supported by a European Commission grant towards improving Maternal and Child health in Kazakhstan, 2009–2011.

Chapter 1
Terms, definitions and concepts

Colin Kennedy

Key messages

- The precautionary principle, first do no harm, was established 2500 years. Justification for the use of a treatment remains the responsibility of the treating physician.
- For many centuries 'ecologies of care' rather than definition of illness was the predominant paradigm of medical practice and this continues to be relevant to the young because the relationships between a child, the family and the wider environment remain important determinants of health outcomes, especially in infancy.
- Discussion of management of disease is greatly facilitated by internationally agreed definitions of disease and these are available as the ICD-10 (www.who.int/classifications/apps/icd/icd10online).
- Evidence-based medicine provides an objective method for the systematic evaluation of the evidence of benefit and harm of medical interventions.

Common errors

- Use of imprecise terms for which international agreement is lacking, for example raised intracranial pressure, hydrocephalus syndrome, myotonic syndrome, hyperexcitability syndrome.
- Imprecise or incorrect use of terms for which precise definitions exist, for example perinatal encephalopathy, epilepsy.
- Generalization of uncommon conditions to common clinical situations, for example attributing trembling of the chin, or feeding problems, or excessive crying, or febrile seizures to neurological disorders.

When to worry
- Separation of infants from their families (one should facilitate bonding between an infant and their main carer).
- Use of poorly evaluated, potentially harmful, interventions in many infants to treat rare neurological problems (one should use common sense, and look at international recommendations of good practice).
- Resistance to evaluation of the benefits and harms of current treatments (one should consider all interventions for potential benefits and risks).

The basis of medical practice

This book offers knowledge, only some of which is truly evidence-based, and a framework for incorporating evidence into the clinical care of infants in whom there is concern about neurological function or developmental progress. Historically, the starting point was myth and wise myths will continue to have their place in medical practice. According to the ancient Greeks, Apollo was the god of healing and Asclepius, his son, was rescued by Apollo from the womb of his dying human mother, Coronis. Asclepius' daughters were Hygeia, the goddess of health, and Panacea, the goddess of cures. Asclepius also had sons and Hippocrates, according to myth, was a descendant of one of those sons. Hippocrates was a practising physician nearly 2500 years ago and author of the Hippocratic Oath (www.pbs.org/wgbh/nova/body/hippocratic-oath-today. html), the most famous text in Western medicine.

The most widely quoted section of that oath states: 'I will use treatments for the benefit of the ill in accordance with my ability and my judgement, but from what is to their harm and injustice I will keep them.' In addition to this statement of the precautionary principle (i.e. 'first do no harm'), other sections of the oath bind the practitioner to resist all temptations that their privileged position as physician offers, to acknowledge the limits of their competence and refer to specialist practitioners when necessary, to leave surgery to the surgeons, to respect patient confidentiality, to treat one's professional teachers as one's parents and to pass on the art of medicine to the next generation. Thus many of the issues of key importance to clinical practitioners and the health systems within which they work are identified within the oath.

Precautionary principles in the context of neurological problems in infancy

The precautionary principle is especially relevant in the assessment and management of neurological and neurodevelopmental problems in infancy when medical intervention may unwittingly hinder the role of the parents in the development, whether typical or impaired, of the child: hospitalization or other institutionalization should be avoided whenever possible (Chapters 2 and 4). Any system of medical activity that involves surveillance of typically developing children should be based on explicit principles of screening (Chapter 6), including evidence that benefit of early intervention, whether special investigation (Chapters 7–9) or treatment (Chapters 10 and 11), outweighs the potential for harm. The range of 'normal', better termed 'typical', neurological development in infancy is broad. In cases of doubt, continuing clinical surveillance and support for normal parenting is needed. This has less potential for harm than enthusiastic separation into medical categories in the border zones of normality and the use of treatments for which benefit is not established or is outweighed by risk of harm. Any system of practice that categorizes more than a few per cent of infants as neurologically abnormal must itself be suspect. Such a system is incompatible with the epidemiology of neurological disorders in childhood and will, by definition, expose many normal children to the risk of being wrongly categorized as impaired. This is, in effect, a particular example of the need for screening, in this case secondary screening, to fulfil a number of criteria additional to those that apply to the treatment of illness (Chapter 6).

Neurological and developmental assessment of the infant is a practical skill of central importance (Chapter 5) that requires hands-on experience as well as knowledge. The importance of the physiological state of the infant (hungry or fed, wakeful or drowsy, contented or distressed), the need to rely on best performance and the extent to which clinical features are consistent over time are more important to bear in mind at this age than at any other. Almost any finding with respect to the deep tendon reflexes, other than complete absence of them, for example, is within the typical (i.e. normal) range in some physiological states or at some age within the first year.

Ecologies of care and categories of illness
On the foundations expressed by Hippocrates, the art of clinical practice in Western countries evolved in the pre-scientific era using a system of knowledge based on the eminence and experience of senior practitioners. For many centuries prior to the more modern description of categories of illness as the basis of medical practice, ecologies of care for maintenance of health and for the treatment of illness acknowledged the importance of the relationship between the patient and the wider environment and provided the predominant paradigm of care. In the case of the child patient, family relationships are of primary importance and are fundamental to the Head Start (USA) and Sure Start (UK) programmes for the improvement of the health and well-being of young children (Blair and DeBell, 2011). These issues are discussed in Chapters 2, 4 and 6 of this book.

The international classification of diseases
The World Health Organization was founded by international treaty in 1948 as a specialized agency of the United Nations with unique authority to establish global health standards and to secure international agreement on defining disease. The 193 member states of the WHO have agreed to use the International Classification of Diseases (ICD) and the updating of ICD-10 is expected to be completed and lead to

the publication of ICD-11 in 2014. Classification of mental disorders, which include neurological disorders, is complex and controversial both because underlying pathophysiology cannot be observed directly and because many symptoms are continuous with normal phenomena. Nowhere are these issues more relevant than in the neurology and neurodevelopment of infants. The ICD-10 classification is predominantly driven by the clinical utility and public health outcomes of the disease entities and, in spite of these controversies, is therefore an appropriate framework for clinical practice (Reed et al., 2011).

The ICD-10 provides the basis of the discussion for classifying the phenomena observed in the clinical contexts that are discussed in Chapters 12 to 24 of this book. A number of entities (e.g. brain tumours of infancy) are included in the differential diagnosis but not covered in detail in this volume for lack of space. Other entities do not appear because they are based on classifications of disease other than ICD-10. Such diagnostic classifications, including some listed in the paragraphs below, may claim to identify disease entities requiring active management in a substantial percentage of neonates or infants. In some cases, the criteria for making such diagnoses are vague, their relationships with disorders of later childhood unknown and the rationale for intervention is obscure.

International clinical guidelines depend upon this shared nosology and classification of illnesses and disease: the foundation for rational management requires knowledge of what treatments are of benefit and what are harmful which in turn requires specific disease definitions that are shared by all those involved in providing care.

Relevant terms and definitions

The brief discussion of terms below is intended to help the reader to navigate through later chapters of the book but is not intended to be exhaustive.

Encephalopathy is defined as 'a disease in which the functioning of the brain is affected by some agent or condition' (*New Oxford Dictionary*). Because this definition is so inclusive, it is of little practical value in clinical medicine. While 'acute' means 'of short duration' or 'experienced to an intense or severe degree' (*New Oxford Dictionary*), the medical definition of *acute encephalopathy* includes alteration in conscious level as an essential criterion (Chapter 14) and to that extent is more clinically useful for the formation of a plan of investigation and management.

The term *perinatal encephalopathy* does not indicate either whether the observed effect on the functioning of the brain is of short duration or whether it involves an alteration of conscious level. Furthermore, the infant's level of consciousness prior to birth is usually not known to the clinician. However the general term encephalopathy is no more useful in the perinatal period than it is generally, especially since there is often disagreement as to whether or not commonly observed neonatal or post-neonatal behaviour (e.g. tremor of the chin) indicates abnormal brain functioning. This carries important potential for harm in exposing many infants, the vast majority of whom will have no known subsequent medical disorder, to the risks associated with medical diagnoses of doubtful validity. In practice, therefore, the definition of perinatal encephalopathy includes alteration of level of consciousness (Chapter 12). It is, in effect, the special case of 'acute encephalopathy' in an individual within the perinatal age group. Other more inclusive uses of the term perinatal encephalopathy are to be avoided and will not be further discussed here.

Hydrocephalus is used to mean an excess of cerebrospinal fluid within the head but excluding those situations where that situation has arisen purely from atrophy or failure to develop of the brain substance (sometimes called hydrocephalus *ex vacuo*). The presence of hydrocephalus cannot be confirmed or excluded from consideration, in isolation, of the dimensions of the third cerebral ventricle. See Chapter 18 for further discussion.

Hydrocephalus and *raised intracranial pressure* frequently co-exist and specific clinical signs, often including disturbed consciousness, can be combined with cranial imaging to provide evidence for the presence of both entities (see especially Chapters 14 and 18) but there is no internationally recognized entity of 'hydrocephalus-intracranial-hypertension syndrome'.

A *seizure* may be epileptic (Chapter 16) or non-epileptic (Chapter 17). Epilepsy is defined as recurrent unprovoked epileptic seizures. Febrile seizures are provoked by a rising fever and are not conventionally regarded as falling within the above definition of an epilepsy. Chapters 16 and 17 provide further discussion of these definitions and of the syndromes that constitute disease entities within them.

Myotonia is defined as the inability of muscle fibres to relax after muscle contraction and can be demonstrated by myotonic discharges on electromyography. This is a very rare phenomenon in infancy and even in an infant with congenital myotonic dystrophy (Chapter 20), myotonia is usually only demonstrable in an affected parent. The term '*myotonic syndrome*', in which abnormality of muscle tone is the dominant feature, is not a recognized diagnostic entity in infants.

'*Hyperexcitability syndrome*' is not a generally accepted diagnostic disease entity term in infancy and internationally accepted criteria for its definition are lacking. Associations between problems with crying, sleeping and/or feeding in infancy and long-term behavioural outcomes in childhood, including attention-deficit-hyperactivity disorder, exist. Meta-analysis suggests that these so-called *early regulatory problems* can have an adverse effect on behavioural or cognitive development but findings have been inconsistent. The risk is highest in those with multiple regulatory problems in infancy in multiple-risk families. These problems are attributable partly to biological predisposition in the infant, partly to parenting behaviours and partly to interactions between the two. Interventions that alter parenting behaviour are followed by a reduction in regulatory problems (Hemmi et al., 2011).

Twenty per cent of infants show early regulatory problems and their predictive value for behavioural problems later in childhood is low. Most cases may therefore be regarded as falling within the spectrum of typical development and need not be conceptualized as indicating an underlying neurological disorder. In a minority, an underlying psychiatric, neurological or other medical disorder could, of course, present with early regulatory problems. Support to parents to help prevent or reduce early regulatory problems is therefore typically given in the context of general paediatric nursing or medical assessment of the infant and advice to families rather than as treatment of a disease entity.

Evidence-based medicine

The accumulated wisdom of previous generations of medical practitioners, has since the nineteenth century, been progressively supplanted by the concept of 'evidence', of greater or lesser quality, to support the use of treatments. Myth has been progressively replaced by evidence although the process has sometimes been hindered by political interference (McKee, 2007). Hopefully the value of certain myths, starting with Hygeia and Panacea, will continue to be recognized.

Evidence-based medicine has only emerged within the second half of the 20th century and has been an increasing influence on medical practice in the 21st century. It is, as described in Chapter 3, the systematic construction of a body of knowledge about interventions for medical illnesses with explicit, objective criteria for rating the quality of the evidence upon which that knowledge is based. The great strength of evidence-based medicine lies in its capacity for constant improvement as new *information* comes to light and without *ad personam* arguments about the authority of the *individuals* advocating any particular treatment, which had dominated previous medical thought since Hippocrates, sometimes referred to as 'eminence-based medicine'.

Unfortunately, the quality of much of the evidence upon which we must currently rely for guidance in the treatment of neurological disorders in infancy is poor. Furthermore the traditional measures of quality of evidence are sometimes difficult to apply when studying rehabilitation including physiotherapeutic interventions (Rosenbaum, 2010; Autti-Ramo, 2011). The methodology of evidence-based medicine can also help us to identify those situations where evidence is lacking and serve to remind us that justification is always required for medical intervention, especially in an infant, and the responsibility for this rests with the physician.

References

Autti-Ramo I. Physiotherapy in high-risk infants – a motor learning facilitator or not? *Developmental Medicine and Child Neurology*, 2011, 53: 200–201.

Blair M, DeBell D. Reconceptualising health services for school age children in the 21st century. *Archives of Disease in Childhood*, 2011, 96: 616–618.

Hemmi MH, Wolke D, Schneider S. Associations between problems with crying, sleeping and/or feeding in infancy and long-term behavioural outcomes in childhood: a meta-analysis. *Archives of Disease in Childhood*, 2011, 96: 622–629.

McKee M. Cochrane on communism: the influence of ideology on the search for evidence. *International Journal of Epidemiology*, 2007, 36: 269–273.

Reed GM, Dua T, Saxena S. World Health Organization responds to Fiona Godlee and Ray Moynihan. *British Medical Journal*, 2011, 342: 1380.

Rosenbaum P. The randomised controlled trial: an excellent design, but can it answer the big question in neurodisability. *Developmental Medicine and Child Neurology*, 2010, 52: 111.

Resources

Edelstein L. The Hippocratic oath. Text, translation and interpretation by L. Edelstein, 1943, p. 56. www.pbs.org/wgbh/nova/body/hippocratic-oath-today.html

ICD-10 codes, www.who.int/classifications/apps/icd/icd10online

Chapter 2

Interprofessional working: user and carer involvement

Audrone Prasauskiene and Maryze Schoneveld
van der Linde

Key messages
- Be aware of the social and cultural environment of the child, such as nationality, language dependence, religion, family situation, etc.
- Use all possible means to avoid separating the child and parents.
- Inform and talk to parents about their child's health problems.
- Inform the child about their health condition in an age-appropriate manner.
- Listen to parents' feelings regarding their child's condition.
- Include parents in the treatment plan for their child, so they have some control over their child's problem.
- Encourage parents to develop a good, strong emotional bond with their child.
- Provide parents and children with a window of hope without denying the seriousness of the child's health situation.
- Life with a disability is certainly possible but needs creativity and flexibility of approach. If parents are having difficulty finding the way forward, try to assist them to find perspectives on life with their child from which they could derive pleasure and satisfaction.
- Discuss with the professional healthcare team their ideas, solutions and feelings regarding the health of the patient.

Common errors
- Being too focused on the medical aspects of treatment and forgetting the psychological and emotional well-being of the affected child, of the parents and sometimes also of healthcare professionals confronted by very difficult situations.
- Forgetting that the patient is not only a sick body, but also a human being with social, emotional and psychological needs.
- Forgetting that parents are the main carers of the child and therefore must be included in the child's treatment plan.

When to worry
- Signs of depression in parents and/or the child.
- Parental interest in orphanages that take care of disabled children. This can indicate that a family plans to leave their disabled child in an orphanage.
- Denial by parents that the child has a health problem.
- Parents avoiding their child. This can be a sign of psychological difficulty in coming to terms with the child's health problems.

The holistic approach to childhood development

Holism comes from the Greek word *holos*, which means 'all' or 'total'. The term 'holistic' means looking at something as a whole, rather than in separate parts. This approach is often linked to health, where the patient may be treated holistically, in the sense that mental, physical, emotional and spiritual well-being are all considered.

Holistic care is based upon valuing the whole child and endeavours to understand the young child as an individual in the context of family, community and culture. It is impossible to separate the normal physical and emotional development of the child from their place in their family. From the first hours of life of the newborn it is very important to ensure that – notwithstanding the need to use all available technologies – infants have close contact with their parents.

The so-called kangaroo care technique was developed for newborn infants. Kangaroo care is the term used for maintaining skin-to-skin contact between the infant and mother (or father) for several hours each day over a period of days or weeks following birth. Typically the infant, wearing only a nappy, is held against the mother's bare chest, with the mother's shirt or hospital gown wrapped under and around the infant's bottom for support. Maternal contact appears to have a calming effect on the newborn in addition to enhancing bonding. For preterm infants the benefits can be even greater, with the mother's body directly responding to the infant's and helping to regulate temperature, for example, more naturally and smoothly than an incubator.

Kangaroo care has also been shown to help stabilize a preterm infant's heartbeat and breathing. Physicians have found that kangaroo care can help to wean an infant off a ventilator sooner than might otherwise be possible.

Another worldwide initiative supported by the WHO and United Nations Children's Fund (UNICEF) is development of infant-friendly hospitals. In these hospitals close contact between mother and infant is maintained and breastfeeding is supported by all means possible.

A child, especially in the early years and particularly when developmental problems are suspected, should not be separated from his or her parents or carers, even if the child is sick and has to be hospitalized. There is scientific evidence that long-term continuity of parental care is very beneficial to all children except, of course, in the cases of those few parents who abuse their children. Long-term hospitalization with isolation from parents during the first year of life may have the same consequences for psychological and emotional development as institutionalization and can cause

- social and behavioural abnormalities (aggressive behavioural problems, inattention/hyperactivity, delays in social/emotional development, syndromes mimicking autism);
- poor growth: institutionalized children cared for without involvement of the family lose 1 month of growth every 3 months; and
- decreased emotional reactivity: children living outside of family care demonstrate deficient sensory perception, including understanding and responding to facial emotion.

As highlighted above, the holistic point of view is a means to better understand a child's individual needs and the many factors which are likely to affect growth and development. So child care has to be based on four main principles:

- client-centred, with the child's and family's needs prioritized;
- strength-focused, based on strengths of the child and family rather than on their weaknesses;
- solution-oriented, based on eliciting a child's strengths and abilities rather than focusing on the roots of his/her deficits; and
- in partnership with the family, irrespective of the child's diagnosis or cultural background.

User and carer involvement
Before discussing the importance of user and carer involvement in health care, it is important to note that there is more than one definition of the concept of disability. One definition of (developmental) disability is a lack or limitation of competence.

Usually disability is seen in contrast to an ideal of normal capacity to perform particular activities and participate in social life. Sickness inhibits ability, but is temporary (whether ending in healing or death), whereas disability is chronic. Disability is used to refer to limitations resulting from physical or cognitive dysfunction. The notion of impairment raises moral and metaphysical problems about personhood, responsibility and the meaning of differences. Questions about autonomy and dependence, capacity, identity and the meaning of loss are central.

In Western cultures, the conceptualization of disability is that of dependency and loss of autonomy but, when looked at more closely, dependence and autonomy are universal in social relationships. Reliance upon another person may be encompassed by love and a feeling of mutuality. Dependency therefore can have different meanings and implications. In some cultures, family and community membership may outweigh individual ability as a value. Dependency also varies according to the characteristics of those with whom a person with a disability lives, and the ability of the person with a disability to develop as an individual (Ingstad and Reynolds Whyte, 1995).

To clarify and specify the concept and the impact of disability, the WHO created the International Classification of Functioning, Disability and Health (ICF) in 2001 (WHO, 2001). The ICF is related to health and health-related domains. It acknowledges that *every* human being can experience a decrement in health and thereby experience some degree of disability. Disability is not something that happens only to a minority of humanity. The ICF thus brings disability into the mainstream of experience and recognizes it as a universal human experience. The ICF takes into account the social aspects of disability and does not see disability only as a medical or biological dysfunction. By including contextual, including environmental factors, the ICF allows recording of the impact of the environment on a person's functioning.

In 2007 the ICF for Children and Youth (ICF-CY; WHO, 2007) was developed from the ICF. The ICF-CY can assist clinicians, educators, researchers and parents to document and measure health and disability in children and youth populations (see Chapter 21, Box 21.1, p 280). The WHO ICF/ICF-CY classification enables disability to be seen as part of life and thus a social responsibility of every society as a whole.

The needs of the child

Children who have a developmental disability or any other health problem early in life need all the support they can get. In many situations healthcare providers such as nurses and treating physicians are the people who can identify the needs of these children and signpost possible problems. All children, regardless of their health situation, need to feel safe, be able to play and thus develop and enjoy life, and to receive unconditional love, respect, care, attention and explanations about what they may be experiencing. Of course it is difficult to explain to an infant about medical treatment, but it is possible to offer some explanation about their treatment to children whose cognitive ability is above the level of a 2-year-old. This can be done via play, using dolls or another toy that a child loves. Explaining to the child what is happening or going to happen shows the child that his feelings, questions, fear, anxiety and pain are being acknowledged.

Family needs

Evaluating a family's situation

The needs of a family whose child has a health problem will vary greatly between families, not only according to the severity of the child's disability but also according to the econonomic and social situation of the family, the parents' personal characteristics, the type of family, etc. A period of great uncertainty is common in families whose child has an unexpected health problem. Whatever their social background or religious beliefs, all parents feel that they are responsible for what has happened to their child. Depending on the nature of health problems, parents also might feel the need to mourn since the future they had hoped for their child will not become a reality because of their child's disability. This is a natural feeling, but it is important that the people around these parents, and not the least the healthcare professionals, support them in perhaps one of the most difficult periods of their lives.

Healthcare professionals and social workers should try to evaluate a family's situation and the way parents can deal with their child's disability, taking into account the parents' educational background, social support and care they can get from the extended family, their need for information, the relations within a family and whether any conflicts exist that could jeopardize a child's health and social situation. This evaluation is important to determine what needs a family has and in what areas they need support.

The contribution of healthcare professionals

Needless to say, healthcare professionals cannot do everything, but they can make a positive difference to the lives of families with a child with a neurodevelopmental problem. Giving parents time, attention or a shoulder to cry on can have a positive impact. Parents in this situation find it important to get good, honest information in their own language about their child's disability, even when the information may not be positive. Information in written form and in the local language(s) is an important resource and enables parents to read about and discuss the health problem of their child at home in their own time. Parents want to know what they can do for their child. Are there therapies, or physical or speech exercises they can help their child to do? Would it be helpful for them to start to learn sign language if their child has a hearing impairment? Healthcare professionals can advise parents on these issues and allow parents to participate in the treatment of their child so that they feel included.

It is important for health professionals always to be honest, not to promise anything and not to offer a negative prognosis too quickly, especially when uncertainty remains. Also, although it seems contradictory, the health professional should give hope by drawing attention to positive experiences the child and parent can both look forward to enjoying in the future. Without hope it will be difficult for parents to find energy to continue to support their child as best as they can. Providing a window of hope for whatever kind of future the child has is essential. Tell parents that there will be reasons that their child will be glad to be alive, even if they are severely disabled and can be expected to do little except to share in family life. It can be helpful to seek connection with them via their spiritual faith. Although providing information, respect, support and explaining the medical cause of the child's disability is very important, *compassion* is essential. It is good to show parents that as well as being a healthcare professional, you empathise with them in their situation.

Team needs
The team working together on the care and management of child with a disability or other health problem may experience a wide range of emotions. Team members need a means to vent their feelings and team meetings provide an opportunity to do this. This requires good collaboration and mutual trust within the team. Good team working will help team members support the parents and the child, address problems, communicate with each other regarding the treatment of the child and focus on the child's future with parents and family, even when the child will be severely disabled.

Team work
The development of the child is a complicated and diverse process, influenced by multiple factors. To provide professional and effective care for the child and family, several professionals should be involved. It is very important that the professionals involved in taking care or providing health care or habilitation/rehabilitation services can to work as a team. There are three types of cross-professional working (Thylefors et al., 2005), as detailed below.

- Multiprofessional: each team member is focused on their own tasks and not on collective working. Contributions are made either in parallel or sequentially to each other with minimal communication. Each contribution stands alone and can be performed without input from others. Independent contributions have to be coordinated. Traditionally, the physician takes the lead. This type of cross-professional work is often the method used in Eastern European countries. In this type of the team the members rely on their own individual assessments to deduce the needs of the family, while the parents stay outside the team.
- Interprofessional (the product is more than a simple sum of its parts): outcome requires interactive effort and contribution of the professionals involved. This model implies a high level of communication, mutual planning, collective decisions and shared responsibilities. Everyone involved in the process must take everyone else's contribution into consideration. This type of teamwork involves all the staff members working with a particular child and parents. This team is more likely to concentrate on needs and goals of the child and the family than on purely medical goals.

- Transprofessional: the opposite end of the continuum from multiprofessional working. The team uses integrative work process so that disciplinary boundaries become partly dissolved. Professionals, by close interpersonal and interprofessional communication, become more sensitive to the needs of the child and the family; they can build treatment strategies that help to achieve functional goals. Communication also helps to share knowledge, solve conflicts and, in general, improve services.

Team work in caring for children with developmental disabilities
The team members that may be involved in the care of a child with developmental disability are listed below.

- Paediatrician: diagnoses and treats infants and children with all kinds of illnesses, sometimes including metabolic diseases. Gives advice regarding feeding, respiratory problems, catheterization, bowel evacuation, etc.
- Neurologist or paediatric neurologist: diagnoses and treats neuromuscular diseases, epilepsy, developmental disorders (including delayed speech, motor milestones and coordination issues), cerebral palsy, myelomeningocele, intellectual disability, traumatic brain injuries, metabolic and progressive disorders and childhood variants of neurological diseases that also affect adults.
- Orthopedic surgeon: treats scoliosis, contractures and other joint or bone problems related to muscle weakness.
- Speech therapist (logoped): helps to diagnose and treat a variety of speech, voice and language disorders. Deals with feeding difficulties.
- Ear, nose and throat (ENT) specialist: treats ear, nose and throat disorders such as a hearing impairment. Every child with developmental disability should be examined for hearing disorder.
- Ophthalmologist: treats diseases of the eye and visual impairments. Every child with developmental disability should be examined for vision disorder.
- Dietician: creates eating plans to manage weight loss and swallowing problems.
- Social worker: helps parents cope with practical concerns such as school, education and financial issues.
- Psychologist: helps parents with their fears and worries and tries to find a way to deal with the new situation of having a child with a developmental disorder. Evaluates the child's cognitive and other abilities to identify the profile of cognitive strengths and weaknesses.
- Occupational therapist (ergotherapist): helps parents to learn new ways to do everyday tasks, adjust home for the needs of the child and deals with fine motor problems. Advises on aids and equipment, including wheelchairs.
- Physical therapist (kineziotherapist): helps the child to do physical exercises, to strengthen weak muscles, prevent contractures, improve stamina, improve motor abilities and reach specific functional goals.

- Special needs teaching assistant or special pedagogue: helps to evaluate and develop the child's educational and developmental skills to ensure the maximum is done to support the child with a disability to be as independent as possible.
- Genetic counsellor: discusses issues related to family risk and family planning and arranges for prenatal diagnoses when applicable and wanted by the family.
- Clinical geneticist: recognizes patterns of malformation and recurrence risk. Advises on diagnostic genetic testing, including prenatal testing in cases where future children are at risk of a genetic condition.

The term developmental disability refers to lifelong disabilities attributable to mental and/or physical impairments, manifested prior to age 18 years. Developmental disabilities can be a single event in a family or can have a genetic background in a family. If the developmental disability of a child is related to a genetic mutation inherited from one parent or both parents, it is important to be aware that this may create a complex emotional and social situation. For the affected family this may create a feeling of guilt for having passed on their 'weak' gene: parents want the best for their child and the knowledge that they are responsible for the child's health problem can be devastating. Recognition, acknowledgement and discussion between the healthcare team and the parents of the resulting feelings of grief and guilt will facilitate their acceptance of the situation. A genetic counsellor can explain to the parents genetic inheritance, why their child is affected by a genetic condition and also what this means for future children. A genetic counsellor or psychologist can help parents to deal with emotional problems and to look at the situation from a different perspective. No one should be blamed for passing on the genetic basis of a disease to a child. It is no less natural than the determination of a child's eye colour.

Whether or not the disorder is genetically determined, parents need to understand that their child has different life opportunities. Having a disability, whether mild or severe, does not mean that a child has no future. A family and community can create an environment at home and at school where a child can be safe, grow and thrive physically and emotionally. When the child gets the necessary support, their full developmental potential can be realized. Many children with a mental and or physical impairment can work, albeit at a very low level in some cases. When they get the support they need, they can have a good life among the people they love, trust and care about.

When a child with a developmental disability grows up, however, the needs of both the child and the parents may change. Every stage in a child's life will involve change for the child and the parents. This means that it is important that child and parents are followed-up well by the healthcare team. The team can identify what additional support or services a child and their parents need. For parents it can be good to be closely involved in the treatment plan for their child. For them, knowing what is done, why it is done and what healthcare professionals hope to achieve can be important.

Taking care of a child with a developmental disability is a lifelong commitment, but the commitment of parents, healthcare professionals and society – and the child themselves – can enable a child to live life to the fullest, within their own capabilities.

References

Ingstad B, Reynolds Whyte S. *Disability and culture*. Los Angeles, University of California Press, 1995:3–11.

Thylefors I, Persson O, Hellstrom D. Team types, perceived efficiency and team climate in Swedish cross-professional teamwork. *Journal of Interprofessional Care*, 2005, 19(2):102–114.

WHO. *International Classification of Functioning, Disability and Health (ICF)*. 2001 resolution WHA 54.21, 2001 (http://apps.who.int/classifications/icfbrowser/).

WHO. *International Classification of Functioning, Disability and Health – Children and Youth Version*. ICF-CY. Geneva, WHO, 2007.

Chapter 3
Clinical epidemiology and evidence-based medicine

Andrew L. Lux

Key messages
- A good understanding of evidence-based medicine and clinical epidemiology is essential for the effective practice of all clinicians.
- Although there are good sources of aggregated data and clinical practice guidelines, effective clinical practice often requires decisions based upon small studies or series of descriptive data, and the ability to interpret those studies reliably.
- You can adopt your own ABC for the evaluation and interpretation of reported clinical studies by considering assumptions, bias, confounding and chance.

Common errors
- We are all prone to recognizing causal patterns from associations where effects are due to chance or other factors, such as bias and confounding.
- Many reported studies force the reader to 'lose touch' with the data by reporting modelled and adjusted effect estimates without first reporting the crude or unadjusted effect estimates.
- Published reports tend to have a 'positive' finding and similar studies that fail to detect an important or significant difference are less likely to get submitted and published. This leads to a further source of bias: publication bias.

> **When to worry**
> – When published evidence contrasts with your personal experience. The definitions and ideas in this chapter should help you determine why your experience is so different, and also to assess the validity of the reported findings.
> – When published evidence is based on *p* values and hypothesis testing alone rather than on reported effect estimates and confidence intervals. This latter approach allows the clinician to assess better the magnitude and importance of any reported effect.
> – When effect estimates, confidence intervals or *P* values are reported without clear reference to the statistical tests from which they are calculated.

Introduction

Epidemiology is the study of the distribution and causes of disease in populations. In *clinical epidemiology* the principles and techniques of epidemiology are applied to clinical settings. It is concerned with activities such as defining cases and exposures, assessing measures of risk, identifying patterns of prognosis in the context of risk-modifying factors and assessing the impact and effects of treatment interventions. It has been described as 'a marriage between quantitative concepts used by epidemiologists to study disease in populations and decision-making in the individual case which is the daily fare of clinical medicine' (Paul, 1938). In other words, its key function is to provide tools allowing the clinician to make good decisions.

Evidence-based medicine is a movement that provides a context for clinical epidemiology and espouses 'the conscientious, explicit, and judicious use of current best evidence in making decisions about the care of individual patients' (Sackett et al., 1996). It attempts to take into account the patient's physical and clinical circumstances, and the beliefs and values of the patient or the patient's family.

This chapter provides an overview of some key elements of clinical epidemiology and evidence-based medicine, but it is by no means a comprehensive or systematic review.

Some basic definitions for clinical epidemiology

Case definition   The features of a disease or condition that make it reasonable to consider that the patient is affected by that condition. These features can be necessary, sufficient, or merely consistent with the diagnosis. In defining cases, it is often necessary also to define exclusion criteria.

Classification and categorization   A classification is an organizing system, and categorization is the process of fitting cases within the classification system. An example of a multi-axial classification system is the International League Against Epilepsy proposed diagnostic scheme for people with epileptic seizures and epilepsy, which has axes for phenomenology, seizure types, epilepsy syndrome, underlying etiology and comorbidity (Engel, 2001).

Syndrome   A confluence of features. For example, onset of focal motor seizures in middle childhood with sleep-activated epileptiform discharges in the central-midtemporal area would be consistent with the epilepsy syndrome of 'benign childhood epilepsy with central-midtemporal spikes'. However, if the patient has a focal neurological or a cognitive deficit, and a temporal lobe tumour, it would be inappropriate to use this syndromic label since we would have identified clear exclusion criteria (see 'Case definition').

Bias   A factor or process that makes results, analyses or their interpretation (the 'inference') deviate from the truth. Systematic bias affects validity. There are many potential forms of bias: for example, Sackett (1979) identified 35 forms relating to sampling and measurement. In spoken presentations, the term 'bias' is often confused with 'skewness', which is a measure of asymmetry of a probability distribution.

Publication bias   The distorting effect of studies being more likely to be accepted for publication when there are positive findings than when no association or causal relationship is identified. This will affect the inferences derived from aggregated data since the published literature is then biased towards positive results. There are techniques for analysing data aggregated from multiple studies, such as funnel plots (Sterne & Egger, 2001) that can identify the presence of publication bias.

Regression to mean effect   Another form of bias. The degree or severity of a condition will tend, over a period of time, to a certain average value. An apparent treatment effect might be falsely attributed to an intervention – for example, the addition of a new antiepileptic drug added at a time at which seizures are particularly frequent or severe – where there is no true effect, since what is observed is the condition tending back to its baseline (mean effect) with respect to frequency or severity, also known as regression to the mean.

Confounding   A form of bias that confuses the effects of the exposure of interest with other effects that might be operating to influence the outcomes. The defining characteristic of a confounding factor is that it is associated both with the exposure being studied and the outcome of that exposure. For example, the severity of hearing impairment would be expected to be associated with age at diagnosis of the impairment (with more severe impairments being diagnosed earlier) and with subsequent language abilities (with more severe impairments being associated with poorer language). In this example the association between early diagnosis and later language skills is said to be confounded by severity of hearing impairment.

Association and causality   Statistical tests can identify associations between random variables (study factors) but clinicians and researchers need to exercise reason and judgement to decide whether such relationships are likely to be causal. Hill's criteria

Table 3.1 Sir Austin Bradford Hill's causal criteria (Hill, 1965)

Criterion	Features
Strength	Strong associations are more likely to be causal but weaker associations are more likely to be due to unidentified biases.
Consistency	The same association is found in different populations and in different circumstances.
Specificity	The cause leads to a single effect rather than multiple effects.
Temporality	The cause necessarily occurs prior to the effect.
Biological gradient	The presence of a dose-response effect, either linear (monotonic) or with threshold effects.
Plausibility	The causal relationship makes sense in terms of current knowledge of biological and social systems (although this is not an absolute requirement: the explanatory mechanism may follow the epidemiological finding).
Coherence	The causal interpretation aligns with what is known about the biological or social system.
Experimental evidence	It might be better to regard this as a means of testing a causal hypothesis.
Analogy	A criterion that seems to lend support to plausibility.

(Hill, 1965) are useful for investigating possible causality (see Table 3.1). It is important to consider the possibility of *reverse causality*.

Bayesian statistics   A Bayesian approach to biostatistical analysis uses clinician or investigator knowledge or belief as the basis for a probability distribution that forms a *prior probability* which is updated by new data to produce a *posterior probability*. Although this approach is said to use a paradigm of *subjective probability*, which to some has connotations of lacking scientific rigour and objectivity, it should not be considered arbitrary or lacking empirical evidence. It forms a coherent and consistent method of statistical inference. Prior probabilities are usually derived from data from earlier studies, but it is also possible to produce 'priors' based on uniform functions that represent a state of prior equipoise in belief about a potential treatment effect. *Classical (frequentist)* statistics have analogous techniques to those used in Bayesian statistical analyses and it can be argued that frequentist statistical analyses are based on implicit assumptions about a prior probability distribution.

Validity   The extent to which something measures what it purports to measure.

Precision   The extent to which measurements are reliable and repeatable; the degree of freedom from random error.

Type I error (alpha)   A 'false positive' study conclusion in which the null hypothesis of a test is rejected where in fact no true association exists; equals the significance level of the statistical test.

Type II error (beta)   A 'false negative' study conclusion in which the null hypothesis of a test is accepted where in fact a true association exists. For a given strength of association between study factors, a larger study will have a smaller beta. Power calculations (see below) are based on achieving an acceptably low chance of failing to detect a true association.

Statistical power   A measure of the study's sensitivity to detect a genuine association or causal relationship; the complement of the Type II error rate (that is, one minus the Type II error). A power of 90% means a 10% chance (beta = 0.1) of failing to detect a true association. Such calculations should be undertaken *before* embarking on a study.

Significance versus importance   In general, it is prudent to reserve the term 'significant' to refer to statistical and analytical elements of a study, and to discuss the clinical 'importance' of the findings independently. A large study, for example, might find a statistically significant difference in mean blood pressure outcomes of 2 mmHg between two groups, but the clinical importance of this finding would be questionable. Another study might find a 15-point (1 standard deviation) difference in mean developmental quotients between two groups that could be clinically important but is not statistically significant because the study is underpowered or did not enrol sufficient participants before study completion.

Confidence interval (CI)   In classical (frequentist) statistics, a 95% CI is calculated from the sample observations and forms the range of values that would be expected to contain the true parameter value 95% of the time if repeated on samples from the same population. In other words, the CI provides a measure of the precision of the best estimate of the value of the parameter. This conveys more information about the potential range of size of an association than does a *P* value and for this reason should be included in clinical research reports. Bayesian statistical methods generate an analogue of the CI that is termed a 'credible interval'.

Table 3.2 Contingency table showing relationships between clinical investigation results and the presence or absence of a disease or condition

		Disease or condition		
		Present	Absent	
Test result	Positive	a *True positive*	b *False positive*	$a + b$
	Negative	c *False negative*	d *True negative*	$c + d$
		$a + c$	$b + d$	$a + b + c + d$

Measures of disease frequency   *Prevalence* is the amount of a disease or condition present in the study population at a given time, whereas *incidence* refers to the number of newly identified cases over a given period of time. These measures depend upon how common the condition is and how long the condition lasts. In Table 3.2, *prevalence* is represented by the ratio $(a + c)/(a + b + c + d)$. In terms of Bayesian probabilities and clinical reasoning, the prevalence proportion can be used as the *prior probability* for a disease or condition, representing the clinician's belief, informed by data, about the probability that the condition is present before any clinical tests are performed.

Sensitivity   True positive rate, $a/(a + c)$; probability that the test result is positive when the disease is present.

Specificity   True negative rate, $d/(b + d)$; probability that the test result is negative when the disease is absent.

False positive rate   Probability of a positive test result when the condition is not present, $b/(b + d)$, which is the same as $(1 - \text{specificity})$.

False negative rate   Probability that the test result is negative when the disease or condition is present, $c/(a + c)$, which is the same as $(1 - \text{sensitivity})$, this latter term being the complement of the specificity.

Positive predictive value   Probability that the disease is present if the test is positive, $(a)/(a + b)$.

Negative predictive value   Probability that the disease is absent if the test is negative, $(d)/(c + d)$.

Odds and odds ratios   Odds are the ratio of one probability to its complement. For example, the *prior odds* of the disease in Table 3.2 is (prevalence)/(1 − prevalence); that is, the probability of the disease being present divided by the probability of the disease being absent. *Posterior odds* are useful to represent the clinician's belief about the probability of the disease being present, updated to take into account information from clinical tests. Odds can be converted to probabilities from the relationship (probability) = (odds)/(1 + odds).

Likelihood ratios (LRs)   These link prior and posterior odds, taking into account the sensitivity and specificity. For a positive test result, (posterior odds) = (prior odds × LR+). For a positive test, the *positive likelihood ratio* (*LR+*) is given by (sensitivity)/(1 − specificity); and for a negative test, the *negative likelihood ratio* (*LR−*) is given by (1 − sensitivity)/(specificity). Another way of looking at likelihood ratios is to consider LR+ as (sensitivity)/(false positive rate) and LR− as (specificity)/(false negative rate). An example of the application of likelihood ratios to indicate the predictive value of particular clinical or imaging features following intraventricular haemorrhage in infancy is given in Table 3.3.

Receiver-operating characteristic (ROC) curves   These can be used to compare the diagnostic power of different tests using information that is independent of the underlying disease prevalence. In effect, it is a graph of sensitivity, $(a)/(a + c)$, on the y axis, against the complement of the specificity, $(1 − ((d)/(b + d)))$, on the x axis, for the test at different levels of diagnostic confidence in discriminating true positive (a) and true negative (d) cases. Points higher in the upper-left corner of the curve represent higher levels of predictive value.

Statistical models   Mathematical equations that generally describe possible relationships between an outcome (dependent) variable and predictor variables. These variables are related to each other by *parameters*, unknown values that are estimated from the data acquired in the study. For example, a *linear regression model* describes a mathematical relationship between an outcome variable (often represented as Y) and the combination of a constant parameter (say a) and one or more predictor variables (X_1, X_2, etc.) that are multiplied by parameters (b_1, b_2, etc.) that are referred to as *regression coefficients*. The simplest form of linear regression model, with a single predictor variable, is shown in Figure 3.1. An example of a relationship that might be (over) simplified into such a form would be postnatal height in centimetres (on the y axis) against age in months (on the x axis) so that height in centimetres equals a constant, a (equal to height in centimetres at birth) plus a coefficient, b, multiplied by age in months.

The linear regression method models continuous data that follow a *normal distribution* but there are other statistical regression models for data modelled by other probability distributions. For binary outcome (Yes/No) data, for example, we can use a logistic regression model, where the regression coefficients represent estimated values for the logarithm of the odds ratio adjusted for the effects of other predictor variables in that model; in other words, adjusted odds ratios. Poisson regression models permit analogous

Table 3.3 Prediction of abnormal neuromotor function by cranial ultrasound. An example of an analysis using prior and posterior probabilities (from Nongena et al., 2010 with permission)

| Ultrasound test result | Cerebral palsy | | | |
	Pre-test probability	Likelihood ratios (95% CI)	Post-test probability (95% CI)	Heterogeneity among studies (I2)
Normal scan	9%	0.5 (0.4–0.7)	5% (4–6%)	90%
Grade 1 or 2 IVH	9%	1 (0.4–3)	9% (4–22%)	88%
Grade 3 IVH	9%	4 (2–8)	26% (13–45%)	82%
Grade 4 haemorrhage (any)	9%	11 (4–31)	53% (29–76%)	84%
Cystic PVL	9%	29 (7–116)	74% (42–92%)	90%
Ventricular dilatation	9%	3 (2–4)	22% (17–28%)	0%
Hydrocephalus	9%	4 (1–13)	27% (10–56%)	97%

Normal scan refers to absence of haemorrhage within the brain parenchyma or ventricles, cysts or ventricular dilation. The grade of intraventricular haemorrhage (IVH) is given according to the Papile classification. Ventricular dilation indicates moderate to severe ventricular dilation not meeting the criterion for hydrocephalus. Hydrocephalus indicates massive ventricular dilation >4 mm above the 97th centile. Pre-test probability refers to the prevalence of cerebral palsy based on the Epipage study (Larroque et al., 2008). The likelihood ratio is the probability that a patient with cerebral palsy has a positive test (abnormal ultrasound result). Post-test probability is the probability that a patient with a specific abnormality on cranial ultrasound will have abnormal neuromotor function. Heterogeneity is a measure of similarity between studies and the validity of statistical pooling. PVL, periventricular leukomalcia.

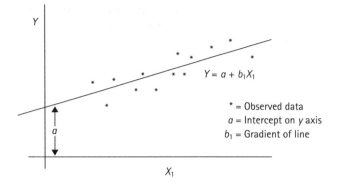

Figure 3.1 Representation of a simple linear regression model relating an outcome variable *Y* to a single predictor variable X_1.

analyses for data describing the rate of events over time, and Cox (proportional hazards) regression models permit analysis of data describing survival times (that is, intervals of time to a specific event, such as a recurrence of an epileptic seizure).

Decision analysis   A collection of methods for combining estimated probabilities of certain outcomes with their *utilities*, which are mathematical functions representing the value or impact of those outcomes for key stakeholders, typically patients or families.

Study design

Observational study   The participants' lifestyle or care pathway is not affected by being part of the study (e.g. the investigator does not determine whether or not participants receive or do not receive a particular treatment). For an observational study, the investigator observes the outcome of participants following their exposure (or non-exposure) to a particular intervention or lifestyle. Interventions observed may include disease screening processes, surgical procedures and lifestyle factors (e.g. smoking) and may be studied prospectively or retrospectively. Classic types of observational studies are cohort studies and case control studies. In observational studies, the intervention is usually being given as part of the standard care pathway and in this respect the clinical element of the study protocols tend to be simpler.

Interventional study   The participants' exposure to a particular intervention (e.g. care pathway or lifestyle) is influenced by participating in the study (e.g. whether or not a participant receives a particular treatment will be determined by the research protocol). Interventions observed may include disease screening processes, surgical procedures and lifestyle factors (e.g. exercise). These studies are prospective. Clinical trials are the most common type of interventional study. Clinical trials of drug interventions are usually categorized by phase (Phase I, II, III, IV). This categorization does not generally extend to types of intervention such as radiotherapy, surgery or medical devices. 'Before-and-after studies' are another type of interventional study as they assess participants before and after introducing a particular intervention (i.e. the participants' exposure to the intervention is again influenced by the research protocol).

Randomization and cluster randomization   Randomization is a process for assigning a treatment interventions to study participants in a predictable and equal way. This is usually an equal chance of receiving an active treatment or a placebo. Cluster randomization is a process in which participants are sampled or given treatments in groups rather than as individuals.

Blinding and masking   These terms are generally used synonymously and refer to the state of knowledge of study participants, healthcare providers and investigators assessing outcomes for a randomized intervention. Although terms such as single-blind, double-blind and triple-blind have been used traditionally, the CONSORT statement (Schulz et al., 2010) recommends instead giving a description of which study members were unaware of treatment assignment.

Cohort study   A form of longitudinal study in which a sample group of participants, the cohort of interest, is studied systematically over time with collection of data at more than one point in time. The cohort shares important and relevant common characteristics or a common experience, such as exposure to a suspected risk factor.

Case control study   A form of study that is usually retrospective but can be prospective and in which participants with a disease or condition are compared with control cases without the disease. Data from such studies can be used to estimate relative risks for exposures or risk factors of interest but they need to be combined with cohort or population data in order to estimate absolute risks.

Systematic reviews and meta-analysis   A systematic review is a method for identifying, collecting, appraising, selecting and synthesizing published evidence relating to a specific clinical or research question. Where relevant unpublished evidence can be identified, this might also be included in order to reduce the effects of publication bias. Meta-analysis is the body of statistical methods used to combine and summarize the results of relevant studies. It produces summary statistics that, because they contain more data than the original individual studies, usually have smaller measures of dispersion (variance) and greater precision.

Some myths

'Only researchers need to be interested in statistics'
Most medical research leads to innovations in practice by clinicians other than those undertaking the research. Therefore all clinicians should have a working knowledge of statistical reasoning.

'P values are best used to accept or reject a treatment choice'
In practice, deciding upon a treatment relies on knowledge estimates of effect size and clinical judgement about the impact and clinical importance of such an effect. A formal decision analysis can be built up from subjective probabilities relating to specific outcomes and the utilities placed upon those outcomes by decision-makers, patients or

families. *P* values are continuous and can be used with three different inferential paradigms: significance testing, hypothesis testing and Bayesian probability. Therefore, the hypothesis test approach is only one way to use the data. Also, the clinician may need to consider several dimensions of a decision-making problem. Knowledge exists on a continuum from explicit to tacit, and the nature of this knowledge affects the style and nature of decision-making. Confidence intervals convey information about the precision of a study finding that *P* values do not.

'There is only one way to approach a clinical study, and all factors need to be closely controlled'
Clinical studies can be performed with an emphasis on one of two paradigms: *efficacy* or *effectiveness*. With the former, the study design does attempt to control factors closely but with the latter, sometimes referred to as a *pragmatic study*, the emphasis is on real-world effects and the study attempts to look for evidence of benefit of an intervention in the setting of clinical practice that will include factors such as diagnostic misclassification and non-adherence to treatment in some study participants.

The four steps of evidence-based medicine

Step 1 Formulate a clinical question
One approach to this uses the PICO acronym: patient, intervention, comparison, outcome (Haroon & Phillips , 2009). An important consideration is the specificity and context of the question. Your question relates to a specific patient or group of patients, but the evidence you might find will relate to different patients. This is the 'generalizability' of study findings. Will you restrict your search to certain features? It is very likely that you will use some form of age restriction, since infants are likely to behave quite differently to adults.

A well-formulated question has an appropriate degree of specificity (Counsell, 1997). Compare (a) 'Is vigabatrin useful in the treatment of infantile spasms?' with (b) 'Does vigabatrin, compared with ACTH or corticosteroid treatments, improve neurodevelopmental and later seizure outcomes in infantile spasms where the underlying etiology is tuberous sclerosis?' Question (a) is too vague to inform an evidence-based search. Question (b) is more specific and appropriate, but it might be necessary to broaden the scope of the question if few relevant studies are identified.

Step 2 Find appropriate evidence
In general, this means identifying appropriate online resources, such as trial registers and metasearch engines. Good places to start looking for data are SUMSearch and TRIPdatabase. SUMSearch is a metasearch engine that searches several databases, including Medline, Database of Abstracts of Reviews of Effectiveness (DARE) and the US National Guidelines Clearinghouse (NGC), for relevant papers, and refines and re-runs the search if there is an inappropriately high or low number of hits.

TRIPdatabase searches systematic reviews, other primary research study databases, and synopses. Databases of systematic reviews, such as the Cochrane Library and DARE, are relatively small. One of the most commonly searched data sites is Medline, which is accessed via the PubMed website and is run by the US National Library of Medicine. There is a range of new sources of clinical evidence, such as Clinical Evidence, Pier, and UpToDate. However, even with such user-friendly sources, most clinicians find that there are significant barriers to using evidence-based medicine. The main barriers are lack of time and lack of skills (Van Dijk et al., 2010).

A pragmatic approach is to look first for published guidelines from bodies such as the UK National Institute for Health and Clinical Excellence (NICE) or professional organizations, and then to search the Cochrane Database of Systematic Reviews. If there are no systematic reviews, or if those reviews do not seem to address the question in the relevant patient group, it is necessary to search primary research publications using PubMed or a similar database. If such primary research is not found, it will be necessary to do a more general internet search or to ask the opinion of a local, national or international expert, though of course such evidence will be less reliable.

Haynes (2006) suggests a hierarchical relationship between sources of evidence, building upwards: studies, syntheses, synopses, summaries, and systems. Since systems collate evidence from summaries, and summaries collate evidence from synopses, etc., the most efficient searches are made on systems.

Step 3 Synthesize and evaluate the evidence
Although it is the responsibility of the clinician to make a specific decision for a particular patient, evidence has sometimes been organized into a guideline. Such guidelines can be found at NICE, the Scottish Intercollegiate Guidelines Group (SIGN), and the NGC.

LEVELS OF EVIDENCE
These are graded differently but generally follow the pattern (from highest to lowest level):

1. Systematic reviews of randomized controlled trials, including meta-analyses;
2. Randomized controlled trials;
3. Controlled observational studies (cohort and case-control studies);
4. Uncontrolled observational studies (case series and case reports);
5. Expert or consensus opinion: sometimes lightheartedly referred to as 'eminence-based medicine'.

Some systems include subdivided gradings according to the risks of bias associated with study design, but this is in itself subjective to some degree. For example, SIGN suggests Level 1++ for meta-analyses or systematic reviews with a 'very low risk of bias', and 1− for meta-analyses or systematic reviews with a 'high risk of bias'.

SCOPE AND FOCUS

Depending upon the scope and focus of the original clinical question, full evaluation of the evidence usually requires consideration of the synthesized data from the guideline or systematic review, and also some consideration of data and argument from some of the original papers. Factors to consider include the following.

1. Is the conclusion and message important, credible and consistent with other research in this area?
2. Are there any ethical or design problems with the research?
3. Are the study objectives and methods clear?
4. Are there any sources of funding that might bias the reporting and conclusions?
5. Are there any authorial competing interests that might affect the authenticity and reliability of the research?

Step 4 Apply the evidence to your specific clinical question

Quantitative evidence does not require a single decision based on acceptance or rejection of a single hypothesis, but rather a decision about which intervention is likely to provide most benefit. At this level, one needs to consider the beliefs and values of the patient. Although it is rare to elicit explicit mathematical utilities for a potential outcome or event, it is possible to make tacit judgements that combine quantitative data about the probability of outcomes with the patient or family's ideas about the impact of such outcomes.

In deciding about the applicability of the search findings to a specific patient, the clinician needs to consider the following questions:

● Is the patient so different from those reported in the studies that the results do not apply?
● Is the treatment feasible and appropriate to my setting?
● What are the likely benefits and harms from the intervention?
● How do the values and beliefs of my patient or the family influence my decision?

After completing an evidence-based medicine process, we should be in a position to state whether there is strong, moderately strong or weak evidence supporting a particular clinical decision. This grading of evidence is based upon factors such as study design, data quality, the sizes of any relevant effects identified in these studies and the validity of interpretations made by study investigators. We also need to consider the clinical relevance of outcome measures used in the studies, which will influence our interpretation of the clinical importance of the effect and its magnitude.

In the field of neonatal and paediatric neurology, there are relatively few randomized controlled trials. It is therefore difficult to synthesize data. Other historical problems in this field of study are that there has tended to be weak reporting of factors such as comparison groups and co-interventions, related but different outcome measures, and the rationale for, and presumed clinical relevance of, clinical studies. Other historical problems have been short-term follow-up in conditions where longer-term outcomes are more important, and a lack of information about patient values and preferences for different outcomes, and about how the interventions might be implementable in daily life.

One of the challenges for future studies is to involve children and families more in formulating study questions so that studies of clinical effectiveness genuinely address the needs of those closest to the disease condition.

An ABC checklist for interpreting studies

(A) Assumptions Are the data and units of randomization valid? For example, has lack of blinding (masking) provided an opportunity or incentive for an assessor, consciously or subconsciously, to report an outcome in a biased fashion? This would affect the validity of the data. A study measuring the effects of a drug on, say, arthropathy and joint swelling would have an inappropriate unit of randomization if the reported outcomes were the number of affected joints since we would not reasonably expect a number of bony joints to react in an independent fashion in a single study participant. Using the bony joint as a unit of randomization would constitute a methodological error called *trial inflation*.

Has the study used appropriate probability distributions on which to base any statistical testing or modelling? There is a variety of probability distributions on which statistical analyses can be performed, and these distributions relate to different processes and scenarios. For example, analyses of a cohort study, which describes events occurring over time, would require an analysis using a probability distribution that handles the time element, such as a Poisson distribution. In this case, crude data would be reported in a unit such as number of cases per patient-year of study follow-up, and an analysis with adjustment for other potential predictor variables might use Poisson regression analysis. In contrast, studies with binary (Yes/No) outcomes determined by cross-sectional measurement, such as a case control study, might be modelled by statistical techniques making reference to the binomial distribution. Even with basic analyses on continuous data, it is necessary to consider whether the data conform to assumptions such as being normally distributed

(B) Bias and confounding Are there factors that dilute, exaggerate, distort or generate any apparent or true effects?

(C) Causality and chance Are the effects in fact due to chance? This is always possible with studies using statistical inference. If there is an association that is proven statistically, is it genuinely causal? See Table 3.4.

Table 3.4 Key questions for different types of primary and integrative study (adapted from Oxman et al., 1993)

Primary studies	
Treatment	Was patient assignment to treatment groups randomized? Were all enrolled participants accounted for and attributed at the end of the study ('intention to treat' and follow-up)?
Diagnosis	Was there an independent, blind comparison with a reference standard? Did the patient sample contain an appropriate spectrum of cases to which the test might be applied in everyday practice?
Risk of harm	Were there clearly identified comparison groups that were similar in all respects except exposure to the intervention under investigation? Were outcomes and exposures measured in the same way in exposed and comparison groups?
Prognosis	Was there a representative patient sample at a well-defined point in the course of the disease? Was follow-up sufficiently long and complete?
Integrative studies	
Overview	Did the review address a clearly focused question? Were there appropriate selection criteria for the included articles?
Practice guidelines	Were the options and outcomes clearly specified? Did the guideline use an explicit process to identify, select and combine evidence?
Decision analysis	Did the analysis model a realistic and clinically important decision? Were baseline probabilities and utilities based on valid evidence?
Economic analysis	Did the analysis compare two or more clearly described alternative interventions? Were the expected consequences of each alternative intervention based on valid evidence?

Summary and conclusion

Clinical epidemiology and evidence-based medicine underpin all good clinical practice. In all clinical practice, quality and improvement are dependent upon appropriate research and innovation. Clinical epidemiology and evidence-based medicine provide the basic tools for organizing our thinking, and for designing, performing and interpreting such research. Interpreting clinical studies and other clinical information is as important as the producing the original studies.

References

Counsell C. Formulating questions and locating primary studies for inclusion in systematic reviews. *Annals of Internal Medicine*, 1997, 127:380–387.

Engel J. A proposed diagnostic scheme for people with epileptic seizures and with epilepsy: report of the ILAE Task Force on Classification and Terminology. *Epilepsia*, 2001, 42:796–803.

Haroon M, Phillips R. 'There is nothing like looking if you want to find something' – asking questions and searching for answers – the evidence based approach. *Archives of Disease in Childhood Education and Practice Edition*, 2009, 95:34–39.

Haynes RB. Of studies, syntheses, synopses, summaries, and systems: the '5S' evolution of information services for evidence-based healthcare decisions. *Evidence-Based Medicine*, 2006, 11:162–164.

Hill AB. The environment and disease: association or causation? *Proceedings of the Royal Society of Medicine*, 1965, 58:295–300.

Larroque B, Ancel PY, Marret S et al. EPIPAGE Study group. Neurodevelopmental disabilities and special care of 5-year-old children born before 33 weeks of gestation (the EPIPAGE study): a longitudinal cohort study. *Lancet*, 2008, 371:813–820.

Nongena P, Ederies A, Azzopardi DV, Edwards AD. Confidence in the prediction of neurodevelopmental outcome by cranial ultrasound and MRI in term infants. *Archives of Disease in Childhood Fetal and Neonatal Edition*, 2010, 95:F388–F390.

Oxman AD, Sackett DL, Guyatt GH for the Evidence-Based Medicine Working Group. Users' guides to the medical literature: I. How to get started. *Journal of the American Medical Association*, 1993, 270:2093–2095.

Paul JR. Clinical epidemiology. *Journal of Clinical Investigation*, 1938, 17:539–541.

Sackett DL. Bias in analytic research. *Journal of Chronic Diseases*, 1979, 32:51–63.

Sackett DL, Rosenberg WM, Gray JA et al. Evidence based medicine: what it is and what it isn't. *British Medical Journal*, 1996, 312:71–72.

Schulz KF, Altman DG, Moher D, CONSORT Group. CONSORT 2010 statement: updated guidelines for reporting parallel group randomised trials. *British Medical Journal*, 2010, 340:698–702.

Sterne JAC, Egger M. Funnel plots for detecting bias in meta-analysis: guidelines on choice of axis. *Journal of Clinical Epidemiology*, 2001, 54:1046–1055.

Van Dijk N, Hooft L, Wierenga-de Waard M. What are the barriers to residents' practising evidence-based medicine? A systematic review. *Academic Medicine*, 2010, 85:1163–1170.

Resources

Everitt BS. *The Cambridge dictionary of statistics in the medical sciences*. Cambridge, Cambridge University Press, 1995.

Garrido MV, Kristensen K, Nielsen CP, Busse R. *Health technology assesssment and health policy-making in Europe*. Copenhagen, WHO, 2008.

Hunink M, Glasziou P. *Decision making in health and medicine: Integrating evidence and values*. Cambridge, Cambridge University Press, 2001.

Rothman KJ, Greenland S, Lash TL. *Modern epidemiology*. Philadelphia, Lippincott, Williams & Wilkins, 2008.

Chapter 4
Promoting child development

Boika Rechel and Dainius Puras

Key messages

- Every child has a basic human right to a standard of living adequate to ensure the child's physical, cognitive, emotional and social development.
- Parents and other family members play a central role in their child's development.
- Parents should be supported through accessible community services, affordable health care, decent housing and good-quality early education.
- Every child has a right to a family life and protection from abuse and neglect.
- Institutionalization can have severe detrimental consequences for child development.

Common errors

- Many incentives for institutionalization still remain in government funding schemes in countries of Central and Eastern Europe.
- Institutionalization of infants and young children affects brain development in the most crucial first years of life.

When to worry

- Physical and emotional abuse and neglect, and lack of involvement in children's activities, are associated with emotional and behavioural difficulties in childhood and later antisocial behaviour.
- Extreme emotional deprivation, neglect and abuse can suppress physical growth and development.

> **Box 4.1 Domains of development**
>
> ● *Physical development:* changes in body size, proportions, appearance, functioning of body systems, perceptual and motor capacities, and physical health
>
> ● *Cognitive development:* changes in intellectual abilities, including attention, memory, knowledge, problem solving, imagination, creativity and language
>
> ● *Emotional and social development:* changes in emotional communication, self-understanding, interpersonal skills, friendships, intimate relationships, moral reasoning and behaviour
>
> Adapted from Berk (2005).

Domains of development

Child development is the subject of interdisciplinary study from the perspectives of psychology, sociology, health and education. For convenience, development is often divided into three broad domains: physical, cognitive, and emotional and social. (See Box 4.1).

These domains are not distinct categories, and each of them influences and is influenced by the others. This chapter focuses mainly on child development in the first years of life, and we adopt a holistic view on child development, recognizing that it is a result of interplay between inherited personal characteristics, parenting, social support outside the immediate family and the wider community.

The right to development

The United Nations Convention on the Rights of the Child (UNCRC) sets out children's basic rights as the right to life, survival and development to their full potential (UN, 1989). National governments that have ratified the Convention are obliged to ensure that children survive and develop healthily. Every child is entitled to a standard of living adequate for the child's physical, mental, spiritual, moral and social development.

Children who have any kind of disability have the right to special care and support, as well as all the rights in the UNCRC, so that they can live full and independent lives. Article 23 of the Convention stipulates that 'every mentally or physically disabled child should enjoy a full and decent life, in conditions which ensure dignity, promote self-reliance and facilitate the child's active participation in the community'. Governments need to ensure that every disabled child has effective access to and receives education, training, healthcare services, rehabilitation services, preparation for employment and recreation opportunities in a manner conducive to the child's achieving the fullest possible social integration and individual development, including his or her cultural and spiritual development. Children have the right to the highest attainable standard of health and to facilities and services for the treatment of illness and rehabilitation of health (Article 24).

Factors promoting development

The central role of parents

In order to develop, young children need appropriate stimulation from their surrounding environment through interactions with caregivers, other adults and children. The role of a primary caregiver (usually the mother) who talks to, responds to and handles the infant in a sensitive, consistent and predictable manner is central to the development of the infant's brain. As children grow and acquire new skills, their parents adjust the way they interact with their toddler or preschool child. They devote less time to physical care and more time to talking, playing games or reading books together. This interaction stimulates the child's cognitive, emotional and social development. Attachments to parents, siblings and family members have a strong influence on the child's development and psychological well-being. These first relationships form models for social relationships and interactions with other children and community members outside the immediate family circle.

Social networks and community support

The family's socioeconomic status and their links with other members of the community also influence children's health and emotional well-being. Poverty has a detrimental impact on children through complex pathways of family functioning, parent–child interactions, educational opportunities, inadequate nutrition and physical illness. Poor children are more likely than their rich peers to suffer from long-term illness or disability, deficits in cognitive development, school failure and behavioural problems. Community resources can mitigate the impact of poverty on child health. Neighbourhood organizations and schools can engage children and adolescents in meaningful activities that can contribute to favourable development including the development of self-esteem and educational aspirations.

Physical development

Physical growth is influenced by the interplay of heredity and a range of environmental factors. Children's rate of growth and final height and weight are related to those of their parents. Genes regulate the production of hormones that affect children's growth, mainly the growth hormone and thyroid-stimulating hormone, produced by the pituitary gland. Environmental factors such as healthy, varied nutrition, sufficient sleep, emotional well-being and physical activity are essential to promote growth. The diet of toddlers and preschool children needs to include milk and dairy products, meat, eggs, pulses, fruit and vegetables. Foods high in sugar, salt and fats should be avoided. Caregivers need to establish a regular bedtime to ensure that children have sufficient sleep which contributes to body growth and children's ability to play and learn. Emotional well-being is important for growth and development. Extreme emotional deprivation, neglect and abuse can suppress the production of growth hormone and lead to short stature. The physical environment in which children play can influence the development of motor skills. For example, playgrounds with a range of appropriate equipment can encourage running and climbing, while play involving drawing, puzzles and construction sets stimulates fine motor development.

Cognitive development: language acquisition and literacy skills
At around 2 months, infants make vowel sounds or coo. From 4 months on, infant babble includes many sounds of spoken language and repeating syllables. Children say their first word at, on average, between 8 and 18 months of age. Language develops rapidly thereafter and by the age of 6 years children have a rich vocabulary and can construct complex sentences. The natural need of children to connect socially to others drives their language learning. Adults encourage children to talk by listening, elaborating on children's talk and responding appropriately. The quality of child care for infants and toddlers has a major impact on cognitive, social and emotional development. Conversational exchange at home and in preschool settings is associated with progress in language development. Exposure to a rich language environment and interactions with adults foster language acquisition in early childhood (Table 4.1).

Social and emotional development: prevention of behavioural and psychological disorders
Parents who are involved in children's activities, and are sensitive and responsive to their children's needs, foster secure parent–child attachment and nurture feelings of

Table 4.1 Promoting early language acquisition

Strategy	Consequence
Caregiver responds to coos and babbles with speech sounds and words	Provides experience with turn-taking in human conversation; encourages experimentation with sounds
Caregiver establishes joint attention, comments and verbally labels what the child is looking at	Fosters learning of words and development of vocabulary
Play social games, such as peekaboo	Provides experience with turn-taking in human conversation
Engage toddlers in joint make-believe play	Promotes development of verbal communication
Engage toddlers in frequent conversations	Predicts faster early language development and academic competence in school
Read to toddlers often, engaging them in dialogues about picture books	Provides exposure to many aspects of language, including vocabulary, grammar, communication skills and information about story structures
Adapted from Berk (2005).	

confidence and security. On the other hand, physical and emotional abuse and neglect, harsh discipline and lack of involvement in children's activities are associated with emotional and behavioural difficulties in childhood and later antisocial behaviour. Children witnessing domestic violence and experiencing family disharmony are more likely to display aggressive behaviour, difficulties in relating to their peers and academic failure.

Children with disabilities

There are various definitions of disability in children. Most of them include children with longstanding illnesses, conditions or impairments which affect them over a period of time and result in significant difficulties with normal daily activities, or would cause significant problems if the children were not taking medication. Children with disabilities are sometimes referred to as children with 'complex needs'. A complex need may be defined as

- a need arising from both a learning disability and from other difficulties such as physical and sensory impairment, mental health problems or behavioural difficulties; or
- a condition implying both breadth (more than one need) and depth (profound, serious or intense need).

Disabled people face a wide range of barriers (e.g. attitudinal, physical and social), the effect of which is to marginalize them within mainstream society. Moreover, compared to people without disabilities, disabled individuals are less likely to have qualifications, and more likely to live in poverty and experience problems with housing, employment and transport. These combined adverse outcomes reduce the quality of life for disabled children and young people and their families.

Families with disabled children require support in many areas of their life: physical environment, finances, social and emotional skills, promotion of developmental progress and management of day-to-day family life. The development of specialist services is vital to help meet the needs of disabled children and their families, thereby improving their well-being and ensuring that they are not excluded from the opportunities available to non-disabled children. High levels of unmet needs of disabled children are more common among families who are poor, from ethnic minorities and those who have a severely disabled child or more than one disabled child.

In the UK, the National Service Framework (NSF) for Children, Young People and Maternity Services (Department of Health, 2004) established standards for promoting the health and well-being of children and young people and providing them with high quality services. Standard 8 of the NSF for disabled children and young people and those with complex health needs states: 'Children and young people who are disabled or who have complex health needs receive co-ordinated, high-quality and family-centred services which are based on assessed needs, which promote social inclusion and, where possible, which enable them and their families to live ordinary lives.'

Child protection

In cases where the family circumstances present a threat to the safety and development of children, the state has a responsibility to intervene and ensure a suitable environment where children can grow and develop. Conditions which may necessitate intervention from the state are wide-ranging and include extreme poverty and poor nutrition, domestic violence, illness, imprisonment, disabled child or parent, child neglect and abuse. Whenever possible, the best option for the child is to be cared for in their natural family, if the state can provide social and other support needed by families in difficulties. In other circumstances, however, children need to be taken away from the natural family for shorter or longer periods of time until the crisis in the family is resolved. In such cases efforts should be made to assist the family so that the child can return to their family as soon as possible.

Models of protective care

There are different models of protective care that have emerged around the world, with the main types being state-supported parental care, foster care, adoption and institutionalization.

STATE-SUPPORTED PARENTAL CARE

Parents receive support from the state in provision of care, but maintain custodial rights.

FOSTER CARE

In foster care the custodial rights are granted temporarily to adults who take on the role of parents. Foster care may take place in a family, among relatives of the child or in small group homes.

ADOPTION

Adoption is an option for protective care in cases where the biological parents have died or there are serious problems in the family resulting in the state revoking custodial rights from the biological parents. It provides children with stability and the opportunity to form lasting relationships with the adoptive parents. Domestic adoption should take priority over international adoption.

INSTITUTIONAL CARE

In Western Europe, most large children's institutions closed during the last quarter of the 20th century, in favour of foster care. These developments occurred under the influence of the attachment theory by Bowlby (1969) which demonstrated the importance of attachment to a primary caregiver for children's psychological and social development. In residential care children lack the opportunity to form an attachment to a parent figure. Institutionalization of infants and young children affects brain development in the most crucial period of the first years of life. The attachment theory had less influence in the countries of Central and Eastern Europe (CEE). In these countries the predominant model of protective care, inherited from the communist regime, was long-term placement in institutions. The approach to care in institutions followed a 'medical model' focused on meeting the physical needs of children, provision of food and clothes, and on the infrastructure of facilities, but little attention was paid to the social and emotional development of children, their quality of life and the social care aspects. Children and their parents had little say in the running of the institutions and the provision of care. The system fostered dependency on the state for care of children of families in need, weakened the family bond and detached the children from their communities. The institutional model of care was both more expensive and much less effective with regard to children's outcomes and their preparedness for independent life in society.

The adverse impact of institutionalization on development
Young children placed in institutional residential care without parents are at high risk of developmental delay and cognitive, social, behavioural and emotional disorders (Dixon, & Misca, 2004). In particular, children who have been raised in institutions more often present with problems with social competence, and peer and sibling interactions (Browne et al., 2005). Furthermore 'quasi-autistic' behaviours have been observed in severely deprived institutionalized children, associated with prolonged experiential and perceptual deprivation, cognitive impairment and lack of opportunity to develop social interaction (Rutter et al., 1999). Prospective studies of Romanian children adopted in the UK have found that the length of time spent in institutional settings was the primary predictor of the prevalence and persistence of behaviour and developmental problems (Beckett et al., 2002). Children who have spent their early years in institutions are more likely to manifest social problems in adolescence.

In CEE, the numbers of children living in institutional care at the end of the 1990s were higher than in 1989 (UNICEF, 2001). The regional average rate was 1441 per 100 000 aged 0–17, a rise of 20% compared to 1194 in 1989 (UNICEF, 2003). Of special concern are the rising rates of infants entering institutional care, in contrast with the overall decline in the infant population in the region. The increase has been particularly steep in Latvia, Bulgaria and Romania, but is also significant in Estonia, Kazakhstan and other former Soviet Union countries (UNICEF, 2003). Most of these children have been abandoned for economic or social reasons, some are physically or mentally disabled and few are orphans.

Carers in institutions in CEE usually have a poor knowledge of children's health needs and whether children suffer from a disability or behavioural problem (UNICEF, 2003). In Romania, the children's institutions had a strong medical orientation. They provided little intellectual or social development activities and the only care revolved around basic medical needs (Zamfir, & Zamfir, 1996). In the worst care homes in Bulgaria, such as those for disabled children, the ratio of caregivers to children could be as high as 1:40 (Save the Children, 2002). Children living in institutions are cut off from society and rarely receive visitors. Children's institutions often discourage links with parents or extended family (Rechel, 2008). See Box 4.2.

Developing community-based models of care: challenges and opportunities for the CEE region
Analysis of the situation of services for children with disabilities and other children with risk factors in the CEE region has revealed that both the historical context and the

---

Box 4.2 Negative effects of institutionalization

- Often, children reared from an early age in institutions fail to learn to sit, stand, walk and talk by the age of 4 years.
- In institutions, children cannot attach securely to a significant adult. As a result, many institutionalized children show indiscriminate affection to adults, exhibit low self-confidence and negative behaviours, lack empathy and are prone to non-compliance and aggressive behaviour.
- Basic human rights cannot be ensured in institutions. The UNCRC asserts the right of children to a family life and protection from abuse and neglect.
- Children in institutions are more likely to have low educational attainment and poor employment prospects.
- Institutions leave children ill-prepared to live in the outside world.
- Institutions often discourage contact with family and deprive young people from social networks.

Adapted from UNICEF (2004).

---

resulting attitudes of service providers are factors tending to obstruct the smooth transition from excessive institutional care for children to community-based and family-focused care. Even after 20 years of transition, many countries in the CEE region are still heavily reliant on institutional care that encompasses newborns to developmentally disabled adults. The problem is exacerbated by the fact that many children who are institutionalized during their first months of life do not have developmental disabilities. However, in the infant homes, which are usually part of the healthcare system, they are labelled as having developmental delay or some other 'medical' problem, to justify their admission to and continued residence in a medical institution. Having stayed in institutional care for the first 2 or 3 years of life, their perceived developmental delay turns into a genuine arrest of development as a consequence of their institutionalization and denial of their basic right to holistic development. A large group of children with mild developmental disabilities can thus be said to have had their rights violated by the system managed by national governments.

The legacy of institutionalization of children with real or perceived developmental disability in the CEE and former Soviet Union stemmed from two prevailing concepts. One of them was the concept of 'defectology' (see below). The other one was the concept of child psychoneurology. A further problem of the former system is that the concept of parent training and psychosocial support for families with disabled children have been non-existent. Clinical social work and child protection services and family support services never having existed in this region, there is a huge vacuum where there might be community-based services.

After the dramatic political changes in CEE in the early 1990s, 30 new democracies emerged and, with them, many new possibilities and opportunities to develop much needed services and concepts. With varying degrees of success, community-based services have been piloted with the support of international foundations. However, these initiatives were often unsustainable without support from governments and local authorities. Instead of prioritizing investment in new community-based services, governments have been more willing to support the traditional infrastructures of residential institutions, such as the system of infant homes for children from birth to 3 years. Even after the need for a child with or without disability to grow up in his or her family has been officially recognized, incentives for institutionalization still remain in government funding schemes in many countries.

Many developed countries have found that the involvement of the parents of children with disabilities is a crucial precondition for the establishment of modern services that promote the development of disabled children. Parent organizations when they are supported by governments, become powerful and constructive partners in changing the system so that instead of being self-serving, the systems of care start to meet the needs of the children.

In the CEE region it is the countries with strong non-governmental parent organizations that move ahead in providing modern services for disabled children while those that do not have such organizations lag behind. An example from Lithuania may reflect both the achievements and challenges of the CEE region in this regard. In 1989, a national organization of parents who have children with developmental disabilities, *Viltis* (which means 'hope'), was founded. Over a period of more than 20 years, this organization has developed into a powerful non-governmental organization undertaking both advocacy and provision of modern policies and services for children and adults with developmental disabilities. Viltis has lobbied effectively for development of early intervention services for children from 0 to 3 who have developmental disabilities or risk factors which might affect their development. A Child Development Centre has been established as a consequence of this lobbying, with a demonstration clinic where children and their parents are involved in developing individual plans for holistic promotion of their development and further integration in society. The next step was to establish early intervention outpatient teams throughout the country so that these services, can be accessed by families in need. This new network of services in which the medical model is combined with strong psychosocial and educational components and parents are involved as equal members of multidisciplinary team, could not happen without active pressure and involvement from interested citizens. Despite all these achievements, many children and adults with developmental disabilities in Lithuania still remain in institutional care. The parents' organization continue to work with politicians and the general public on the need to develop family-oriented and community-based services so that use of institutional care, especially for children from 0 to 3, can be stopped.

Similarly, involvement of parents as equal partners is crucially important at the level of management of children with disabilities in, for example, the early intervention services. After many years of paternalistic relations between doctors and patients or, in the case of children with disabilities, their parents, a paradigm shift in the training of medical doctors and other professionals was needed in this field. In the former system, the information on diagnosis and management provided for parents was minimal: the prevailing ideology was that the less parents knew, the better. In the new system of services, parents are equal partners with doctors and other professionals, and professionals learn a lot from parents as the parents are uniquely expert on the subject of their own child. However, as this shift of paradigm in the mentality of professionals is so huge, there is still a great deal of resistance to these modern approaches among health service providers and medical education systems: modernization is perceived by those who are reluctant to accept it as depriving them of their monopoly of power in making decisions.

In the experience of the UN Committee on the Rights of the Child (UNCRC) in CEE countries, the transition from institutional care to modern care for children with disabilities has been extremely complicated and the need to facilitate change remains urgent. The UNCRC, in its Concluding Observations, when considering reports from the countries of the CEE region, has expressed concerns on the continuing overuse of institutional care for children with disabilities and has recommended to many countries in this region that they should invest in early intervention and family support services and stop the tradition of institutionalization of children with disabilities which is harmful both for children and for the society.

The obstacle to effective implementation of the UNCRC policies posed by the system is the tradition of protecting and promoting economic and social rights (i.e., to protect the right to life and survival) at the expense of civil rights. In this regard, institutional care is classical example of 'protection' in the narrow sense. But in a broader and modern sense, this is also a deprivation of liberty and is contrary to the right to holistic development. This seems to be a barrier to progress in the CEE region where, after some years of enthusiasm, criticism of liberal democracy and nostalgia about the totalitarian past is becoming increasingly prevalent.

Conclusions

The physical, cognitive and emotional development of a child is the result of a complex interplay between genetic and environmental factors. Growing in an optimal environment enables children to achieve their full potential and is a basic human right of all children. Parents play a central role in their child development but need to be supported by wider society in fulfilling this role through accessible community services, affordable health care, decent housing and good-quality early education. In cases where families experience substantial difficulties and are unable to look after their children, foster care and adoption are the second best options for child rearing. Institutionalization can have severe detrimental and irreversible consequences for child development, particularly when children are placed in institutions in infancy or before the age of 3 years. There have been growing efforts in CEE to develop community-based services and to decrease the number of children in institutions. However, socioeconomic and political circumstances as well as the strong tradition of institutionalization have been obstacles in this process.

References

Beckett C et al. Behavior patterns associated with institutional deprivation: a study of children adopted from Romania. *Journal of Developmental and Behavioral Pediatrics*, 2002, 23(5):297–303.

Berk L. *Infants, children and adolescents*. Harlow, Pearson Education, 2005.

Bowlby J. *Attachment and loss, vol. 1: attachment*. London: Pimlico, 1969.

Browne K et al. *Mapping the number and characteristics of children under three in institutions across Europe at risk of harm*. European Commission DAPHNE Programme in collaboration with WHO Regional Office for Europe and the University of Birmingham, 2005.

Department of Health. *National Service Framework for Children, Young People and Maternity Services*. London, Department of Health, 2004.

Dixon L, Misca G. *Mapping the number and characteristics of children under 3 in institutions across Europe at risk of harm*. Copenhagen, WHO Regional Office for Europe, 2004.

Rechel B. Access to care and the right to life of disabled children in Bulgaria. In Clements L, Read J, eds, *Disabled people and the right to life: The protection and violation of disabled people's most basic human rights*. Abingdon, Routledge, 2008.

Rutter M et al. Quasi-autistic patterns following severe early global privation. *Journal of Child Psychology and Psychiatry*, 1999, 40(4):537–549.

Save the Children. *Continuing misuse of children's institutions in Bulgaria*. Sofia, Save the Children UK, 2002.

UN. *Convention on the Rights of the Child*. New York, United Nations, 1989.

UNICEF. *A decade of transition, Regional Monitoring Report No 8*. Florence, UNICEF Innocenti Research Centre, 2001.

UNICEF. *Changing minds, policies and lives. Improving protection of children in Eastern Europe and Central Asia. Gatekeeping services for vulnerable children and families*. Florence, UNICEF Innocenti Research Centre, 2003.

UNICEF. *De-institutionalisation of children's services in Romania: A good practice guide*. Publication of the High Level Group for Romanian Children, 2004.

Zamfir C, Zamfir E. *Children at risk in Romania: Problems old and new*. Innocenti Occasional Papers, Economic Policy Series, 56. Florence, UNICEF Innocenti Research Centre, 1996.

Resources

Browne K, Hamilton-Giachritsis C, Johnson R, Ostergren M. Overuse of institutional care for children in Europe. *British Medical Journal*, 2006, 332:485–487.

Ginsburg KR and the Committee on Communications and the Committee on Psychosocial Aspects of Child and Family Health. The importance of play in promoting healthy child development and maintaining strong parent-child bonds. *Pediatrics*, 2007, 119:182–191.

Hall D, Williams J, Elliman D. *The child surveillance handbook*, 3rd edn. Radcliffe Publishing, Oxford, 2009.

Hall DMB, Elliman D. *Health for all children*, 4th edn. Oxford, Oxford Medical Publications, 2003.

UNICEF Innocenti Research Centre. *Children and disability in transition in CEE/CIS and Baltic States*. Florence, UNICEF Innocenti Research Centre, 2005.

Chapter 5

Neurological and neurodevelopmental assessment

Leena Haataja, Vittorio Belmonti and Giovanni Cioni

Key messages
- Distinguish deviant development from normal variation.
- Use standardized protocols for neurological and neurodevelopmental assessments.
- Realize that there is no criterion standard: different protocols have different goals.

Common errors
- Misinterpreting a normal variant as abnormal.
- Suspecting neurological disorders without comprehensive examination.
- Failing to adapt the neurological examination derived from adult neurology to the examination of infants.
- Delaying diagnosis and intervention.

When to worry
- Abnormal quantity or quality of movement repertoire.
- Deviant neurological findings.
- Late developmental milestones.
- Loss of developmental skills at any age.
- Concerns about vision or hearing (parental or professional).

Normal neurological development

Wide individual variation is the key feature in normal neurological development. Typically developing infants spontaneously show a large range of complex movement activities and an innate interest in new stimuli which allows them to discover, over time, the most efficient way to move and behave in a given environment. There is also a wide biological variation in attaining developmental milestones; for example, walking independently in neurologically normal infants may happen at any given time between 8 and 18 months of age or even beyond the age of 2 years in 'bottom-shufflers'. Another characteristic feature of normal development is the general forward direction of development with the various developmental skills usually appearing in a predictable sequence. Typically, there are periods of rapid progress in attaining a new skill alternating with developmentally stable periods. Even though normal development allows discontinuity, the typically developing infant does not lose learned skills. Normal development is a dynamic and multifaceted process which is a challenge to accurate measurement. Nevertheless, the use of formal developmental screening tools improves the early identification of infants with developmental problems, thus improving the prospects for interventions.

Main features of typical neurological development

Morphological and functional development

This paragraph is not intended to give a detailed description of the embryogenesis and maturation of neural structures, but some points which are critical for clinical assessment will be highlighted. The main stages of the development of the central nervous system (CNS) and the corresponding abnormalities shown in Table 5.1.

The key message is that morphological disorders (i.e., CNS malformations) may arise at any moment from a variety of causative factors, not only genetic but also external ones. These factors are complex and largely unknown, while the timing (phase of onset) of each pattern of malformation (phenotype) is rather consistent. Therefore, all traditional classification schemes are mainly based on phenotypical and temporal criteria (e.g. disorders of proliferation, migration, organization, etc.) This approach to CNS malformations has recently been replaced with an integrated one, including etiological criteria (especially genotype) whenever possible. In a clinical context, however, the dependency of the nature of morphological abnormalities, including those resulting from perinatal or postnatal brain injuries, on the age at onset seems to provide easier and more general guidance than etiology. This, for instance, is one of the bases of most modern classifications of the cerebral palsies, which include the timing of the lesion as a fundamental criterion.

Even if neurons in most brain regions do not continue to proliferate after birth, it is now clear that maturational processes extend far into postnatal life, even into adult life. Brain plasticity and reorganization after insults are surely the most desirable consequences of such a prolonged maturation: the immature brain is capable of impressive rearrangements of pathways and of regional specialization. For example,

Table 5.1 The main stages of central nervous system development and peak gestational age for their occurrence and the main disorders which may arise (adapted from Aicardi, 2009)

Gestational age	Stage of CNS development	Disorders that may arise
2 weeks	Formation of the neural plate	Enterogenous cysts and fistulae
3–4 weeks	Dorsal induction/neurulation (the neural tube and crest are formed)	Blastopathies (e.g. anencephaly, encephaloceles, spina bifida, meningoceles)
4–7 weeks	Dorsal induction/caudal neural-tube formation	Diastematomyelia, Dandy-Walker syndrome, cerebellar hypoplasia
5–6 weeks	Ventral induction (forebrain and face emerge; cleavage of the forebrain into two cerebral vesicles, formation of optic and olfactory placodes and of diencephalon)	Disorders of ventral induction (holoprosencephaly, median cleft face syndrome)
8–16 weeks	Neuronal and glial proliferation (cells proliferate in ventricular and subventricular zones; early differentiation of neuroblasts and glioblasts)	Disorders of proliferation (microcephaly, megalencephaly)
12–20 weeks	Migration (mainly radial migration of neurons towards the cortex)	Disorders of migration (e.g. lissencephaly–subcortical band heterotopia–pachygyria spectrum, nodular heterotopias), agenesis of corpus callosum
24 weeks onwards	Organization (alignment, orientation and layering of cortical neurons, synaptogenesis, programmed cell death, glial proliferation and differentiation)	Disorders of organization (e.g. polymicrogyria, focal cortical dysplasias)
24 weeks gestational age to 2 years post-term	Myelination	Dismyelination, clastic insult (24–36 wks GA: typically deep white matter damage; 36 wks GA–early post-term age: cortical–subcortical damage)

language areas may shift from the dominant to the contralateral hemisphere, while the damaged primary motor area may reorganize either around the lesion or contralaterally, depending on timing and extent of the lesion.

Nature or nurture

Researchers have long been engaged in a sterile debate on whether all individual features were due to 'nature' (hereditary and constitutional factors) or, at least with regard to behavioural differences, to 'nurture' (breeding, environment, society). Most researchers in the field now believe in an interplay between the two.

A crucial question is how such a wide variation as that found in normal neurological development could be explained. The major developments in imaging and neurophysiological techniques during the last few decades have allowed us to understand that infant motor activity is a complex process driven by the CNS and involving interaction between afferent information, and spinal and supraspinal controlling networks. The current prevailing neuronal group selection theory (NGST) is based on the synergy between genetic and environmental determinants of activity that influence the maturation of infant development. According to NGST the abundant variation in the repertoire of motor behaviours is expressed from fetal life onwards and continues through infancy when selection of the functionally most effective motor pattern happens at a particular age that is specific to the motor function.

Norms and variability

Child development consists of gross motor, fine motor, language, cognitive and social-behavioural domains of development. Taking into consideration the wide normal variation in attaining any developmental milestone it is important to emphasize that the available different norms for developmental screening are more in the form of reference ranges than clear-cut differences between normal and abnormal. Above all, an abnormal developmental finding implies the need for close follow-up and, depending on the case, the need for further consultation and intervention to enable all the available developmental potential to be realized. Late developmental milestones or loss of developmental skills act as red flags that suggest abnormal development to the assessor. The references for developmental milestones, which should be regarded as for guidance rather than absolutely invariable, are given in the subsections that follow. In particular, it is important not to place too much reliance on a single milestone falling outside the reference ranges provided.

GROSS MOTOR MILESTONES

The WHO Multicentre Growth Reference Study (2006) collected longitudinal data on the attainment of six gross motor milestones (sitting without support, hands-and-knees crawling, standing with assistance, walking with assistance, standing alone and walking alone) in a total of 816 children aged 4–24 months in Ghana, India, Norway, Oman and the United States (these growth charts are reproduced in Appendix 1 of the report and can be downloaded from http://www.who.int/childgrowth/standards/en/). The normal variation in the ages of mastering any given milestone was described with a concept of 'a window'; that is, a time interval during which normal, typically

Table 5.2 The upper age limits for attaining motor milestones during infancy

Milestone	Age (months)
Sitting without support	9
Hands-and-knees crawling	14
Standing with assistance	11
Walking with assistance	14
Standing alone	17
Walking alone	18

developing infants learn a specific motor task. It is also of interest that 4.3% of infants never crawled on hands and knees, which is also reported in other studies as the milestone often missed out as a variation of normal. In 90% of infants the milestones were achieved in a fixed order, the most common sequence, seen in 42% of infants, being sit, crawl, stand, assisted walking then unassisted walking. It has also been reported that there is no significant difference in attainment of different motor milestones between girls and boys, and they can therefore share a common reference range. If the infant has been born preterm, it is common practice, although not uniformly accepted, that the performance of the infant is compared to the infant's corrected age – that is, age from the expected date of delivery – for the 2 years after birth. The upper age limits for attaining the six main motor milestones in typically developing infants are given in Table 5.2 and the range is shown in Figure 5.1. A simplified rule of thumb is that infants should sit independently by 10 months and walk independently no later than at age 18 months.

FINE MOTOR MILESTONES
Separating fine motor function from gross motor development is somewhat arbitary during the first year of life since developmental changes happen in interplay, for example attaining posture control and independent sitting position are prerequisites for the most efficient development of hand function. The upper age limits of attaining fine motor milestones in typically developing infants are presented in Table 5.3. A simplified rule of thumb is that the infant should voluntarily grasp an object by 5 months and show pincer grasping by 10 months of age.

LANGUAGE AND SOCIAL MILESTONES
Typically developing infants produce different reflexive sounds associated with internal states (e.g. crying for hunger) from birth onwards. The vowel sounds are increasingly produced between 2 and 6 months, and canonical babbling (babbling long utterances

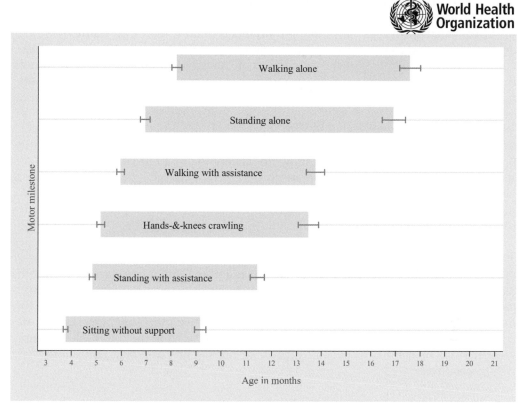

Figure 5.1 Windows of achievement for six gross motor milestones. Source: WHO Multicentre Growth Reference Study Group. WHO Motor Development Study: Windows of achievement for six gross motor development milestones. *Acta Paediatrica Supplement*, 2006, 450:86–95. Reproduced with permission of John Wiley & Sons Inc.

Table 5.3 The upper age limits for attaining fine motor milestones during infancy

Milestone	Age (months)
Reaches for an object	4
Grasps using whole hand	5
Changes object from one hand to another	7
Pincer grasp	8–10

including consonants) begins between 6 and 10 months. Laughing aloud is usually present by 6 months of age. The comprehension of spoken language precedes expressive language in early development. Infants recognize their own name by 8 months of age, and start understanding single words between 8 and 10 months of age. Normally hearing infants start the production of true words – that is, verbal utterances used consistently to indicate specific stimuli in the external world – by 10–12 months of age.

The general rule of thumb is that by 8 months of age, the infant should produce canonical babbling and show consistent reaction when called by name. By 12 months of age, normally developing infants show understanding of a few words. If there is a suspected delay in sound production and/or receptive language it is always advisable to have the child's hearing checked. If their hearing is normal, this would then raise the question of whether the infant shows signs of a specific language or autistic-spectrum disorder or a significant general impairment of early development.

Typically developing infants show a smile in response to external sensory stimuli by 2 months of age, and a selective social smile, for example to their caregiver, by 3 months of age. Around 7 months of age infants start distinguishing between familiar persons and strangers, and they start showing anxiety when approached by strangers. By 8–10 months of age infants start showing attempts at interactive play. They typically first start to release or cast toys with the expectation of somebody giving the toys back to them. By 12 months of age infants become capable of playing give-and-take games and waving goodbye.

Absence of the smile response is a red flag for the need of visual assessment. The absence of any attempt at interactive play and joint engagement by 12 months requires a thorough investigation of the psychosocial environment of the child in addition to the medical differential diagnostic work-up according to the lines of speech delay outlined above.

Main items of clinical neurological examination and available standardized protocols

Clinical neurological assessment always comprises three main aspects: history taking, physical examination and neurological assessment. Systematical history taking should include items listed in Table 5.4.

Physical examination including growth pattern (see growth charts, Appendix 1, especially the increase in head circumference over time plotted on a growth chart with z scores or centiles for age (see growth charts), may give a crucial 'diagnostic handle' in cases of abnormal development (see especially Chapters 18, 19, 21 and 24 in this volume).

The examiner has to be sensitive to both the state and clinical condition of the infant, especially those under the age of 1 year. The optimal timing of the neurological examination relative to the infant's state is important and findings in a crying, irritable infant may be misleading. In neonatal examinations it is advisable to assess the newborn infant in the middle third of the time interval between feeds to avoid disturbing the infant's sleeping cycle and to make the assessment before the infant becomes hungry for the next feed.

The widely used Dubowitz examination is taken as an example of a structured neonatal assessment. The Dubowitz examination includes 34 items, and the list of main item headings is presented in Table 5.5. This method provides reference ranges for typically

Table 5.4 Items included in systematic history taking

- The course of pregnancy and birth

- Achieved developmental milestones (e.g. first smile, rolling onto side)

- Enquiry about any unusual behaviour patterns

- Previous and current health problems

- Previous and present medications

- Parental concerns about the child

- Social situation of the family

- Family history of neurological disorders

Table 5.5 The main item headings included in the neonatal examination

- Orientation and behaviour

- Tone and tone pattern including assessment both prone and supine

- Neonatal reflexes:
  tendon reflexes, suck and gag
  palmar/plantar grasp, placing and Moro reflexes

- Movements: quantity and quality

- Abnormal signs:
  abnormal hand/toe posture, excessive tremor, startle

Table 5.6 Clinical signs suggesting central nervous system involvement

- Altered state of consciousness

- Convulsions

- Abnormal tone patterns

- Abnormal movements

- Abnormal auditory or visual responses

- Sucking/swallowing difficulties

- Abnormal posture of hand or toes

developing term infants tested during the first days after birth. The same method can be applied to preterm infants. However, preterm infants show less limb flexor tone and poorer head control at term age than infants born at term. Furthermore, preterm infants have a tendency to be more hyperexcitable (brisk reflexes, startles, tremors) and have less mature visual behaviour compared with term infants. The normal reference ranges for preterm infants assessed at term are available elsewhere (see Cioni and Mercuri, 2007; Dubowitz et al., 1999).

Isolated abnormal clinical findings in the Dubowitz examination have little diagnostic value, but merely indicate the need for later reassessment. Abnormal findings that usually require further assessment are listed in Table 5.6.

The Hammersmith Infant Neurological Examination (HINE) is taken as an example of a structured infant assessment. HINE is based on the same methodological principles as the neonatal Dubowitz examination, and it has been developed for use after the neonatal period up to 24 months of age. This method can be used to make a distinction between normal and abnormal development and to predict future outcomes. The examination includes 26 items evaluating posture, active and passive tone, assessment of cranial nerve function, movements, reflexes and protective reactions (Table 5.7). The examination has been standardized on the basis of findings in a cohort of low-risk term infants at 12 and 18 months. The infant examination can be performed in preterm infants as early as 6 months of corrected age, and the neurological findings at 9 months of corrected age have been shown to predict motor function at 2 years of age.

In addition to the items listed in Table 5.7, it is advisable to assess systematically, at least in infants with suspected neurological problems, hearing, visual function and

Table 5.7 Items included in the Hammersmith infant examination

- Assessment of cranial nerve function:
  facial appearance, eye appearance, auditory response,visual response, sucking/swallowing

- Posture:
  head and trunk in sitting, arms, hands, legs, feet in supine sitting and standing

- Spontaneous movements:
  quantity and quality

- Tone:
  scarf sign, passive shoulder elevation, pronation/supination, adductors, popliteal angle, ankle dorsiflexion, pull to sit, ventral suspension

- Reflexes and reactions:
  tendon reflexes; protective upper limb reflexes on falling from sit (lateral propping); arm extension on moving head toward floor (forward parachute)

growth, and physical abnormalities that could be related to neurological diseases, such as axial, proximal and distal muscle bulk, tone and power (see also Chapter 20 in this volume).

Complementary approach to neurological evaluation in the first year of life

Background
In the 1980s Heinz Prechtl outlined the basic requirements for a new method of neonatal assessment: to be non-invasive, rapid and sensitive to variations of the age-specific functional repertoire. The observation and categorization of spontaneous movements in the first months of life then led to the identification of several normal and abnormal motor patterns. Among others, the so-called general movements (GMs) were identified as ongoing global movements involving all body parts and appeared particularly suitable for assessment. This gave rise to Prechtl's Method on the Qualitative Assessment of General Movements in Preterm, Term and Young Infants (Einspieler et al. 2005).

GM assessment: methodology and purposes
Although based on global and qualitative judgements, GM assessment has proven to be reliable and to have predictive value not only for later cerebral palsy, but also for minor neurological disorders, Rett syndrome, cognitive and autistic-spectrum disorders.

Table 5.8 Typical time course of the normal patterns of general movements

Pattern	Age (weeks post-menstrual age)	Description
Writhing movements (WMs)	Range: 9–49 Peak: 40 (term)	Variable amplitude, slow to moderate speed, typically ellipsoid limb trajectories lying close to the sagittal plane with superimposed rotations.
Fidgety movements (FMs)	Range: 46–64 Peak: 52	Smaller than WMs, moderate average speed with variable acceleration in all directions, migrating through all body parts as an ongoing flow of movement. Continual in the awake infant, except during fussing, crying and focused attention.

Normal GMs involve the whole body in a complex sequence of arm, leg, neck and trunk movements. They wax and wane in intensity, force and speed, and have a gradual beginning and end. Rotations along the axis of the limbs and slight changes in the direction of movements make them fluent and elegant and create the impression of complexity and variability. GMs appear as early as 9–12 weeks post-menstrual age and continue after birth without substantially changing their form, irrespective of when birth occurs. The typical time course of normal GM patterns is described in Table 5.8.

GMs of infants with cerebral impairment lack complexity, fluency and/or variability. Abnormal GM patterns are sorted into two groups depending on whether they are observed in the writhing movements (WMs) or in the fidgety movements (FMs) period (Table 5.9). In the FM period, various other motor patterns gradually emerge and mingle with GMs, thus building up the so-called associated motor repertoire, whose richness and age-adequacy have been related to the optimality of later motor coordination.

The 'global' visual perception of movement quality (Gestalt perception) has proven a powerful and reliable instrument, but only if carefully applied after specific training in this form of assessment. A thorough description of the standardized assessment procedure can be found in Einspieler et al. (2005). Notably, the standard GM assessment is based on video recording, but it has also proven reliable (especially in the FM period) when employed by examiner's observation as a part of neurological examination.

Table 5.9 Main abnormal patterns of general movements

Pattern	Description
(a) Writhing movements (WM) period	
Poor repertoire (PR)	Monotonous sequences, few movement components, repetitive and not so complex as in normal WMs. Fluency may be reduced too (but usually more spared than complexity and variability).
Cramped-synchronized (CS)	No complexity, fluency and variability: all limb and trunk muscles contract and relax almost simultaneously.
Chaotic (Ch)	Large amplitude, high jerk and chaotic order without any fluency or smoothness. Rare, often evolving into CS.
(b) Fidgety movements (FM) period	
Absent FMs	FMs are never observed in the whole period.
Abnormal FMs (AF)	Fidgety-like movements, but amplitude, average speed and jerkiness are exaggerated.

Diagnostic and prognostic validity of GMs assessment
Although several developmental disorders are related to GM abnormality, the most reliable GM markers concern the prediction of cerebral palsy. These markers are (1) a consistent cramped-synchronized (CS) pattern throughout the WM period and (2) the Absent FM pattern. Consistent CS, though not common, has a 100% specificity for the diagnosis of cerebral palsy, while the absent FM pattern has both a high sensitivity and specificity for cerebral palsy. The other abnormal patterns are less reliable, possibly leading to a normal neurological outcome. In unilateral cerebral palsy, additional assessment of selective distal movements will identify the laterality of the lesion.

Structured neurodevelopmental scales
There is a wide selection of neurodevelopmental scales available, and the goal of the assessment should guide the selection of a specific scale (e.g. whether used as a screening tool by a community paediatrician or as a detailed standardized scale for an infant at high risk for developmental problems). Unlike the tools of neurological examination, neurodevelopmental scales are not aimed at a categorical diagnosis (e.g. of cerebral palsy or behavioural disorder), but at an assessment of the infant's functioning on certain dimensions of development. Most scales are multidimensional and provide a developmental profile, but there are also unidimensional ones,

specifically for motor function, cognition or language. All structured scales must be administered by a specifically trained examiner. They are usually relatively time-consuming compared with neurological examination. They are, however, important for the assessment of high-risk infants: poor functioning in one or more developmental areas, and especially in cognitive, perceptual-motor and visual-spatial abilities, language and/or behaviour, is much more common than a definite neurological disorder at toddler and school age. Moreover, neurodevelopmental assessment allows the planning and monitoring of intervention protocols, individualized to suit the infant's strengths and weaknesses and prioritized to achieve functional goals.

One of the key characteristics of standardized tests is the derivation of standardized scores, based on a previous standardization process involving a large sample of typically developing infants. Importantly, the standardization of a test does not guarantee properties such as validity and reliability, which vary greatly among the tests. Screening tools are on average far less reliable and predictive for later functioning than detailed scales. However, the selection of a particular scale may also be determined by other considerations than its psychometric properties, such as availability, proven validity for a specific class of disorders or risk factors (e.g. preterm infants, visual or auditory defects, etc.), or personal experience. A crucial feature that should always be checked, is whether standardized scores for a given population (e.g. non-English-speaking populations) are provided. The standardized scales for assessing development from birth to 2 years are given in Table 5.10.

Practical conclusions

Modern techniques of exploration of the nervous system, such as genetic tests, electrophysiological measures (EEG, evoked potentials) and neuroimaging, cannot replace the essential contribution of neurological clinical examination to diagnosis and prognosis of neurodevelopmental disorders in the young infant. The examiner should be competent in the assessment of 'normal' or, more precisely, 'typical' development, to be able to distinguish between the normal biological variation and abnormal development. The essential items to be examined and the red flags to be taken into account have been described in this chapter.

The use of comprehensive and standardized protocols is always preferable to limited and personal lists of items. There is no consensus for a unique criterion standard, and the examiner should be aware of the advantages and limitations of the assessment method applied. Spontaneous and elicited gross and fine motor skills, perceptual, social and attentional functions should be included in a comprehensive assessment. The appropriate use of neurological comprehensive assessment is not a single event, but it has the great advantage of being easily repeatable to obtain developmental trajectories, which are much more informative than a single assessment. They can be used either to reassure doctors and parents by detection of positive changes in development or, on the contrary, to lead to suspicion of static or delayed development or a progressive neurological disorder. In these situations they may help to identify appropriate investigations or treatments for the underlying cause.

Table 5.10 Standardized scales for assessing development from birth to 2 years (adapted from Johnson and Marlow, in Cioni and Mercuri, 2007)

Name	Age range	Duration	Domains
Bayley Scales of Infant Development, 2nd ed. (BSID-II)	1–42 months	25–60 min	Mental Development (MDI), Motor Development (PDI), Behaviour Rating Scale (BRS)
Bayley Scales of Infant and Toddler Development, 3rd ed. (Bayley-III)	1–42 months	30–90 min	Cognitive, Language, Motor, Social-Emotional (parent report), Adaptive Behaviour (parent report)
Griffiths Mental Development Scales–Baby Scales (Griffiths Scales: 0–2)	Birth to 23 months	35–60 min	Locomotor, Personal-Social, Hearing and Language, Eye-hand Coordination, Performance
Mullen Scales of Early Learning (MSEL)	Birth to 5 years 8 months.	15–30 min (depends on age)	Gross Motor, Fine Motor, Visual Reception, Receptive Language, Expressive Language
Battelle Developmental Inventory II (BDI-II)	Birth to 8 years	1–2 h	Personal-Social, Adaptive, Motor, Communication, Cognitive
Merrill-Palmer Revised (M-P-R)	1 month to 6 years 6 months	30–40 min	Cognitive, Fine Motor, Receptive Language, Memory, Visual-Motor, Speed of Processing, Expressive Language, Gross Motor, Social-Emotional, Self-Help/Adaptive Temperament
Alberta Infant Motor Scale (AIMS)	Birth to 18 months	20–30 min	Gross Motor Skills (assessed in four postures)
Peabody Developmental Motor Scales, 2nd ed. (PDMS-2)	Birth to 5 years 11 months	45–60 min	Gross and Fine Motor

References

Aicardi J. *Diseases of the nervous system in childhood*, 3rd ed. London, Mac Keith Press, 2009.

Cioni G, Mercuri E. *Neurological assessment in the first two years of life. Clinics in developmental medicine 176*. London, Mac Keith Press, 2007.

Dubowitz LMS, Dubowitz V, Mercuri E. *The neurological assessment of the preterm and fullterm newborn infant. Clinics in developmental medicine 148*, 2nd ed. London, Mac Keith Press, 1999.

Einspieler C et al. *Prechtl's method on the qualitative assessment of general movements in preterm, term and young infants. Clinics in developmental medicine 167*. London, Mac Keith Press, 2005.

WHO Multicentre Growth Reference Study Group. WHO Child Growth Standards. *Acta Paediatrica Supplement*, 2006, 450.

Resources

Heinemann KR, Hadders-Algra M. Evaluation of neuromotor function in infancy. A systematic review of available methods. *Journal of Developmental and Behavioral Pediatrics*, 2008, 29(4):315–323.

WHO. *The WHO Child Growth Standards report.* www.who.int/childgrowth/standards/en/

Chapter 6

Prevention of neurological disease in infants

Jane Williams and Colin Kennedy

Key messages

- Screen only for disorders that meet screening criteria (see Table 6.1).
- Antenatal screening for fetal infection, Down syndrome.
- Neonatal screening includes physical examination, hearing screen and heel-prick blood tests.
- Prevent neonatal hypothermia and treat neonatal hypoglycaemia or eye infection early.
- Monitor neonatal bilirubin.
- Breastfeeding is best.
- Iron supplementation for high-risk groups (preterm <37 weeks, low birthweight, feeding difficulties).
- Immunize systematically.
- Monitor growth on appropriate centile charts.
- Consider screening for anaemia at 9 months particularly in high risk groups.

Common errors

- Screening without defining precisely the cut-off for a positive screen.
- Screening for target conditions in which the benefit of early diagnosis is doubtful.
- Neglecting the need for counselling before and after screening.
- Over-interpretation of a single late milestone.

When to worry

- Developmental quotient <70 (i.e. less than 70% of mean reference level).
- Persistent primitive, asymmetric, very brisk or absent reflexes with abnormal tone.
- Loss of acquired skills.
- Lack of visual fixing or following at 6–8 weeks.
- No response to voice at 6–8 weeks.
- Family history or syndromic features that increase risk of childhood deafness.

Primary prevention, screening and surveillance

Although screening programmes have been in place for many years in several European and non-European countries there is still confusion as to what they can and cannot achieve. It is hoped that screening tests will pick out individuals who are at highest risk of having the disorder in question before they become symptomatic and discriminate between those who truly have a disorder from those who do not.

The term screening programme includes screening tests, diagnostic tests and any treatment or action that follows on from these. It is important to remember that a screen is usually not a diagnostic test but rather identifies those at high risk of a medical condition and whose families should then be offered the diagnostic test. A screening programme should lead to an improvement in the quality of life of the person being screened, or their family. This is an especially important issue in those who screen positive for a target condition, some of whom will be true positives and some false positives. Families whose child has a false-positive result (i.e. who screens positive but does not have the target condition) may be exposed to significant harm, including unnecessary anxiety. The design of screening programmes should be scrutinized by experts and service users offering a wide range of perspectives to guarantee that the positive impact of the test itself outweighs the possible negative effects, including the emotional cost of any screening programme. Screening programmes can be universal; that is, for the whole population (e.g. measurement of haemoglobin in all pregnant women to detect anaemia) or targeted to high-risk groups (e.g. infants of parents known to be carriers of a genetically inherited condition).

Possible benefits of a true positive screen could include the early treatment of a disease so that its adverse effects are minimized or, in the case of prenatal screening, lead to confirmatory tests that show that the fetus has a serious medical condition, enabling a pregnant woman to make an informed choice whether or not she wishes to continue with the pregnancy. The success of such a programme must be evaluated the basis of the proportion of women who feel that they have received enough information and support to allow them to proceed to an informed choice. This is a different criterion than the number of pregnancies affected by the target condition that are terminated.

The Wilson–Jungner criteria (Wilson & Jungner, 1968) to evaluate a screening programme, updated in 2003, are shown in Table 6.1.

Information and counselling

The provision of up-to-date information and high-quality/professional counselling and support enables individuals to make the choices that they consider best. In regard to antenatal screening, the United Kingdom Royal College of Obstetricians and Gynaecologists (1995) recommend the following.

- Women and their partners should feel free to make the decision they feel most appropriate from the options they are given.
- Screening and diagnostic tests must only be undertaken with the knowledge and consent of the individual woman.

Table 6.1 Criteria to consider in a screening programme (Wilson & Jungner, 1968)

The condition

- An important health problem

- A simple, safe, precise and validated screening test

- The natural history including from latent to declared disease, should be adequately understood and there should be an early presymptomatic stage.

- Intervention at the presymptomatic stage should be cost-effective.

- If the carriers of a genetic mutation, as well as cases of the disease, are identified as a result of screening, this impact must be considered.

The test

- Know the distribution of test values in the target population and agree the cut-off point separating positive from negative screening results.

- Acceptable

- Agree policy on further diagnostic investigation of those with positive results.

- If testing for mutations, select and provide information to enable interpretation of test results that is appropriate to the subset of mutations screened.

- An effective treatment or intervention for patients identified and evidence of early treatment leading to better outcome

- Evidence-based policies covering treatment

- All healthcare providers should optimize care for the condition prior to participation in a screening programme.

The screening programme

- Evidence from high-quality randomized controlled trials that the screening programme is effective in reducing mortality or morbidity

- The programme is clinically, socially and ethically acceptable to health professionals and the public.

Table 6.1 *Continued*

- Benefits of test outweighing harm of test (including psychological harm)

- 'Value for money'

- Agreed plan for monitoring programme

The treatment

- Adequate staffing for carrying out programme and treatment

- All other options for managing the condition should have been considered.

- Information from a reliable evidence base available for participants

- Anticipate public pressure for widening the eligibility, reducing the screening interval and increasing the sensitivity of the testing process.

- If screening is for a mutation, the programme should be acceptable to people identified as carriers and to other family members.

- For all aspects of antenatal screening, women and their partners must be given verbal information on the screening supported by suitable written or audiotape/audiovisual information, if required.
- For all aspects of antenatal screening, women and their partners should be aware of the risks and benefits associated with each test.
- It is suggested that there should be a policy on how, and when, women and their partners are given results. Results of specific tests, such as those for fetal abnormality or human immunodeficiency virus (HIV), should be given in person.
- Individuals should be informed of all the results of any tests undertaken.
- Women should be fully supported and offered access to specialist advice and support if required. This may include counseling or specialist advice for genetic disorders, HIV or haemoglobinopathy. It should also include referral to self-help groups.
- Women should be satisfied with the service offered. This can be audited.

In order to minimize the emotional distress often associated with screening programmes, individuals may be offered accurate and sensitive counseling at various stages including the following:

- prior to screening, during which individuals are given the opportunity to make an informed choice about whether or not to have particular tests;

- after screening, during which individuals are given the results of investigations and presented with the options for future action. At this time, support is offered to individuals for decision making;

- post-decision making, during which information from subsequent investigations is given, support is offered concerning the decision about what action is to be taken, whether this relates to the continuation of a pregnancy or the provision of specialized treatment for a neonatal problem; and

- prior to a subsequent pregnancy, where parents are helped to make decisions about antenatal diagnostic tests, where available, and cope with the anxiety that often accompanies subsequent pregnancies.

Antenatal screening is undertaken for a number of conditions in the mother and unborn infant. For conditions in the mother, for example anaemia and raised blood pressure, treatment is available during the antenatal period to improve her health and indirectly that of the infant. For conditions in the infant, the screening test may enable a mother to make an informed choice about continuation of the pregnancy or allow treatment to improve the infant's health to be started as early as possible. (See Table 6.2).

Screening for maternal disease
Screening for maternal disease involves monitoring pregnancies to try to select those where, even though the pregnant woman appears well, she has a condition such as anaemia, hepatitis B, syphilis, HIV infection or high blood pressure, which could be harmful to the unborn infant. Once the condition has been discovered, treatment can be started to reduce the effect of the condition on the unborn infant. Immunity to rubella is checked, so that any non-immune mothers can be offered vaccination with two doses of measles, mumps and rubella (MMR) vaccine after delivery. If a mother is found to be infected with hepatitis B, then her infant can be immunized soon after birth to reduce the chances of becoming infected.

Screening for abnormalities of the unborn infant
Screening for fetal abnormality is offered to pregnant women as part of routine maternity care. Screening is based on either ultrasound examination or blood tests. (See Table 6.2).

Neonatal screening and perinatal care

Neonatal screening
Neonatal screening is offered so that the presence of a congenital disorder in the newborn may be identified as soon as possible after birth and treatment offered. Neonatal screening aims to ameliorate disabling conditions that impair a child's quality of life. The timeliness of screening ensures that appropriate treatment may begin and lead to the maximum possible reduction of the adverse effects of the condition. Screening takes a number of forms in the neonatal period, as follows.

Table 6.2 Antenatal screening

Gestational age	Screening test	Comments
Preconception		Folic acid prophylaxis of neural tube defects Targeted advice to women with epilepsy in relation to anticonvulsant choices, diabetics in relation to control of blood sugar, chronic illness groups
8–12 weeks	Rubella, VDRL, HIV, hepatitis B, blood group, Rhesus antibody, FBC, red cell alloantibodies, haemoglobinopathies	
11–13 weeks	USS USS for nuchal translucency	To establish gestational age and screening for more than one fetus For women >35 years: positive in 80% infants with Down syndrome
16–18 weeks	Triple test: alphafetoprotein, human chorionic gonadotrophin and unconjugated oestriol (uE3)	The triple test can detect 69% of trisomy 21 pregnancies; false-positive rate of 5%. The likelihood of a fetus having trisomy 21 in a patient with a negative test is about 2%. A normal result reduces the likelihood of trisomy 21 but does not exclude it.
18–20 weeks	Quadruple test: as above plus inhibin A Detailed USS	Quadruple test detection rate for Down syndrome: detects 81% of true cases if screen referral threshold set for false-positive rate of 5% for fetal anomalies

FBC, full blood count (maternal for check for anaemia); USS, fetal ultrasound scan; VDRL, Venereal Disease Research Laboratory test (blood test for syphilis).

- A very small quantity of blood is taken from the infant's heel between 5 and 8 days after birth. Currently all infants in the United Kingdom are tested for phenylketonuria, congenital hypothyroidism, cystic fibrosis, sickle-cell disorders and medium-chain acyl-CoA dehydrogenase deficiency (MCADD), an inborn error of metabolism.
- All infants are recommended to have a routine detailed physical examination within 72 h of birth. A general examination ensures that there are no visible malformations and, more specifically, the eyes are examined for conditions such as cataracts, the heart for heart defects, the hips for developmental dysplasia and the testes for cryptorchidism.
- All infants have their hearing tested in the first few weeks of life.

Monitoring of the mother and unborn infant at the time of delivery is crucial by a competent birth attendant or midwife. High risk factors for the subsequent health of the infant would be in particular maternal ill health (that hopefully would have been excluded, treated or planned for from the antenatal programme), preterm labour and unrecognized obstetric factors, such as breech presentation.

After delivery the immediate care of the infant, maintaining body temperature and access to intensive neonatal care for those infants born preterm or who are manifesting signs of ill health, are vital to the subsequent health and neurological health of the child.

Infant screening and health promotion after the neonatal period

Universal screening physical examinations of infants vary between countries. In the United Kingdom all infants have a physical examination at 6–8 weeks. This takes the same form as that in the neonatal period; in particular, infants should be seen to exclude prolonged jaundice. More than one post-neonatal examination in the first 6 months in term infants who are healthy at post-neonatal discharge has been evaluated as providing very little additional net benefit.

Growth monitoring

The weight, length and head circumference of all infants should be measured and plotted on a standardized growth chart. We recommend this should happen at birth and at intervals over the first year of life. Accurate and calibrated tools for measuring weight and length are essential. All the processes of growth and development are dynamic and a single point on a growth chart is less useful than serial measurements (see Appendix 1 in this volume).

Developmental surveillance

UNIVERSAL SURVEILLANCE

It is usual to examine an infant in the first 24 h of life to look for any obvious structural abnormalities or features that may indicate congenital problems. Some of these will have developmental consequences. For the majority of newborn infants no abnormality is found. The child will be offered routine review at the ages shown below when developmental progress will be reviewed. The age ranges for developmental progress in typically developing infants are discussed in Chapter 5.

It is recommended in many countries to routinely review a child's development as follows:

- newborn review
- examination at 14 days to exclude jaundice
- 6–8-week check, including fundoscopy
- before 1 year; consider haemoglobin check
- at approximately 18 months.

TARGETED SURVEILLANCE
Infants with known illnesses with developmental consequences are required to have developmental follow-up in order that early intervention with therapy, support and teaching can be initiated if developmental problems occur, for example post hydrocephalus or a known chromosomal abnormality. Children who have been diagnosed as blind or deaf will also require vigilant developmental follow-up as additional developmental problems can follow either as a consequence of the sensory problem or as an association. This may lead to further investigations to clarify an all-embracing diagnosis (e.g. Usher syndrome) but it is more usual that an infant will present with late attainment of developmental milestones and later be found to have a visual- or auditory-associated finding. In fact, it may then lead to targeted investigations and an all-embracing diagnostic conclusion.

Infants with known parental genetic illness will also need relevant targeted screening – for example, deafness, thalassemia, sickle-cell disease – but also those with homes or parental lifestyles that may contribute to adverse environmental circumstance for optimum growth and development, such as violent situations or parental drug abuse.

Outlines of universal and targeted testing are given in Table 6.3.

Developmental screening tests
Identifying a measurement to reliably assess development and give a prognostic indicator is not as easy as it would seem. Various screening tests have been validated. Each has inherent difficulties when applied to a population, not least in relation to the practicalities of assessing development in a child's local circumstances (see Chapter 4 in this volume).

The most commonly used specific tests include the DENVER II test and the Clinical Adaptive Test/Clinical Linguistic and Auditory Milestone Scale (CAT/CLAMS), which is heavily language-orientated. There are also tests reliant on parent or teacher questionnaires, such as the Parents' Evaluation of Development Inventory.

Table 6.3 Health promotion programme: what to include and risk factors

Universal	High-risk groups in whom additional targeted screening may be needed
Health and development reviews at birth, day 1, 6 weeks and 1 year	Maternal illness, e.g. diabetes, depression, other maternal mental health problems.
Immunisations	
Promotion of health and well-being	Parental or familial genetic disease
Reduce parental smoking	Maternal alcohol and drug use
Dietary advice (mother and infant)	Poor-quality housing
Promote breastfeeding	Poverty
Keep safe	Single parent Preterm infant
Prevention of sudden infant death (safe sleeping)	Domestic violence
Maintaining infant health	
Promote parenting and child bonding	
Involve fathers	
Maternal mental health	

More detailed assessments of children's developmental performance in comparison to reference ranges for typically developing infants include the Griffiths Mental Development Scales and Bayley Infant Neurodevelopmental Screen (BINS).

Personal knowledge of the spectrum of development in typically developing infants (see Chapter 5) is crucial in neurological examination and will facilitate early detection of preschool children who are late at achieving developmental skills, either generally or in one domain of development.

Infant diet and iron deficiency

Iron deficiency anaemia (IDA) is the most common nutritional deficiency worldwide. Severe or prolonged iron deficiency can cause IDA. Data on the prevalence of IDA in infants 6–12 months are sparse and among term infants younger than 1 year the prevalence of IDA is low but high-risk groups include preterm and low-birth-weight infants with prolonged neonatal stays in hospital. There are also variations on case definitions of IDA (Table 6.4). The risk of IDA is increased if infants are fed on non-iron-fortified milks. Breast milk, even though it has less iron per 100 ml, is by far the best source of iron, as well as having many other nutritional advantages, and is the nutrition of first choice.

IDA has been associated with psychomotor and cognitive abnormalities leading to poor school performance in children and an increased risk of poor pregnancy outcome in pregnant women. However, the relationship between maternal IDA, IDA in pregnancy and birth outcome remains poorly understood and the relationship between postpartum maternal IDA and developmental impairments in the offspring remains unclear.

Screening of haemoglobin and/or haematocrit at 9–12 months of age and then again 6 months later has been recommended by the American Academy of Family Physicians in groups at high risk of IDA. Continuation of breastfeeding for at least the first year of life, while introducing complementary iron-rich foods from 6 months of age and iron supplementation for preterm and low-birth-weight infants are also advised (US Preventive Services Task Force Evidence Syntheses, 2006).

Table 6.4 Percentage of UK infants with iron deficiency using different definitions (from Sherriff et al., 1999)

Criteria	Haemoglobin (Hb)		Hb and ferritin	
	12 months	18 months	12 months	18 months
Hb <100 g/l; ferritin <16 µg/l (Avon Longitudinal Study of Parents and Children)	5%	5%	0.5%	0.6%
Hb <110 g/l; ferritin <12 µg/l (WHO)	18%	17.3%	0.4%	1.7%
Hb <110 g/l; ferritin <10 µg/l (Institute of Medicine, USA)	18%	17.3%	0.1%	1.1%

Screening for hearing

It is recommended that all infants have a hearing screen performed as soon as possible in the infant's life, ideally in the neonatal period, to detect permanent hearing loss and facilitate an early intervention to amplify hearing. It is important to stress that any method used is only a screen and must be followed by an evaluation of hearing before any diagnosis is made.

Otoacoustic emission screening test

The otoacoustic emission (OAE) test is commonly used as the neonatal screening test for hearing. It works on the principle that a healthy cochlea will emit a faint sound, the OAE, detectable by a microphone in the outer ear, when stimulated with a repeated clicking sound presented through a small earpiece containing both a loudspeaker and recording microphone. This test can be done with no equipment other than the earpiece and a small computer to average the OAEs occurring a few milliseconds after the click. A normal recording is associated with normal cochlear hair-cell function and this typically reflects normal hearing.

This is a simple and quick test but can have a relatively high false-positive rate in the first 24 h of life due to amniotic fluid in the ear canal. If this happens the test is usually repeated. OAE detection is a test of cochlear function and will not detect auditory neuropathy, also known as auditory dyssynchrony, a rare cause of hearing impairment in which the impairment is in transmission of signals from the cochlea to the brain. If the infant fails again, an automated auditory brainstem response test (AABR; see below) and full assessment are arranged.

The automated auditory brainstem response test

The AABR test works by recording brain activity in response to sounds. An infant may be sleeping naturally or may have to be sedated for this test. Older, cooperative children may be tested in a silent environment while visually occupied. Earphones are placed in or on the infant 's ear. Usually click-type sounds are introduced through the earphones and the electrical responses to the sounds in the auditory pathway are measured with scalp electrodes. The computer-averaged electrical response is compared with a stored template of a normal ABR. If the recorded and template responses are similar to one another the test is classified as a pass and if dissimilar as a 'refer'. This test has the advantage that it screens the entire hearing pathway from ear to brainstem, but disadvantages include the need to apply scalp electrodes and for the infant to be asleep during the test.

Distraction hearing test

In this test a child (developmental range 6–8 months) will sit on a carer's lap while one tester stands behind making sounds and someone else stands in front to distract the child and to watch the child's reaction. This test is a good indicator of a general hearing problem if the test is carried out properly but most infants screening positive will prove to have temporary conductive losses at this age. Furthermore, several studies have found unacceptably high false-negative results in infants with permanent hearing loss. Both tester and distractor need to be well trained for this screen to perform it adequately and its use is now confined only to those for whom OAE and/or AABR screening is not available.

Hearing impairment

Epidemiology

Hearing impairment is the most prevalent sensory deficit in the human population. There are two main groups: sensorineural hearing loss and conductive hearing loss. In the child under 1 year the former is the main concern but the latter is much more prevalent, especially between the ages of 6 and 12 months when screening leads to detection of many cases of conductive nonpermanent loss for each case of sensorineural hearing loss.

Levels of hearing are described by looking at average air-conduction thresholds; that is, the additional intensity of sound, relative to the normal hearing threshold, required at frequencies of 0.5, 1, 2 and 4 Hz to reach the threshold level of audibility in the affected individual. The degree of impairment may be summarized as the average threshold across these four frequencies (Table 6.5). Bilateral permanent moderate or greater hearing loss leads to well-documented impairment in the development of language and related skills and this impairment can be reduced by universal newborn screening, justifying the introduction of such screening programmes (Kennedy et al., 2006). In individuals affected by this degree of impairment, about half will be moderate, a quarter severe and a quarter profound. Most cases of permanent hearing loss of this degree are congenital and should be detected soon after birth but some children present later either because they are acquired (e.g. following meningitis) or because the condition is late-onset and/or there is a progressive increase in severity over time. The evidence that the benefit exceeds the risk of harm and justifies the cost of newborn screening is less secure for lesser degrees of hearing impairment.

Table 6.5 Sound intensity relative to normal required to reach hearing threshold level

Hearing loss	Additional sound intensity relative to normal required to reach hearing threshold level
Normal hearing	≤15 dB
Mild	15–39 dB
Moderate	40–69 dB
Severe	70–94 dB
Profound	≥95 dB

High-risk groups for hearing impairment are

- family history of hearing loss
- bacterial meningitis or measles encephalitis
- children with developmental impairments
- extreme preterm birth
- congenital infection
- severe neonatal jaundice
- craniofacial syndromes
- children with visual impairment
- head injury with base-of-skull fracture or auditory symptoms
- prolonged course of ototoxic drugs (including oncological drugs)
- history of acute encephalopathy.

Sensorineural hearing loss: etiology and management
The prevention of hearing loss is an important public health issue. Preventative measures include immunization against mumps, measles, rubella and bacterial meningitis, effective management of neonatal jaundice, reducing environmental noise pollution and educating young people regarding the long-term risks of hearing loss from exposure to high-volume noise from electronic devices such as personal music systems. The etiology of childhood sensorineural hearing loss has changed in the new millennium in those European countries with an immunization schedule in that fewer cases are now attributed to childhood infections such as mumps, measles, meningitis or congenital rubella. But in other parts of the world the prevalence of these infections is a major causative factor in sensorineural hearing loss. The successful implementation of vaccination programmes would have a major impact on decreasing the numbers of children affected.

Where immunization programmes are in place, the importance of genetic causes has now grown, with approximately 50% of cases now being attributed to single-gene mutations. The most common genetic cause of sensorineural hearing loss is nonsyndromic or isolated deafness, with no other recognizable features. Multiple different chromosomal loci are associated with this form of deafness. The molecular basis for the deafness has been identified in certain cases. In deafness due to the connexin family of genes, the faulty gene codes for abnormal gap junctions involved in recycling potassium ions in cochlear hair cells. These genes are thought to be responsible for up to 70% of cases of deafness in European populations and are situated at a single locus on chromosome 13q. In Usher syndrome there are 10 possible genes involved, which code for myosin.

There may be a clear environmental determinant such as congenital cytomegalovirus but in other cases genes and the environment interact, causing deafness. For example, carriers of the mitochondrial mutation A1555G in *12srRNA* are predisposed to deafness caused by aminoglycosides. The use of this group of antibiotics should be avoided if there is a family history of aminoglycoside-induced deafness.

The best outcome for sensorineural hearing loss is dependent on early detection and early intervention to maximize hearing. The early years offer an enhanced opportunity for better functional outcome, perhaps because of the sensitive period for language development in the central nervous system at this age. Children who lose their hearing ability after having learned to talk usually retain speech. Addressing educational, social and family issues in conjunction with amplification of residual hearing is essential for optimum prognosis.

Treatment options include education of families regarding communication with the affected child and hearing aids, which can be fitted before 6 months of age. Children with profound loss are often suitable for cochlear implantation at specialized centres.

Vision impairment

Visual development
For the first 4–6 weeks of life eye movements are relatively imprecise and slightly jerky, although some ability to fixate is often apparent. Poor fixation after 2 months of age is pathological. Accurate smooth pursuant eye movements and central fixation then develop and by 2–3 months of age the infant has learned to accurately follow the movement of small objects (Table 6.6).

Infants frequently have variable eye alignment with approximately 70% manifesting transient small, variable squints (exotropia) but by 2–3 months this will have resolved and developing infants will have established normal alignment (orthotropia)

Definition of blindness
Blindness is defined as a corrected visual acuity in the better eye of less than 3/60 or a central visual field loss to less than 10° around the point of central vision. This is equivalent to the ability to identify script 60 mm in size at a distance of 3 m. However, this definition immediately raises difficulties in childhood because accurate measurement of visual acuity in children can be difficult for multiple reasons.

Epidemiology
Data are scarce but Scandinavian registers suggest that visual impairment (visual acuity <6/18) affects 8 in 100 000 children each year but it has been estimated that 500 000

Table 6.6 Early visual development

Birth to 2 months	2–6 months	3–4 years
Short-lasting fixation, some jerky movements and mild exotropia allowed	Accurate fixation Smooth eye movements	Visual acuity 6/9

children worldwide become blind each year. In developing countries this is associated with significant mortality from the most common causes, measles infection and vitamin A deficiency.

Causes of neonatal blindness include

- blurred retinal image, for example cataract
- retinal disease, for example toxoplasmosis, retinitis of prematurity, vitamin E deficiency
- optic nerve disease, for example optic nerve hypoplasia, coloboma
- cortical blindness, for example secondary to hydrocephalus or other structural anomaly; in many countries this has become the most common cause of childhood blindness
- neurogenetic/degenerative disease, for example Leber congenital amaurosis
- delayed visual maturation: this is a more common cause of poor visual attentiveness in infancy and if not associated with seizures or any other central nervous system defect may be followed by normal visual function in later childhood.

Prevention of blindness
Primary prevention of blindness can include

- immunization of the mother against infective disease, for example rubella,
- identification of sexually transmitted disease and HIV of the mother,
- genetic counselling for those with relevant genetic illness,
- health education with regard to adverse effects of alcohol, drugs and X-ray or irradiation exposure in pregnancy, and
- safe food preparations and avoidance of exposure of pregnant women to potential sources of toxoplasmosis from, for example, cat litter.

Secondary prevention of blindness can include

- treatment of disease, for example meningitis,
- early identification of ophthalmia neonatorum,
- prenatal diagnosis on serology and consideration of termination if pregnancy is affected, and
- early identification and treatment, for example congenital glaucoma.

Tertiary prevention of blindness can include

- surgery on cataract, and
- iridectomy for ophthalmia neonatorum.

Conclusion

Screening has significant differences from other clinical practice as it offers to help apparently healthy individuals make better informed choices about their health. There are risks involved in screening and it is important, therefore, that individuals have realistic expectations of what a screening programme can deliver. Although screening may have the potential to save lives or improve quality of life through the early diagnosis of serious conditions, it is not a foolproof process. As such, although screening may reduce the risk of developing a condition or its complications, it cannot offer a guarantee of protection against that condition nor, of course, against other conditions and while a positive screening test can bring benefits, it can sometimes cause harm.

'Routine management' of children judged to be at high risk of neurodevelopmental impairments is, in some instances, targeted screening. The potential of such clinical practice for benefit or harm should be considered against the criteria for screening (see Table 6.1) rather than against the criteria that might be regarded as reasonable in the context of management of an identified medical condition or illness.

References

Kennedy CR et al. Early life detection of permanent hearing loss and subsequent language. *New England Journal of Medicine*, 2006, 354:2131–2141.

Royal College of Obstetricians and Gynaecologists. *Report of the Audit Committee's Working Group on Communication Standards*. London, Royal College of Obstetricians and Gynaecologists, 1995.

Sherriff A et al. and the ALSPAC Children in Focus Study Team. Haemoglobin and ferritin concentrations in children aged 12 and 18 months. *Archives of Diseases in Childhood*, 1999, 80(2):153–157.

US Preventive Services Task Force Evidence Syntheses. *Screening for iron deficiency in childhood and pregnancy*. Report No.: 06-0590-EF-1. Rockville, MD, Agency for Healthcare Research and Quality (US), 2006.

Wilson JMG, Jungner G. *Principles and practice of screening for disease. WHO Chronicle. Public health papers No 34*. Geneva, World Health Organization, 1968. http://whqlibdoc.who.int/php/WHO_PHP_34.pdf.

Resources

Dutton G, Bax M, eds. *Visual impairment in children due to damage to the brain. Clinics in developmental medicine 186*. London, Mac Keith Press, 2010.

Elliman DAC, Dezateux C, Bedford HE. Newborn and childhood screening programmes: criteria, evidence, and current policy. *Archives of Diseases in Childhood*, 2002, 87:6–9.

Healthy Child Programme, www.dh.gov.uk/publications.

National Screening Committee. *Screening tests for you and your baby* (http://www.screening.nhs.uk/getdata.php?id=7885).

Perez EM. Mother–infant interactions and infant development are altered by iron deficiency anaemia. *Journal of Nutrition*, 2005, 135(4):850–855.

Preece PM, Riley EP. *Alcohol, drugs and medication in pregnancy: the outcomes for the child*. London, Mac Keith Press, 2011.

Royal College of Obstetricians and Gynaecologists. *Report of the Audit Committee's Working Group on Communication Standards*. London, Royal College of Obstetricians and Gynaecologists, 1995.

Royal College of Obstetricians and Gynaecologists has a range of useful information in its Guidelines section, including 'Understanding how risk is discussed in healthcare – Information for you' (http://www.rcog.org.uk/understanding-how-risk-is-discussed-healthcare).

Sheridan M, Frost M, Sharma A. *From birth to five years: children's developmental progress*. Windsor, NFER Publishing, 1997.

Skotko BG. With new prenatal testing, will babies with Down syndrome slowly disappear? *Archives of Diseases in Childhood*, 2009, 94:823–826.

WHO Multicentre Growth Reference Study Group. WHO Child Growth Standards. *Acta Paediatrica Supplement*, 2006, 450. Growth charts are reproduced in Appendix X (http://www.who.int/childgrowth/standards/en/).

Glossary

False negative result	A negative result is present as is the condition.
False positive result	A positive result is present but the condition is not.
Negative result (on a screening test)	This is a result which indicates that an individual is at low risk of a condition.
Positive predictive value	The proportion of people with a positive test result who have the condition.
Positive result (on a screening test)	This is a result which indicates that an individual is at high risk of a condition.
Screening programme	This includes screening, diagnosis and the management of a condition.
Screening test	This is a test that is designed to identify those individuals who are at a high enough risk of having a particular disorder to warrant the offer of a diagnostic test. A screening test may be a procedure, such as a blood test, or it may be the asking of a question, such as 'How old are you?'
Sensitivity of a screening test	This refers to the ability of the test to accurately detect those who have a condition. A highly sensitive test has a sensitivity approaching 100%. The consequence of a test that lacks sensitivity is that individuals are informed that they do not have a condition when in fact they do (this is known as a false negative result).
Specificity of a screening tests	The ability of the test to accurately identify those who do not have the condition. A highly specific test has a specificity approaching 100%. The consequence of a test that lacks specificity is that an individual is informed that they have a condition when in fact they do not (this is known as a false positive result).

Chapter 7
Cranial imaging

Brigitte Vollmer

Key messages
- Structural imaging of the brain and spine allows assessment of normal anatomy and brain maturation as well as effects of disease on the brain parenchyma.
- When ordering a neuroimaging assessment formulate a clear question to be answered. Incidental findings are common and usually do not explain the reported symptoms. They can cause confusion to doctors and stress to families if their reporting is not managed well.
- To aid accurate reporting provide the radiologist with details of medical history, clinical findings and results of laboratory investigations to tailor imaging optimally to the individual case.

Common errors
- Imaging the brain for moderate early developmental impairment with normal head size and in the absence of abnormal neurological signs.
- Relying on ultrasound alone for interpretation of changes in brain parenchyma.

When to worry
- No imaging available for a patient with acute undiagnosed neurological illness.

Neuroimaging: principles

Ultrasound is very useful in infants with an open fontanelle. No radiation is involved and it is easily performed at the bedside. Serial cranial ultrasound scans are an essential part of routine neonatal intensive care.

Main indications include

- imaging of intracranial haemorrhage or periventricular white matter abnormalities in the preterm infant (initial diagnosis, and monitoring by serial scanning);
- initial imaging of term infants with neonatal encephalopathy (hypoxic ischaemic changes, focal infarction); should be followed by magnetic resonance imaging;
- imaging of macrocephaly for hydrocephalus; and
- detection of intracranial calcification.

Practical issues include

- cranial ultrasound should be performed according to a standard protocol and include, as a minimum, coronal and sagittal/parasagittal standard views;
- it should be performed serially to evaluate changes in brain pathology; and
- images should be stored so that they are available for review.

Limitations/disadvantages are listed below:

- imaging of posterior fossa abnormalities is limited;
- view of cerebral convexities is limited; and
- in preterm brain injury, ultrasound is good at detecting cystic focal lesions but not sensitive for diffuse white matter injury.

Transcranial Doppler ultrasound is used to assess cerebral blood flow and can also be used when the fontanelle is closed.

Skull radiography is useful in the investigation of craniosynostosis and assessment of fractures in the evaluation of trauma and inflicted traumatic head injury (ITBI). However, if a computed tomography (CT) is performed, then plain skull films should not be routinely carried out in addition as they will not influence management further. For further detail on indications see www.e-radiography.net/technique/skullindications. htm.

Computed tomography (CT) is an X-ray-based imaging modality. Many of the indications for CT have been replaced by magnetic resonance imaging (MRI). However, it remains important because CT can be performed quickly and is sensitive and specific for detection of acute intracranial haemorrhage and secondary low-density tissue changes (oedema, ischaemia, infarction).

Main indications include

- acute neurotrauma and ITBI (detection of haemorrhage and fractures)
- intracranial calcifications
- craniosynostosis
- cerebral venous thrombosis.

Limitations/disadvantages are listed below.

- MRI is superior to CT in defining parenchymal injury in the acute phase of haemorrhage, and more accurate in mapping and detection of subacute and chronic intracranial haemorrhage.
- CT delivers a high dose of radiation to the brain, which is a disadvantage in children.

Structural MRI
Structural MRI is based on the principles of nuclear magnetic resonance. MRI uses a magnetic field (in paediatric neurology, the most common field strengths used are 1, 1.5, or 3 Tesla) to align the magnetization of some atoms in the body, then uses radio frequency fields to alter the alignment of this magnetization systematically. This causes the nuclei to produce a rotating magnetic field detectable by the scanner. This information is recorded to construct an image of the scanned area of the body. MRI does not involve radiation and the main advantage of structural MRI is that it can show different tissue contrasts (T1-weighted, T2-weighted, spin density, diffusion and flow) in multiple planes (sagittal, coronal and axial).

Common MR sequences are listed below.

- T1-w images provide good white and grey matter differentiation and are used mainly for assessment of anatomy.
- T1 inversion recovery (T1 IR) images show very good grey/white matter contrast and are useful, for example, to detect heterotopia. These are useful images for assessment of cortical structures when myelination is not yet completed.
- T2-w images are good for detecting 'pathology' such as infection, inflammation and tumours, which appear bright on T2-w images.
- T2 fluid-attenuated inversion recovery (T2 FLAIR) images suppress the cerebrospinal fluid (CSF) signal and are therefore useful for assessment of tissue close to CSF spaces (e.g. gliosis in periventricular regions).
- T2*-w gradient echo images are sensitive to field inhomogeneity caused by blood products and are useful in imaging vascular malformations or trauma.
- fat-saturation images suppress the signal from fat and are useful in imaging of lesions that contain fat, such as teratomas.
- contrast enhancement with gadolinium given intravenously is useful in imaging of inflammation, acute infection, tumours, neurocutaneous disorders and vascular disorders.

- Diffusion-weighted imaging (DWI) is based on the Brownian motion of water and can quantify the extent to which water diffuses freely within tissues. The main application is very early identification of ischaemic events (before they are visible on T1-w and T2-w images). Acute ischaemic lesions can be distinguished from chronic ischaemic lesions using DWI in combination with T2-w images. The apparent diffusion coefficient (ADC) is a quantitative measure of diffusion imaging and reflects water mobility within the brain. ADC maps are useful in determining the timing of ischaemic injury. The interpretation of ADC has to be done with caution as the coefficient varies with time after injury; the lowest ADC value is usually observed around day 3 after the event, then shows pseudo-normalization between day 3 and day 7, and after day 7 remains high in the injured area.

Magnetic resonance angiography and venography
Magnetic resonance angiography (MRA) and magnetic resonance venography (MRV) are non-invasive and allow quick imaging of the large arteries and veins. MRA/MRV is useful for excluding sinus venous thrombosis and arteriovenous malformations. However, in the neonatal period interpretation of non-contrast-enhanced MRA and MRV can be difficult because of slow flow in sinuses. Contrast-enhanced MRV is therefore preferable.

Imaging protocols
A combination of T2-w images in two planes and T1-w images in two planes is a good basis for an imaging protocol. Additional sequences such as contrast enhancement or diffusion-weighted images can then be added depending on the clinical question.

A basic MRI protocol for children under 2 years of age should include

- axial T2-w images
- coronal FLAIR images (or coronal T2-w images)
- sagittal and coronal T1-w images
- if possible: diffusion-weighted images with calculation of ADC maps.

Main indications are described here.

- MRI is the most useful imaging modality for assessment of central nervous system (CNS) anatomy, maturation and pathology.
- MRI is superior to CT except for imaging of acute haemorrhage, calcifications or bone structures.
- in neonates, MRI provides more detailed information than cranial ultrasound. It is useful in distinguishing pathologies that mimic hypoxic ischaemic encephalopathy (infection, metabolic disorders, venous infarction and malformations).
- neonatal MRI can detect patterns of brain injury, which help with diagnosis of the underlying pathology, timing of injury and prediction of outcome.

Keep the following in mind for MRI in infancy

- MR protocols need to be tailored to the clinical question and take into account that the brain continues to develop during early infancy and childhood.
- in the first 2 years of life water content of the brain decreases and myelination increases, which results in T1 and T2 shortening. Therefore, modifications of sequences are necessary to achieve optimal soft-tissue contrast between normal and pathological structures.
- before the age of 6 months myelin maturation is best seen on T1-w images; after 6 months until about 2 years on T2-w images.
- during myelination there is a time period where grey matter and subcortical structures are iso-intense, which means that subtle grey matter features such as migration abnormalities are difficult to judge in the first 6 months of life.

Practical issues include

- newborns can in the majority of cases be scanned in natural sleep ('feed and wrap'),
- in infants beyond 2 months of age sedation or anaesthesia is often required for MR imaging,
- MRI is very noisy and it is important to provide adequate hearing protection (earplugs and infant earmuffs), and
- cardiorespiratory function has to be monitored during scanning.

Limitations/disadvantages include

- MRI is not good for detection of calcification,
- MRI takes time and requires the patient to lie still for at least 20 minutes,
- movement artifacts are a common problem and degrade images, and
- large metallic implants cause artifacts and smaller metallic devices (e.g. arterial clips) may move during scanning; metal objects can heat up and cause tissue damage.

Spinal imaging
MRI is the main modality for spinal imaging. Ultrasound is useful before the posterior parts of the vertebrae ossify and therefore is a useful screening tool in neonates. However, infants with an abnormal spinal ultrasound or infants with a normal spinal ultrasound but neurological symptoms will still need MRI of the spine.

The most common indications for spinal imaging in the first year of life are

- detection of spinal dysraphism in infants with cutaneous abnormalities,
- in infants with congenital abnormalities of other organs that may be associated with spinal abnormalities, and
- in infants where a tumour is suspected.

MR sequences for spinal imaging should include sagittal and axial T1-w and T2-w images. In infants with suspected dysraphism axial T1-w images through the conus and filum terminale are useful for detection of lipomas. T2-w fat-suppressed images are useful for detection of oedema.

Clinical settings

Neonatal encephalopathy

Neonatal encephalopathy is a clinically defined syndrome of acutely disturbed neurological function in the term infant (see Chapter 12). It is manifested by difficulties with respiration, depression of tone and reflexes, alteration of consciousness and often seizures. Causes include the following:

- diffuse cerebral injury (hypoxic ischaemic insult)
- focal cerebral injury (arterial ischaemic stroke, cerebral venous thrombosis, primary intracerebral haemorrhage)
- metabolic disorders
- infection
- drug exposure (not covered here)
- CNS malformations.

Cranial ultrasound is useful for initial rapid evaluation, for example to detect haemorrhage, oedema or infarct. It does not replace MRI if the infant is stable enough to undergo MRI. Early CT can exclude haemorrhage. However, it has to be kept in mind that CT exposes the infant to a considerable dose of radiation. If possible, structural MRI including a diffusion-weighted sequence should be performed to establish the pattern of injury and aid in prediction of neurological and neurodevelopmental outcome. MR spectroscopy is not covered in this chapter.

The Quality Standards Subcommittee of the American Academy of Neurology and the Practice Committee of the Child Neurology Society published practice parameters on neuroimaging of the neonate (Ment et al., 2002) and recommended the following:

> For infants with a history of neonatal encephalopathy, significant birth trauma, and evidence for low haematocrit or coagulopathy:
>
> First a non-contrast CT should be performed to look for haemorrhage. If the CT findings cannot explain the clinical status of the neonate, MRI should be performed.
>
> For other neonates with acute encephalopathy:
>
> MRI should be performed between days 2 and 8 of life, including DWI and single-voxel MR spectroscopy if available. CT should be performed only if MRI is not available or if the neonate is too unstable for MRI.

Interpretation of MR images obtained in the neonatal period should be done by an experienced person who is familiar with the peculiarities of the neonatal brain and the range of abnormalities seen in neonatal encephalopathy as well as the effect of time from injury to appearance on the images. It is important to consider perinatal and postnatal clinical details for correct interpretation of imaging findings.

DIFFUSE CEREBRAL INJURY: PERINATAL HYPOXIC ISCHAEMIC INSULT

Different injury patterns may be seen, involving both grey and white matter. Patterns of brain injury differ between term and preterm infants and in this section only the term infant is considered.

Ultrasound is useful in the initial evaluation, which – depending on the severity of the insult – may show

- brain swelling
- diffuse hyperechogenicity, loss of sulci and fissures, slit ventricles ('fuzzy brain')
- increased echodensity in the thalami (and relative hypodensity of the caudate)
- early haemorrhage in primary ischaemic areas that subsequently become hyperaemic.

When using ultrasound for aiding in the prediction of outcome, serial examinations up to the fourth week after the insult are recommended.

After disappearance of brain swelling, MRI is superior in more detailed delineation of the injury, in particular for subcortical structures and parasagittal cortical injury. MR spectroscopy, which is useful in early imaging of hypoxic ischaemic encephalopathy (HIE), is not covered in this section.

Structural MRI should include a combination of T1- and T2-weighted imaging and diffusion-weighted imaging. Hypoxic ischaemic injury has characteristic appearances on T1 and T2-w imaging that depend on the severity and duration of the insult as well as the stage of brain development:

- parasagittal cortical injury and subcortical white matter injury ('watershed injury') with relative sparing of the central grey matter structures (basal ganglia, thalami, brainstem), usually bilateral; seen following a prolonged partial hypoxic ischaemic insult; and
- central injury with thalami, basal ganglia (mainly putamen), hippocampi, brainstem, and corticospinal tract involvement (posterior limb of the internal capsule); typically seen after an acute hypoxic ischaemic insult.

Diffusion MRI depicts abnormalities earlier than conventional MRI sequences and should be performed within a week of birth for early identification of ischaemia. If possible, an ADC map should be calculated since this quantitative assessment may help in cases in which the diffusion-weighted image are difficult to interpret or appear normal.

The timing of MRI depends partly on the reason for imaging, i.e. whether MRI is performed to aid in diagnosis or in prediction of outcome.

- On T1 and T2-w images, lesions are obvious 1–2 weeks from delivery and imaging at this time is useful in aiding prediction of outcome (mainly motor outcome).
- In order to clarify the diagnosis or help with regard to clinical management, earlier imaging may be required.
- It is important to keep in mind that on conventional T1 and T2-w imaging performed within a week of birth and the likely insult, subtle abnormalities may be missed. It is therefore useful to include diffusion-weighted MRI in the protocol. Diffusion MRI shows ischaemic injury hours after the insult and this lasts for 7–14 days, by which time conventional T1 and T2-w images will show abnormalities.

FOCAL CEREBRAL INJURY

This includes focal cerebral injury due to arterial ischaemic stroke, cerebral venous thrombosis and primary intracranial haemorrhage.

On ultrasound, focal cerebral injury appears as hyper-echogenic foci. MRI is the imaging modality of choice in neonatal focal cerebral injury.

- In addition to conventional T1 and T2-w sequences and diffusion-weighted MRI (which is the most sensitive sequence to detect ischaemic injury), MRA and/or MRV should be included for detection of abnormalities in the large arteries and the superficial and deep venous system.
- Imaging should not only include the brain but also the neck region.

In *arterial ischaemic stroke*, which in the majority of cases involves the middle cerebral artery, ultrasound abnormalities are seen in a large proportion of cases, in particular when ultrasound is performed 3 or more days after the onset of symptoms. Early findings include areas of increased echogenicity with a normal pattern of gyri and sulci. Subsequently, the affected regions become more echodense and there is loss of white and grey matter differentiation.

MRI can identify the vessel and branch that is involved, delineate the extent of the injury, and help with prognosis. Imaging appearance of ischaemic stroke changes with time.

- In the acute phase the area of infarction may be difficult to visualize on T1 and T2-w images but may be seen as loss of grey/white matter differentiation with increased signal in the affected region on T2-w images and decreased signal on T1-w images.
- Thus in the acute phase, diffusion-weighted MRI is extremely useful because the region of infarction is seen as high signal on diffusion-weighted images and low signal on the ADC map. The high-signal intensity observed on diffusion-weighted images in the acute phase is due to restricted diffusion, caused by cytotoxic oedema.

- A few days after the event there is a decrease in signal intensity on diffusion-weighted images and an increase in ADC values (due to the development of necrosis, cell lysis and cell shrinkage, resulting in an increase in extracellular space and increased water diffusion). The area of injury becomes less obvious on diffusion-weighted images towards the end of the first week after the insult; however, by this time lesions are clearly seen on T1 and T2-w images

In *venous sinus thrombosis* (in the majority of cases the superior sagittal sinus is affected, followed by the transverse sinuses of the superficial venous system and the straight sinus of the deep system) associated lesions such as thalamic haemorrhage, intraventricular haemorrhage or parenchymal haemorrhagic infarction are frequently seen.

- High-frequency ultrasound may identify venous sinus thrombosis, the adjacent area of increased echogenicity in the parenchyma and the secondary associated lesions. However, ultrasound has poor sensitivity for cerebral infarction and should not be used for the primary detection of venous sinus thrombosis and delineation of the extent of injury. Doppler ultrasound can detect absent or reduced flow in the superficial venous sinuses.
- If MRI is not immediately available, ultrasound with Doppler and/or CT venography should be considered.
- MRI (T1 and T2-w images) with MRA/MRV, and including a diffusion sequence, is the method of choice for diagnosis of venous sinus thrombosis and associated injury. MRA/MRV will show reduced flow or no filling in the sinus and diffusion imaging will identify ischaemic tissue. MRI should be repeated after a week to assess thrombus propagation, and again after 6 weeks to assess re-canalization of the vessel.

Primary intracranial haemorrhage, which accounts for up to a third of intracranial bleeding in term-born infants, can be solitary or multifocal.

- Ultrasound will demonstrate the presence and extent of a haemorrhage.
- CT readily identifies the presence and location of subdural, subarachnoid and intracerebral haemorrhage.
- MRI is helpful in more detailed characterization of location and extent of the lesion, and superior to ultrasound regarding the differentiation between a primary parenchymal haemorrhage and non-haemorrhagic infarction. If there is an underlying arteriovenous malformation (which should be suspected in the absence of birth trauma or coagulopathy), MRI is helpful in its detection after the initial oedematous phase.

METABOLIC DISORDERS

Imaging findings in inherited metabolic disorders, which often present with neonatal encephalopathy, will be discussed in detail below. Here, imaging in kernicterus (bilirubin-induced neurological dysfunction, BIND) and hypoglycaemia are discussed.

In kernicterus

- ultrasound can show echogenicity in the basal ganglia and white matter; and
- MRI-detected lesions develop with age and in the neonatal period the most frequent abnormalities are increased signal on T1-w images in the globus pallidus, and less frequently in other regions such as the thalami, hippocampus, substantia nigra and dentate nuclei. Later in infancy these signal changes are mainly seen on T2-w images. Diffusion MRI does not seem to be useful in the diagnosis of BIND kernicterus.

In hypoglycaemia:

- ultrasound can show patchy areas with increased echogenicity in white matter; and
- there is a specific pattern of injury consisting of abnormal signal on T2-w MR images in the occipital and parietal white matter regions. Haemorrhage, middle cerebral artery infarction, basal ganglia/thalamic abnormalities and cortical injury have been described as well. On diffusion MRI, restricted diffusion is seen in affected regions.

Neonatal infections (excluding congenital infections)
Although meningitis is identified through a clinical and laboratory-based diagnosis, neuroimaging is useful in the initial evaluation and monitoring of infants with meningitis and essential for early diagnosis of encephalitis. It is important to remember that imaging appearances, potential complications (which are common in neonatal meningitis) and clinical course can differ in neonates from those seen in older children.

CT should include images with contrast for visualization of meningeal enhancement. Similarly, MRI should include T1- and T2-weighted images and also contrast images and diffusion-weighted images.

Details of imaging for *bacterial meningitis* are described below.

- Cranial ultrasound aids the management of neonatal meningitis as serial examinations at the bedside may monitor the progression of complications. Initial signs of meningitis are brain swelling, wide sulci and increased echogenicity in the cortical grey matter, with areas of hyperechogenicity in the periventricular and subcortical white matter. Intraventricular strands attached to the ventricular surface and echodense ependyma are signs of ventriculitis. Post-infective changes consist of ventricular dilatation, parenchymal cysts and periventricular calcification.
- CT (native and with contrast) is valuable in both the acute stage and long term. Unlike ultrasound it provides information on oedema severity, the location of any obstruction to CSF flow and areas of infarction, and can detect an abscess or subdural collections. Longer term, ventricular dilatation/hydrocephalus, the development of cysts or brain atrophy can be visualized.

- MRI (T1-w and T2-w images, native and with contrast) shows the abnormalities that are seen on CT but provides more detailed information on infarction and haemorrhage. Diffusion MRI will show ischaemic lesions and oedema earlier and more effectively than CT.

Details of imaging for *encephalitis* are given here.

- MRI is very useful for the early diagnosis of encephalitis since it will show patchy signal abnormalities in white matter on T1-w and T2-w images and changes on diffusion MRI before CT becomes abnormal.
- All three imaging modalities (ultrasound, CT, MRI) are suitable for visualizing progression of abnormalities to multicystic encephalomalacia, but MRI is the most useful modality for detection and delineation of white and grey matter injury.

Note: in neonatal herpes simplex virus (HSV) encephalitis there is a more diffuse distribution of brain abnormalities and no predisposition for the temporal lobes, which is typical in older infants and children.

CNS MALFORMATIONS

Here, malformation refers to morphological abnormalities of the CNS that date from the embryonic or fetal period, regardless of the underlying mechanism. One way of categorizing CNS malformations is according to the three phases of CNS organogenesis: (1) neurulation, formation and closure of the neural tube, (2) prosencephalation, development of the forebrain and (3) histogenesis, proliferation and migration of neurons.

- Although ultrasound and CT provide useful information in diagnosing CNS malformations, the best imaging modality for detailed visualization is MRI, in particular for cortical malformations.
- It is important to include a sagittal plane in the protocol for assessment of the corpus callosum, which functions as a 'marker': if there is a malformation of the corpus callosum it is imperative to search for other associated CNS malformations.
- For the diagnosis of disorders of histogenesis (e.g. polymicrogyria) high-resolution MRI may be necessary.
- Progression of myelination makes identification of abnormal patterns of grey matter, such as those suggestive of neuronal migration defects, easier after 18 months of age: it is therefore sometimes necessary to wait until this age before such malformations can be confirmed.

Neonatal seizures

There are multiple causes to be considered in a newborn with seizures (see Chapter 13 in this volume) and any newborn with seizures should undergo imaging. The principles outlined above apply with regard to the application of different imaging modalities and protocols.

Early-onset metabolic and degenerative disorders
MRI is the imaging modality of choice for the diagnosis of metabolic and degenerative disorders of the brain. The minimum imaging protocol includes the standard MRI protocol as outlined at the start of this chapter under Neuroimaging: principles, with the addition of FLAIR images. It is beyond the scope of this chapter to cover in detail the imaging features of the individual early-onset disorders. Rather, a general approach to assessing MR images for signs of metabolic and degenerative disorders is described.

When assessing MR images for metabolic and degenerative disorders it is important to consider the following points in order to classify these disorders based in imaging characteristics.

- Decide *which structure is affected primarily*: cortical grey matter, basal ganglia, white matter, or both grey and white matter.

In assessment of white matter, is there delayed myelination or hypomyelination? It important to know the pattern of myelination in the normally developing brain so that delayed myelination is not confused with hypomyelination. Within the first year of life in normal brain development there is little myelin and it is not possible to diagnose permanent hypomyelination. Hypomyelination can be diagnosed if there is an unchanged pattern of deficient myelination on two MRIs at least 6 months apart in a child older than 1 year.

- Are the abnormalities focal, multifocal or confluent? In leukodystrophies (genetic disorders) abnormalities are mainly bilateral and confluent, whereas in acquired disorders are often multifocal.
- Localization: most localizations are frontal, parieto-occipital, periventricular, subcortical, diffuse cerebral and/or posterior fossa.
- Are there other specific brain abnormalities such as cysts, small haemorrhages, calcium deposits or megalencephaly?

Using such a 'pattern-recognition' approach will achieve a specific diagnosis in a large proportion of patients as described in detail by Schiffmann and van der Knaap (2009).

Trauma (postnatal)
Accidental head injury can lead to epidural, subdural, subarachnoid and parenchymal haemorrhage. In ITBI the most common is subdural haemorrhage.

- CT is the image modality of choice for the quick and initial assessment of traumatic brain injury.
- MRI on days 3–5 after the trauma is useful for assessing the extent of parenchymal injury in more detail. The basic MR protocol should be expanded by sagittal T2-w images to detect injury to the cervical spinal cord. Diffusion MRI will detect ischaemic injury.
- If imaging shows parenchymal injury MRI should be repeated 2–3 months after the trauma to obtain prognostic information, which may aid clinical management.

Post-neonatal epileptic seizures
Neuroimaging in infants with epilepsy is important in those who develop epilepsy before the age of 2 years and in those with focal seizures.

- Imaging is performed to detect cortical abnormalities and the imaging modality of choice is MRI.
- In children with intractable seizures the basic MR protocol (see Neuroimaging: principles) should be expanded by a three-dimensional T1-w sequence for assessment of mesial temporal structures.
- Only in a setting where no MRI is available should CT be performed to exclude gross structural abnormalities and also in situations where there is suspicion that acute illness may be causing the seizures.

Macrocephaly, including hydrocephalus
Macrocephaly is due to either a large brain or large spaces with CSF. Causes of macrocephaly are described in Chapter 18.

- In the neonatal period ultrasound is a good tool for initial evaluation and monitoring of ventriculomegaly.
- CT or MRI is necessary for more detailed investigation of underlying causes following initial evaluation with ultrasound.
- MRI (T1-w and T2-w images) is the method of choice for detailed evaluation of structural brain abnormalities that may cause ventriculomegaly (e.g. aqueduct stenosis, obstruction by a tumour), and for assessment of parenchymal abnormalities that may cause a large brain (see Chapter 18).

Microcephaly, including congenital infections
The etiology of microcephaly is diverse (see Chapter 19). Primary microcephaly has heterogeneous genetic origins. Secondary microcephaly is caused by acquired lesions or pathological processes that affect the developing brain in the first years of life. Neuroimaging plays an important role in identifying possible underlying causes and in differentiating acquired microcephaly from genetic types of microcephaly.

- Structural brain abnormalities such as malformations, hypoxic ischaemic lesions, post-infective lesions and CNS abnormalities in metabolic disorders are best visualized with MRI (see relevant sections above).
- CT is more sensitive in the detection of calcifications (e.g. in congenital infections, Aicardi–Goutières syndrome).

Congenital infections frequently lead to microcephaly. Radiological signs of congenital infections are summarized in Table 7.1.

The floppy infant
The diagnostic approach for the floppy infant (see also Chapter 20) depends on whether there is a suspected central origin or whether the clinical signs point towards a

Table 7.1 Radiological signs of congenital infections

Infection	Findings in CT and/or MRI
Toxoplasmosis	Calcifications in basal ganglia, periventricular white matter and cortical grey matter Ventriculomegaly
Cytomegalovirus	Calcifications in periventricular white matter Neuronal migration abnormalities such as polymicrogyria and lissencephaly Delayed myelination and glial scars in white matter Cerebellar hypoplasia
Rubella	Calcifications in periventricular white matter, basal ganglia, cortical grey matter Ventriculomegaly Delayed myelination Diffuse areas of increased signal on T2-w images
Syphilis	Cerebral infarcts Meningeal enhancement (on contrast-enhanced images)
HIV	Calcifications in periventricular white matter and basal ganglia Brain atrophy, ventriculomegaly Signs of progressive leukoencephalitis with demyelination possible

peripheral origin. In the majority of infants the origin is central and for these infants neuroimaging should be part of the diagnostic process.

- In the neonatal period ultrasound can be used for initial assessment of gross structural abnormalities, the presence of haemorrhage or hypoxic ischaemic injury. Most of the disorders outlined in the section on neonatal encephalopathy can be associated with 'floppiness'.
- MRI (using the basic protocol and additional sequences as clinically indicated) is the method of choice, in particular, beyond the neonatal period, for detection of structural brain abnormalities, signs of neurodegenerative or metabolic disorders of the brain, hypoxic ischaemic injury, infection or trauma.

Early developmental impairment
- Moderate developmental impairment without other clinical features is not an indication for neuroimaging.
- Severe or profound impairment is an indication for neuroimaging.

- If there are clinical signs such as abnormal head size, dysmorphic features, abnormal findings on neurological examination or epilepsy, neuroimaging is likely to be beneficial in establishing the cause.

- MRI is the imaging modality of choice and the basic protocol outlined at the start of this chapter should be used. If possible, a three-dimensional gradient echo sequence should be included.

- CT is preferable for visualization of calcification that is associated with, for example, congenital infections.

Note: delayed myelination (identified on MRI) is a non-specific feature observed in many children with developmental impairment of any cause.

Febrile illness (bacterial meningitis and encephalitis)
For imaging of bacterial meningitis and encephalitis, see the section on neonatal infections (excluding congenital infections) above.

References

Ment LR et al. Practice parameter: neuroimaging of the neonate: report of the Quality Standards Subcommittee of the American Academy of Neurology and the Practice Committee of the Child Neurology Society. *Neurology*, 2002, 58(12):1726–1738.

Schiffmann R, van der Knaap MS. An MRI-based approach to the diagnosis of white matter disorders. *Neurology*, 2009, 72(8):750–759.

Resources

Govaert P, deVries LS. *An atlas of neonatal brain sonography. Clinics in developmental medicine 141/142.* London, Mac Keith Press, 1997.

Lequin MH et al. Magnetic resonance imaging in neonatal stroke. *Seminars in Fetal and Neonatal Medicine,* 2009, 14(5):299–310.

McDonald L et al. Investigation of global developmental delay. *Archives of Disease in Childhood,* 2006, 91(8):701–705.

Rutherford M et al. Best practice guideline. Magnetic resonance imaging in hypoxic-ischaemic encephalopathy. *Early Human Development,* 2010, 86(6):351–360.

Saunders DE et al. Magnetic resonance imaging protocols for paediatric neuroradiology. *Pediatric Radiology,* 2007, 37(8):789–797.

Chapter 8
Neurophysiological investigations

Bernhard Schmitt and Varsine Jaladyan

Key messages
- Normal electroencephalography (EEG) doesn't exclude epilepsy.
- EEG in sleep provides additional information.
- Interpretation of EEG requires knowledge of the patient's clinical condition during the recording.
- Treat the patient, not the EEG.

Common errors
- Mistaking immaturity for burst suppression or discontinuity.
- Mistaking age-specific normal EEG patterns for an EEG abnormality.
- Mistaking artefacts, drug effects or non-cerebral causes for an EEG abnormality.

When to worry
- Isoelectric or low-voltage EEG.
- Burst-suppression pattern.
- Prolonged periodic discharges.
- Lack of sleep cycles and lack of responsiveness on stimulation.
- Hypsarrhythmia.
- Electrographic seizures.

Prerequisites

Qualification of the persons involved

Electroencephalographer: special electroencephalography (EEG) training and experience in neonates and infants is an essential prerequisite. The risk of misinterpretation and doing harm is considerable. The electroencephalographer should know when and when not to perform EEG.

EEG technician: electrode montage (see Figure 8.1) and EEG recording in neonates and infants need a high level of training, experience, patience and empathy. Cooperation with nurses or parents and attention to hygiene, particularly on intensive care, is mandatory.

Environment and condition of the patient

The recording of EEG on intensive care is a challenge even for well-trained EEG technicians. Technical artefacts produced by machines and monitors must be reduced as far as possible. In the EEG laboratory the atmosphere should be quiet and relaxed. The infant should be warm and well fed, and the napkin or diaper changed. To avoid the need for drugs to induce sleep, the time of EEG recording should be scheduled to the usual sleep time and individual sleeping routine should be considered. Interference with the infant during the recording should be avoided. In neonates, all sleep stages should be recorded, which will take at least 60 min. Synchronized video recording is helpful for the interpretation of seizures and EEG abnormalities.

Technical aspects

The International 10–20 System and the standard montages are used. In neonates and infants with small heads the number of electrodes can be reduced to Fp1, Fp2, T3, T4, C3, C4, O1, O2, Cz (see Figure 8.1) and ear (A1, A2) or mastoid (M1, M2) (American Clinical Neurophysiology Society, 2006). In neonates additional polygraphic recordings are necessary to assess accurately the infant's state during the recording. For recording eye movements (electro-oculography), one electrode is placed 0.5 cm above and

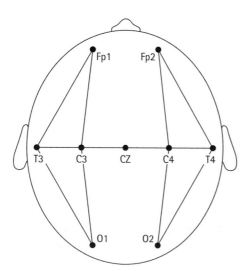

Figure 8.1 Electrode map and neonatal bipolar montage.

slightly lateral to the outer canthus of one eye (E1) and another 0.5 cm below and slightly lateral to the outer canthus of the other eye (E2) and linked either to each other (E1-E2) or to ear or mastoid E1 to A1/M1 and E2 to A1/M1 (or E1-A2/M2, E2-A2/M2). Muscle movements are recorded by submental electromyography (EMG) 1–2 cm from the midline and the heart rate (electrocardiography) by electrodes placed on both arms or precordium. A respirogram can be recorded by abdominal or thoracic strain gauges, impedance pneumogram or airway thermistors. Electrode impedances of less than 5 kohms can usually be obtained, although higher impedances may be allowed to avoid excessive abrasion of skin. Marked differences in impedances among electrodes should be avoided. For filter settings and amplification see Table 8.1.

Information and documentation

Reliable interpretation of EEG requires clinical information about the patient and the conditions during recording. As a minimum, the following information should be carefully documented:

- medical history: family history, pregnancy, birth (Apgar score, umbilical arterial pH), birthweight, head circumference;
- gestational age (GA; weeks from the last menstrual period): preterm ≤37 weeks GA, term >38 weeks GA;
- age at time of recording;
- conditions during recording: vigilance (sleep, awake, drowsy), eyes closed or open, movement (including abnormal eye movements), breathing, artificial ventilation, temperature, responsiveness, skin condition (oedema, haematoma), deformations of the skull, etc;
- time interval from the acute event (seizure, hypoxic ischaemic event, etc.);
- drugs;
- movement or other care given during the recording, technical and other artefacts;
- seizures or abnormal movements.

Steps to interpret the EEG

- Is the EEG activity age-appropriate (continuity, background activity, amplitude, responsiveness to stimulation, sleep/wake cycle, EEG elements, variability, spatial organization)?
- Symmetry and synchrony
- Epileptiform activity (ictal and inter-ictal)

Normal EEG

Neonates

The EEG shows dynamic changes between 26 and 44 weeks GA that parallel brain maturation. Every GA has typical EEG features which allow determination of GA with an accuracy of ±2 weeks.

Table 8.1 Technical parameters in the EEG and polygraphic recording of the newborn

Parameter	Transducers	Electrode placement	Amplification	Filters	
				Time constant (high-pass)	Low-pass
EEG	Silver cups	Fp1, Fp2, C3, C4, T3, T4, O1, O2, Cz (Fz, Pz)	7–10 µV/mm	0.3 s (0.5 Hz)	70 Hz
Electro-oculography	Silver cups	0.5 cm above and 0.5 cm below the lateral outer canthus of the eyes	7 µV/mm	0.3 s (0.5 Hz)	30–70 Hz
Electromyography	Silver cups	Submental 1–2 cm from midline	3 µV/mm	0.1–0.03 s (1.6–5 Hz)	70–120 Hz
Electrocardiography	Disposable electrocardiographic electrodes	Precordial or both arms	200 µV/mm	0.3–0.1 s (0.5–1.5 Hz)	35–70 Hz
Respiration	Strain gauges Thermistors	2 cm above umbilicus Nasal, buccal (airflow)	10 µV/mm	1 s (0.15 Hz)	15 Hz

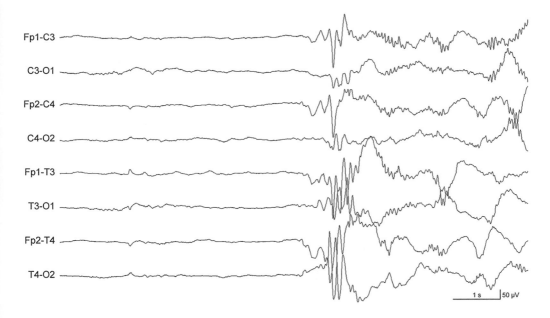

Figure 8.2 Tracé discontinue in a preterm infant (29wks GA): interburst interval up to 10 s.

Continuity: discontinuous activity (tracé discontinu; see Figure 8.2) is the characteristic EEG pattern at less than 30 weeks GA. Bursts of activity alternate with inactivity. The interburst intervals (inactivity between the bursts) decrease from <60 s at 24–27 weeks GA to <26 s at 28–29 weeks GA (Table 8.2). After 30 weeks GA discontinuity occurs only in non-rapid eye movement (NREM) sleep and fall to <10 s at 34 weeks GA. Beyond 34 weeks GA inactivity is replaced by low voltage activity (tracé alternant) which persists until term and disappears before 46 weeks GA.

Sleep/wake cycles can be recognized at later than 30 weeks GA by more continuous activity during rapid-eye-movement (REM) sleep. After 38 weeks GA six sleep states are defined:

- REM 1: continuous delta-, theta- and alpha-activity (40–100 µV)
- NREM 1: continuous high-amplitude (50–150 µV) delta-activity mixed with low-amplitude theta- and beta-waves
- NREM 2: tracé alternant (synchronous high-amplitude delta-/theta-waves alternating with low-amplitude fast activity)
- REM 2: low-amplitude activity (20–50 µV) with intermingled alpha-waves
- indeterminate sleep: activity between sleep states
- awake: continuous diffuse central theta-waves (20–50 µV), occipital delta-waves (20–50 µV), central high-amplitude theta-waves lasting 1–3 s, irregular alpha-/beta-activity (<30 µV).

Table 8.2 Maturation of EEG according to gestational age

EEG activity	Gestational age (weeks)						
	24–27	28–29	30–31	32–34	35–37	38–42	>42
Longest duration of burst	60 s	160 s	Continuous activity awake and in REM sleep				
Longest interburst interval	<60 s	<26 s	8–18 s	4–10 s		<6 s	
Activity in interburst interval	TD	TD	TD	TD/TA	TA	TA	TA
Sleep stages	Not detectable		Awake, REM, NREM		Awake, REM 2, NREM 2	Awake, REM 2, NREM 2, undetermined sleep	
Synchrony of bursts	88%	100%					
Delta brushes		X	XXX	XXX	XX	X	
			REM > NREM	NREM > REM			
Temporal saw-tooth waves	X	XXX	XXX	X	X	X	
Frontal sharp transients					X	X	X
Multifocal spike waves			X	XX	XX	X	X

TD, tracé discontinu; TA, tracé alternant; NREM, non-rapid eye movement; X, occur; XX, occur often; XXX, occur regularly.

REM sleep is the first and dominating sleep state until birth and lasts up to 20 min. After 42–43 weeks GA, NREM replaces REM sleep as the first sleep state and the proportion of REM decreases. Sleep spindles become obvious after 44 weeks GA.

Tactile stimulation causes generalized desynchronization or voltage changes at later than 30 weeks GA.

Delta-waves (100–300 µV or more) are dominant at >24 weeks GA and are uni- or bilaterally synchronous. Occipital delta-waves become longer after 28 weeks GA. Frontal delta-rhythms are obvious in REM sleep at 36–37 weeks GA.

Delta brushes are delta-waves with spindle-like fast activity (8–24/s, 10–25 µV) superimposed on the ascending part of the wave. They occur after 28 weeks GA, are dominant in REM sleep at 31–32 weeks GA and in NREM sleep after 33 weeks GA. After 35 weeks GA they become less and disappear in the first weeks of life.

Theta-waves are often sharply contoured. Between 24 and 40 weeks GA (max 28–32 weeks) they occur uni- or bilaterally over the temporal region (temporal saw-tooth waves). STOPs are sharp theta rhythms on the occipital areas.

Spikes are transients, clearly distinguished from background activity, with pointed peak and a duration from 20 to under 70 ms. The main component is generally negative relative to other areas. Amplitude is variable.

Sharp waves are transients, clearly distinguished from background activity, with pointed peak and duration of 70 to 200 ms. The main component is generally negative relative to other areas. Amplitude is variable.

Spikes and sharp waves occur after 30 weeks GA, become more frequent at 32–34 weeks GA and decrease after 35 weeks GA. High-amplitude (50–200 µV) uni- or bilateral *frontal sharp transients* occur later than 35 weeks GA and persist in NREM sleep after 38 weeks GA. They disappear by the age of 8 weeks.

Infants
- *Background activity*, apparent over the posterior region after eye closure, increases from 2–3/s at age 2 months to 3–4/s at 4 months, 5/s at 5 months and 6–7/s at 1 year. However, this maturation shows distinct variability. Blockade by eye opening is detectable after age 4 months.
- *Shut eye waves* are bilateral high-amplitude (100–200 µV) biphasic transients over the occipital region provoked by eye blinking. They occur after age 6 months.
- *Lambda-waves* (occipital positive, saw-tooth-like waves <50 µV) are provoked by visual exploration and are visible from birth.
- *Photic driving* is detectable at low-frequency stimulation (4–7 Hz) after age 3–4 months.

- *Drowsiness* is characterized by slowing and voltage increase of background activity. Between age 6 and 24 months central beta-activity increases during the transition from wake to sleep.
- *Sleep*: REM sleep decreases from 50% at birth to 30% at age 1 year. Centromedian vertex waves become apparent after age 3 months and K-complexes (vertex waves + spindles) after age 6 months. Rhythmic 13–15/s sleep spindles appear after age 4 weeks. In the first 6 months they have their highest frequency and their duration increases up to 10 s. Most of them occur asynchronously. After age 6 months spindle duration decreases to less than 1 s at age 6 years. Awakening is characterized by voltage attenuation in the first 3 months of life and by more and more serial frontal delta-/theta-waves after 3 months.

Abnormal EEG

Neonates
A single EEG is only conclusive when the abnormality is severe. Repeated recordings may distinguish temporary from persistent abnormalities and may detect ongoing changes in the brain. EEG abnormalities can be divided into acute and chronic, as follows.

- Temporary changes reflect recent or ongoing disturbances of the brain. They are characterized by (1) significant increase in discontinuity, (2) reduction of alpha-, theta- or beta-activity or (3) voltage attenuation (moderate <50 µV, distinct/ extensive <20 µV).
- Persistent changes reflect brain damage in the past. They are characterized by (1) abnormal or delayed maturation, (2) abnormal organization (deformed or abnormal quantities of theta-/delta-waves or delta brushes) or (3) increased sharp-wave activity.

EEG activity can improve or normalize in follow-up, which, however, doesn't exclude later neurological problems. The quality of background activity has more impact on the prognosis than the occurrence of ictal EEG changes.

Continuity is always related to the GA. Age-appropriate interburst intervals are given in Table 8.2; however, absolute limits don't exist. As a general rule, the larger the deviation from age-appropriate values, the poorer the prognosis and the higher the risk of neurological sequelae.

Burst-suppression pattern is characterized by bursts (1–10 s) of high-amplitude synchronous theta-/delta-activity mixed with spike and sharp waves alternating with isoelectric or very low-voltage (<5–15 µV) activity. The pattern doesn't vary during the EEG recording, persisting during both wakefulness and sleep, and is not influenced by stimulation. After 34 weeks GA burst suppression can be easily distinguished from tracé alternant. Before 34 weeks GA distinction from tracé discontinu is difficult. Intoxication (i.e. by barbiturates or lithium) has to be excluded. Burst suppression is the typical EEG pattern of *early infantile epileptic encephalopathy* (EIEE or Ohtahara syndrome) and *early myoclonic epilepsy* (see Chapter 16).

Variability: lack of EEG variability and fluctuation is critical in preterm and term neonates. After 30 weeks GA repeated recordings without sleep/wake cycles indicate poor prognosis. Abnormal sleep architecture is found in neonates from drug-addicted mothers and in neonates with brain malformations or hyaline membrane disease.

Maturation: extrauterine and intrauterine brain maturation follows the same speed and sequence. The EEG activity is immature when the pattern is more than 2 weeks behind the age-appropriate level. Criteria for immaturity are inadequate sleep cycles, prolonged interburst interval and localization and occurrence of delta brushes. Immaturity is a risk factor, but doesn't exclude normal development.

Inactivity is the most severe EEG abnormality in neonates. The term inactivity is more appropriate than isoelectric, because rare bursts of low-voltage activity may occur. Long time constants, maximal amplification, large inter-electrode distances and long-lasting recordings without artefacts are technical prerequisites for the diagnosis. Intoxication, acute hypoxia, hypothermia or post-ictal recordings should be considered. The EEG should be repeated, especially when the inactivity is registered shortly after the critical event. Criteria for the diagnosis of death by EEG criteria do not exist in neonates.

Low-voltage EEG is characterized by amplitudes between 5 and 25 μV, poor variability, lack of sleep cycles and, in preterm, lack of delta brushes. Technical, toxic-metabolic and non-cerebral causes (i.e. subdural haematoma, scalp oedema, caput succadaneum) should be excluded.

Asymmetries: voltage differences of more than 25% registered during the whole recording or asymmetrical occurrence of sustained waveforms indicate a local disturbance. Unilateral delta brushes indicate the less abnormal hemisphere in the preterm and the abnormal hemisphere in the term infant. Transient voltage asymmetries are normal. The EEG is asynchronous when morphologically similar bursts appear with an interhemispheric time difference of more than 1.5 s.

Spike and sharp waves are found in normal term and preterm infants. They might be abnormal when they occur unilaterally and frequently. *Positive Rolandic sharp waves* (positive over C3, C4, Cz) are abnormal before 34 weeks GA or when they occur more than 1–2/min. They indicate periventricular leukomalacia but have no epileptic background. *Positive temporal sharp waves* (positive over T3, T4) are abnormal in term infants when they appear frequently.

Ictal EEG in neonates is variable in morphology and localization. It consists of rhythmic spikes, sharp waves or rhythmic beta-, alpha-, theta- or delta-waves. In preterm infants rhythmic delta-waves are the most common ictal pattern. During the ictal discharge morphology, frequency and localization can change. Sometimes multiple discharges can start simultaneously or sequentially with differing localizations, morphologies and frequencies. Their onset and end are sometimes difficult to determine. Focal clonic or focal tonic seizures exhibit focal EEG discharges while generalized myoclonic jerks are associated with generalized bursts. On the other hand, focal myoclonic jerks and generalized tonic movements may exhibit no ictal EEG changes. Subtle seizures occur with and without ictal changes ('electroclinical dissociation'). Apnea in neonates usually has a non-epileptic etiology but the rare epileptic apnea starts with monomorphic alpha-/beta-activity over the temporal region. Electrographic seizures may have no associated clinical symptoms and be detectable only in the EEG.

Periodic discharges are monomorphic and broad-based complexes with regular intervals of 1–2/s and without variability in frequency and localization. When they last more than 10 minutes they are called periodic lateralized epileptiform discharges (PLEDs). Background activity is always severely abnormal (often low-voltage) and additional ictal discharges might occur. PLEDs have a poor prognosis.

Infants of 1–12 months
EEG abnormalities are divided into two categories: (1) disappearance of normal patterns and (2) appearance of abnormal patterns. Most abnormal patterns are non-specific and not associated with a specific etiology. Interpretation should be made only in the context of the patient's history and the clinical and neuroradiological findings.

Abnormal maturation of background activity should be diagnosed when the frequency deviates by more than 2/s from the age-appropriate values.

Abnormal background activity should be characterized according to the following criteria:

- localization: focal, unilateral, generalized,
- frequency: beta-, theta-, delta-, subdelta-activity,
- continuity: discontinuity, burst-suppression pattern, lack of variability and responsiveness to stimulation,
- sleep: absence or abnormality of sleep cycles or sleep patterns,
- symmetry and synchrony, and
- voltage: asymmetries, high- or low-voltage or isoelectric activity, intermittent voltage depression.

Burst-suppression pattern, low-voltage (<20 μV) and isoelectric EEG are the most severe abnormalities. They can indicate severe brain damage. Before drawing conclusions, technical, non-cerebral and drug-related causes have to be excluded as well as recent acute hypoxic events, seizures or medical interventions. Other EEG risk factors for poor outcome are lack of fluctuation and responsiveness to stimulation, and lack of sleep cycles in prolonged EEG recordings. Background slowing, even when registered over several days, has no prognostic value and doesn't exclude normal outcome.

Focal abnormal background activity is detected by comparison with the contralateral hemisphere. Over the abnormal hemisphere the activity is often slower; the amplitude however, might be higher or lower.

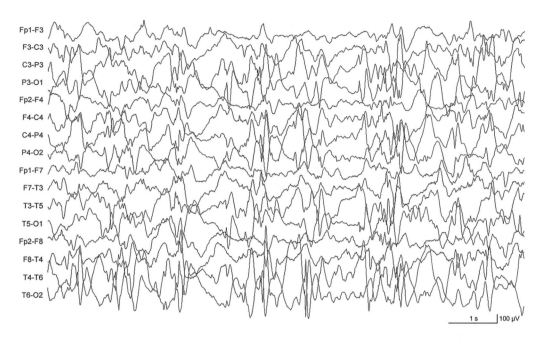

Fp1-F3
F3-C3
C3-P3
P3-O1
Fp2-F4
F4-C4
C4-P4
P4-O2
Fp1-F7
F7-T3
T3-T5
T5-O1
Fp2-F8
F8-T4
T4-T6
T6-O2

1 s   100 µV

Figure 8.3 Classical hypsarrhythmia during waking state. Male, age 5 months with infantile spasms (West syndrome).

Inter-ictal epileptiform activities are focal, multifocal or generalized spikes, sharp waves, polyspikes, spike and polyspike wave complexes, 3/s spike waves and slow-spike wave complexes. They should not be confused with artefacts and physiological sharp elements.

Hypsarrhythmia (see Figure 8.3) is characterized by random high-voltage slow waves and spikes. The spikes vary from moment to moment, both in duration and in location. At times they appear to be focal, and a few seconds later they seem to originate from multiple foci. Occasionally the spike discharge becomes generalized. The abnormality may be confined to the sleeping record but is apparent in the awake record in most cases. Hypsarrhythmia is the characteristic EEG pattern of *infantile spasms* (West syndrome).

Ictal EEG patterns can be associated with symptoms or occur without them.

Focal seizures often start with focal desynchronization and very fast low-voltage spiky activity which gradually rises in amplitude and diminishes in frequency. Sometimes only a focal change of frequency is obvious, which gradually becomes slower and involves adjacent electrodes. Focal seizures often indicate brain lesions or malformation. In *benign localized epilepsies of infancy*, low-voltage spiky activity evolves from the temporal or parieto-occipital region and spreads to the ipsilateral hemisphere.

In *malignant migrating partial seizures*, focal EEG discharges are typically migrating, starting from a cortical area and remaining localized or expanding to contiguous regions whereas others independently develop in different areas of the same or the opposite hemisphere. Three different ictal patterns can be distinguished: (1) rhythmic focal spikes or sharp alpha-theta activity over the Rolandic region; (2) polymorphic theta-delta activity over the temporo-occipital region; and (3) initial flattening or small discharge of fast polyspikes in one hemisphere.

Spasms: the ictal EEG pattern of infantile spasms (West syndrome) consists of (1) a positive-vertex slow wave, (2) sometimes followed by a variable voltage attenuation and (3) a fast spindle-like activity which can precede the slow wave. The spasms usually occur in clusters. Before the first spasm, hypsarrhythmia is often replaced by a mixture of irregular middle-amplitude faster frequencies. This 'relative normalization' of background activity usually persists until the end of the cluster.

Myoclonic seizures are characterized by generalized irregular spike/polyspike waves. They occur in *benign myoclonic epilepsy* and in *severe myoclonic epilepsy* or Dravet syndrome.

Atypical absence seizures show regular and irregular 2–3.5/s spike waves, for example in Dravet syndrome.

Tonic seizures exhibit desynchronization with almost flat EEG and fast, very low-voltage activities which may gradually increase in voltage and decrease in frequencies.

Tonic-clonic seizures: fast rhythmic spikes (tonic phase) which become discontinuous with rhythmic spike or polyspike waves (clonic phase).

Periodic EEG patterns are usually not associated with epileptic seizures. The term includes several patterns of more or less continuous, repetitive, rhythmical monomorphic waves and often indicates a severe ongoing brain disease.

Amplitude-integrated EEG or cerebral function monitoring

Amplitude-integrated EEG (aEEG) allows continuous assessment of brain function in critically ill neonates and is an indispensable diagnostic tool on neonatal intensive care units. It is easy to install and simple pattern recognition allows interpretation by non-electroencephalographers. aEEG is usually recorded from one (P3-P4) or two pairs (C3-P3, C4-P4) of electrodes and amplified and passed through an asymmetrical bandpass filter that suppresses activity below 2 Hz and above 15 Hz. The signal is displayed on a semi-logarithmic scale at slow speed (6 cm/h). A second tracing continuously displays the original EEG.

Assessment of aEEG background pattern
- continuous normal voltage (CNV) pattern: continuous trace with a voltage 10–25 (−50) μV;

- discontinuous normal voltage (DNV) pattern: discontinuous trace, low voltage predominantly >5 μV;
- discontinuous background pattern (burst suppression): periods of low voltage (inactivity) intermixed with bursts of higher amplitude;
- continuous background pattern of very low voltage (CLV; ≤5 μV); and
- very low voltage, mainly inactive tracing with activity <5 μV (flat trace, FT).

Sleep/wake cycling is characterized by semiperiodic variation in bandwidth. Broadening of the bandwidth represents the discontinuity of quiet sleep, narrowing represents the more continuous activity during wakefulness or active sleep.

Neonatal seizures are characterized in aEEG as a transient, sharp rise in the lower margin of the bandwidth often accompanied by a smaller rise in the upper margin, with narrowing of the bandwidth (see Figure 8.4). Neonatal status epilepticus, defined by continuous discharges for 30 min, can present as a 'saw-tooth pattern' or as continuous increase of the lower and upper margin.

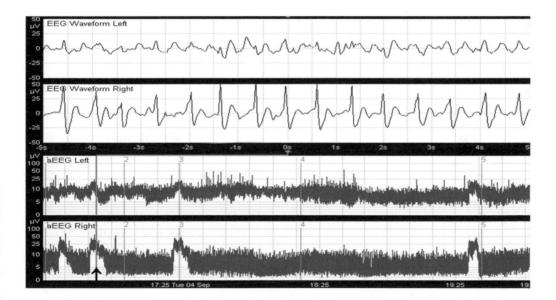

Figure 8.4 Amplitude–integrated EEG (aEEG) in a term newborn with hypoxic ischaemic encephalopathy and seizures. Lower 2 lines: a EEG over 3 h. Line 4, arrow and grey line: transient sharp rise in the lower margin of the bandwidth accompanied by a smaller rise in the upper margin, with narrowing of the bandwidth and in line 2 the respective original right hemispheric epileptiform discharge.

When should EEG or aEEG be performed?

Neonates
EEG and aEEG cannot replace each other. EEG is useful for a detailed analysis of age-appropriate or abnormal EEG pattern, whereas aEEG is useful for monitoring the brain over hours and days to detect changes in cerebral activity or ongoing seizures.

aEEG should be performed in neonates

- who are in poor condition,
- with artificial ventilation,
- with muscle paralysis,
- with suspected seizures,
- with neurological abnormalities.

Video-EEG should be performed in neonates

- who are in poor condition,
- have abnormal aEEG,
- with suspected seizures.

Infants
In addition, in infants in the intensive care unit aEEG is useful for monitoring the brain. Indications for aEEG are the same as in newborns. Video-EEG awake and asleep should be performed in infants

- with suspected seizures (including infantile spasms),
- with acute encephalopathies.

Video long-term EEG is recommended in infants

- with ambiguous paroxysmal events,
- with hypsarrhythmia but no obvious infantile spasms,
- with suspected subclinical seizures (i.e. under treatment with antiepileptic drugs).

When not to do EEG
Inappropriate questions and overuse of EEG may do harm by over-interpretation of harmless abnormalities found by chance and unrelated to the present neurological problem.

- Early developmental impairment as an uncomplicated clinical problem: the diagnostic yield of EEG is very low, approximately 1%.

- Febrile seizures: EEG results have no therapeutic implications.

- Breath-holding spells are caused by an immature autonomic nervous system. They are non-epileptic, benign, age-limited and have an excellent prognosis. Diagnosis can be made by history alone.

- Hyperekplexia, characterized by pronounced startle responses to tactile or acoustic stimuli and hypertonia, is a dysfunction of glycine neurotransmission. EEG is normal and doesn't provide any additional information.

- Shuddering attacks are a benign condition. Diagnosis is based on descriptive history and video review. The attacks are not associated with EEG abnormalities.

- Head trauma: if there are no seizures, EEG is not informative and has no therapeutic consequences.

- 'Cranial hypertension' – if indeed such a thing in neonates and infants exists in any context other than intracranial hypertension in the setting of acute encephalopathy or obstructive hydrocephalus causing excessive head growth, depressed conscious level, vomiting or forced downgaze ('sunsetting') – cannot be diagnosed by EEG.

- Hydrocephalus: EEG does not contribute to diagnosis.

- Headache cannot be diagnosed at this age. If suspected by abnormal behaviour of the infant, EEG is – as in older children and adults – not contributory to the underlying diagnosis.

Reference

American Clinical Neurophysiology Society. *Guideline two: Minimum Technical Standards for Pediatric Electroencephalography*. 2006. www.acns.org/pdfs/Guideline%202.pdf.

Resources

Andre M et al. Electroencephalography in premature and full-term infants. Developmental features and glossary. *Neurophysiologie Clinique*, 2010, 40:59–124.

Hellström Westas L, de Vries LS, Rosén, I. *Atlas of amplitude-integrated EEGs in the Newborn*, 2nd ed. London, Informa Healthcare, 2008.

Hirsch LJ et al. The ACNS subcommittee on research terminology for continuous EEG monitoring: proposed standardized terminology for rhythmic and periodic EEG patterns encountered in critically ill patients. *Journal of Clinical Neurophysiology*, 2005, 22:128–135.

Holmes GL, Lombroso CT. Prognostic value of background patterns in the neonatal EEG. *Journal of Clinical Neurophysiology*, 1993, 10:323–352.

Hrachovy RA, Frost Jr JD, Kellaway P. Hypsarrhythmia: variations on the theme. *Epilepsia*, 1984, 25:317–325.

International Federation of Clinical Neurophysiology. *Recommendations for the practice of clinical neurophysiology: Chapter 3.3 Neonatal EEG*. 1999. www.clinph-journal.com/webfiles/images/journals/clinph/Chapter3-3.pdf.

Niedermeyer E, Lopes Da Silva F. *Electroencephalography basic principles, clinical applications, and related fields*, 5th ed. Philadelphia, Lippincott Williams & Wilkins, 2005.

Petersen I, Eeg-Olofsson O. The development of the electroencephalogram in normal children from the age of 1 through 15 years. Non-paroxysmal activity. *Neuropadiatrie*, 1971, 2:247–304.

Shewmon DA. What is a neonatal seizure? Problems in definition and quantification for investigative and clinical purposes. *Journal of Clinical Neurophysiology*, 1990, 7:315–368.

Stockard-Pope JE, Werner SS, Bickford RB. Atlas of neonatal electroencephalography, 2nd ed. New York, Raven Press, 1992.

Tharp BR, Cukier F, Monod N. The prognostic value of the electroencephalogram in premature infants. *Electroencephalography and Clinical Neurophysiology*, 1981, 51:219–236.

Watanabe K, Hayakawa F, Okumura A. Neonatal EEG: a powerful tool in the assessment of brain damage in preterm infants. *Brain Development*, 1999, 21:361–372.

Chapter 9

Biochemical and haematological testing

Valerie Walker and Mary Morgan

Key messages

- Biochemistry tests are a supportive diagnostic tool.
- Use tests selectively to address specific questions.
- Interpret results within the clinical context.

Common errors

- Inappropriate samples.
- Inappropriate reference ranges.
- Ignorance of test limitations.

When to worry

- Acute encephalopathy.
- Intractable seizures resistant to conventional treatment.
- Hypotonia, dystonia and/or movement disorders.
- Progressive loss of skills.
- Multisystem disorders with neurological abnormalities.
- Macrocephaly or microcephaly with neurological abnormalities.

Cerebrospinal fluid analyses

Cerebrospinal fluid (CSF) is produced primarily by filtration from plasma across the blood–CSF barrier with a small contribution by active secretion. The choroid plexuses are the principal source, with a contribution from the ependyma lining the ventricles. CSF fills the ventricles and cisternae, bathes the spinal cord and is reabsorbed into the blood through the arachnoid granulations in the dural venous sinuses. CSF turnover is rapid, exchanging about four times per day. Changes in CSF biochemical composition occur with altered metabolic activity of the brain, intracranial inflammation, haemorrhage or tumour infiltration, immunological damage, brain trauma, ischaemia and infarction. These changes may be useful diagnostically when interpreted within the clinical context.

Constituents and significance of abnormalities

PROTEINS

More than 80% of proteins in CSF originate from plasma by ultrafiltration through the walls of capillaries in the meninges and choroid plexuses. The remainder are from brain and cells in the CSF. Protein concentrations are higher in lumbar CSF than in ventricular fluid, and many are around 200 times lower than in serum. After concentration of CSF a band of transferrin lacking sialic acid (β-transferrin; tau protein; note that this is distinct from Alzheimer-related tau protein) is a normal finding. Total protein concentrations are high neonatally, due to increased capillary permeability but generally fall to adult levels by 3 months of age (Table 9.1).

CSF proteins are raised for the following reasons:

- increased transudation of plasma proteins across an impaired blood–brain barrier due to: inflammation associated with bacterial or viral meningitis or encephalitis, brain tumours, intracerebral haemorrhage, trauma and mechanical obstruction of CSF circulation. Its severity can be demonstrated by analysis of albumin in paired CSF and serum samples: CSF/serum albumin index (mg/g) <9: intact barrier; 9–14 slight impairment; 14–30 moderate; 30–100 severe; >100 complete breakdown of blood–brain barrier.

- local production of gamma globulins within the central nervous system (CNS). Although mixtures of immunoglobulins, these show restricted heterogeneity and may appear as distinct bands on electrophoresis. It is assumed that they are products of a small number of B-cell clones. They are classed as oligoclonal bands if there are two or more bands, shown to be IgG, which are not found in paired serum. To demonstrate local production of IgG, albumin and IgG are analysed in paired CSF and serum samples to calculate the IgG index which excludes or corrects for leakage through a defective blood–brain barrier: the reference value is 0.30–0.70; more than 0.70 is evidence of intracranial IgG synthesis although this method will lead to some false positive and false negative results.

Table 9.1 Reference ranges: lumbar CSF

Constituent	Reference ranges	Comments
Volume (ml)	Infants: 40–60 Young children: 60–100	
White blood cell count (cells/ml)	Infants: preterm 0–25, term 0–22; Post-neonatal infants <5	
Glucose (mmol/l)	2.5–4.5 Neonates: 60–80% of blood glucose Older: approx. 60% of blood glucose; GLUT1 transporter deficiency: <46%	Varies with blood glucose; may take up to 4 h to equilibrate. False +ves at age <3 months
Protein (mg/l)	Neonates <1200; VLBW <3700 1–3 months: <800 >3 months: <500	Variable in neonates, higher in preterm; ranges also depend on analytical method
CSF/serum albumin index (mg/g)	<9 BBB intact; 9–14 slightly,14–30 moderately and 30–100 severely impaired; >100 complete breakdown	
IgG index	0.30–0.70; >0.70 suggests intrathecal IgG synthesis	CSF IgG x serum albumin/ serum IgG x CSF albumin. False +ves and false –ves occur.
β2-Transferrin (desialated transferrin; mg/l)	3–5	Collect a paired plasma to exclude a genetic transferrin variant
Lactate (mmol/l)	<2.0	
Pyruvate (μmol/l)	70–140	
CSF/plasma glycine ratio	<0.04; >0.06 consistent with nonketotic hyperglycinaemia	Possible increases from valproate therapy and blood contamination

Table 9.1 *Continued*

Constituent	Reference ranges	Comments
Lactate/pyruvate ratio	<20	If raised lactate, ratio >30 significant; 20–29 grey zone; spurious increase if pyruvate degrades (unstable)
Bilirubin (umol/l)	Neonates 0.7–7.5; higher in preterm Older: not detectable	High in neonates with severe hyperbilirubinaemia
Serum/CSF β-HCG ratio	>60	Ratio <60 indicative of intracranial germ-cell tumour
AFP (KU/l)	After 1 month <2 May be detectable in normal neonates;	Check for leaky BBB with CSF/serum albumin index
β2-Microglobulin	2–3 mg/l	Check for leaky BBB with CSF/serum albumin index
Neuron-specific enolase (μg/l)	<10	Check for leaky BBB with CSF/serum albumin index

AFP, α-fetoprotein; BBB, blood–brain barrier; GLUT1, glucose transporter 1; β-HCG, β-human chorionic gonadotropin.

IgG index = CSF IgG (mg/l) × serum albumin (g/l) serum IgG (g/l) × CSF albumin (mg/l)

CSF is also analysed by electrophoresis for oligoclonal bands.

Note: patients with total CSF proteins within the normal range may have abnormal transudates of plasma proteins or intrathecal IgG synthesis.

Causes of increased total protein in CSF include most cases of bacterial (including tuberculous) meningitis, cryptococcal, leptospiral and sometimes viral meningitis, encephalitis, neurosyphilis, poliomyelitis, brain abscess, lymphomatous, leukaemic or carcinomatous infiltration of the leptomeninges, cerebral haemorrhage, Guillain–Barré syndrome after the first week and spinal cord tumours or prolapsed intervertebral disc (protein may exceed 20 000 mg/l in Froin syndrome).

Disorders with intrathecal IgG synthesis and oligoclonal bands include multiple sclerosis (more than 90% if clinically definite), subacute sclerosing pan-encephalitis (SSPE; 100%), viral encephalitis (35%), meningitis (including cryptococcal; 33%); neurosyphilis (55%), systemic lupus erythematosus, Guillain–Barré syndrome, sarcoidosis and tumours. Their likelihood is governed by age.

GLUCOSE

The glucose concentration in CSF is regulated by facilitated diffusion across the blood–CSF barrier. In neonates, concentrations in newly secreted CSF may approach 80% that of plasma. Thereafter they are around 60%. This fraction may fall in the presence of hyperglycaemia because of saturation of glucose transport. Paired blood and CSF samples are essential for interpretation and, in general, the blood sample should be obtained immediately prior to the procedure for lumbar puncture. However, equilibration between plasma and CSF glucose may take up to 4 h, and the ratio is less reliable during states of metabolic flux.

Causes of low CSF glucose include hypoglycaemia; most, but not all, cases of pyogenic bacterial and tuberculous meningitis; around half with fungal meningitis, but few (<5%) with viral meningitis; neurosyphilis; Lyme disease; meningoencephalitic mumps; leukaemic, lymphomatous or carcinomatous infiltration; subarachnoid haemorrhage; neurosarcoidosis; systemic lupus erythematosus and the rare inherited deficiency of GLUT1 glucose transporter of the brain. Their likelihood is governed by age.

LACTATE AND PYRUVATE

The CSF concentrations of lactate and pyruvate largely reflect production from CNS glycolysis and hence, indirectly, the redox potential of the brain. Inflammatory, malignant and red blood cells in the leptomeninges or subarachnoid space are other sources. At physiological pH lactate is ionized and crosses the blood–brain barrier slowly. CSF levels are therefore independent of serum lactate if the barrier is intact. CSF lactate is analysed to investigate for respiratory chain or tricarboxylic acid cycle defects, pyruvate dehydrogenase deficiency and pyruvate carboxylase (and biotinidase) deficiencies.

Causes of raised CSF lactate include *spurious increases* due to blood contamination from traumatic lumbar puncture or delayed analysis if the CSF cell count is raised; *true increases* due to inherited defects of pyruvate metabolism, the respiratory chain and tricarboxylic acid cycle; bacterial meningitis; brain trauma and/or ischaemia; intracranial haemorrhage; brain abscess; cerebral leukaemia; lymphoma or carcinomatous infiltration of the leptomeninges and thiamine deficiency.

AMINO ACIDS

Glutamine concentrations are normally similar to plasma levels. Concentrations of the other amino acids are much lower, due partly to restricted entry from blood and partly to active transport from CSF to blood by carrier-mediated mechanisms.

Causes of abnormal CSF amino acid concentrations include: *generalized increases* due to breakdown of the blood–brain barrier, for example severe hypoxia/ischaemia; autopsy samples (generally uninterpretable); intracranial haemorrhage; bacterial meningitis or cerebral abscess; *increased glutamine*: hyperammonaemia in hepatic encephalopathy and inherited urea cycle defects; *increased glycine* with a high paired CSF/plasma glycine ratio: nonketotic hyperglycinaemia; *increased glycine, threonine, histidine, taurine and low arginine (variable mix)*: pyridox(am)ine 5′-phosphate oxidase (PNPO) deficiency; *low serine* 3-phosphoglycerate dehydrogenase deficiency (serine deficiency); *increased phenylalanine and low tyrosine*: poorly controlled phenylketonuria.

NEUROTRANSMITTERS AND RELATED METABOLITES

Dopamine, 5-hydroxytryptamine (5HT), noradrenaline, and their metabolites homovanillic acid (HVA), 5-hydroxyindoleacetic acid (5HIAA) and 3-methoxy-4-hydroxyphenylethylene glycol, respectively, do not readily cross the blood–brain barrier. They are actively transported out of the CSF. CSF concentrations are assumed to reflect changes in the brain, particularly of the striatum which can discharge neurotransmitters into adjacent ventricular fluid. These compounds, together with biopterins needed for their biosynthesis, are measured in CSF for diagnosis of inherited defects causing dystonia or severe seizures.

Causes of abnormal neurotransmitters and their metabolites include inherited tyrosine hydroxylase deficiency; aromatic L-amino acid decarboxylase deficiency; defects of biopterin metabolism; poorly controlled phenylketonuria; Menkes disease.

TUMOUR MARKERS

The main types of CNS malignancies are primary brain tumours, brain metastases, lymphomas and leukaemia. Identification of tumour cells in CSF is the most specific test, short of biopsy, but is insensitive, detecting only some tumours which involve the leptomeninges or lie close to the ventricles, but not deep-seated primary malignancies. It may be difficult to identify tumour cell origins, or to differentiate them from inflammatory cells. β-Human chorionic gonadotropin (β-HCG) and α-fetoprotein (AFP) are valuable when measured together for diagnosis of germ-cell tumours of gonadal or extragonadal origin (excluding dysgerminomas). Neither is normally expressed in brain.

β-HCG must be measured in paired blood and CSF samples to correct for spillover from high blood levels. A serum/CSF ratio of less than 60:1 strongly suggests intracranial germ-cell tumour. A low ratio may precede radiological evidence of metastases. Causes of intracranial HCG synthesis include primary choriocarcinoma, malignant teratoma, embryonal carcinoma and pineal germ-cell tumour; metastatic teratomas or trophoblast tumours.

AFP is produced by yolk-sac elements. The CSF/albumin index should be measured (see above) to correct for increased blood–CSF barrier permeability. AFP may be detectable in neonatal CSF because of high serum levels (Table 9.2) and the permeable

Table 9.2 Reference ranges: blood

Constituent	Reference ranges	Comments
Acid/base Hydrogen ions (nmol/l) pH pCO2 (kPa) Derived (actual) Bicarbonate (mmol/l) Base excess (mmol/l) Anion gap (mmol/l), = $[Na^+] - ([Cl^- + HCO_3^-])$	38–48 7.35–7.42; neonates 7.32–7.42 4.5–6.0; neonates 4.0–5.5 22–27; neonates 17–25 −4 to +4 7–16	
Albumin (g/l)	Neonates 28–44; then 35–48	Lower in preterm neonates; ranges vary with method
α-fetoprotein (KU/l)	At birth 50 000–150 000; 4 weeks: 1500–2500; 8 weeks: 50–100; 10 weeks 6–12; from 3 months: 3–8	Higher in preterm neonates; plasma half-life approx 5 days
Ammonia (μmol/l)	Neonates: healthy <110; sick <180; if >200 metabolic disease strong possibility; from 1 month: healthy <40; if >80 metabolic disease strong possibility	
Total bilirubin (μmol/l)	<18 μmol/l (conjugated <10%); neonates up to 10 days: <200 μmol/l; 14–28 days: <50; (conjugated <20 μmol/l)	Higher in preterm neonates
Total calcium (mmol/l)	Neonates 0–5 days: 1.95–2.65; then 2.15–2.55	
Ionised calcium (mmol/l)	1.13–1.32	
Chloride (mmol/l)	95–110	
Caeruloplasmin (mg/l)	250–450; neonates 50–260	Ranges vary with method

Table 9.2 *Continued*

Constituent	Reference ranges	Comments
Copper (µmol/l)	0–6 months: 3–11; then 12–26	
Cortisol (nmol/l)	After approx 6 weeks: 09.00 h: <100 consistent with adrenal insufficiency; >500 adrenal insufficiency excluded; >600: good response to stress	No diurnal rhythm until around 6 weeks and random levels often low-do synacthen test if deficiency suspected
Creatine kinase (IU/L)	Neonates: in first 2 weeks up to 3 times or more higher than normal paediatric ranges, then rapid fall.	Peak is at 24–48 h; ranges are method dependent-wide variation among laboratories
Creatinine (µmol/l)	0–2 days: 40–100; 3–14 days: 30–65; 14 days–3 months:10–60; 3–6 months: 10–50; 6 months–1 year: 10–60	
C-reactive protein (mg/l)	<10	
Glucose (random) (mmol/l)	3.5–5.5	Hypoglycaemia: 2.5 mmol/l or less
Lactate (mmol/l)	<2.1	
Lactate/pyruvate ratio (mmol/mmol)	<20	If raised lactate, abnormal if >30; 29–29: grey zone-may not be significant
Lead (whole blood; µmol/l)	<0.5	

Table 9.2 *Continued*

Constituent	Reference ranges	Comments
Magnesium (mmol/l)	0.74–1.03	Ranges vary with method
Osmolality (mmol/kg water)	275–295	
Phosphate (mmol/l)	Neonates: 1.80–2.78; then falling to 1.29–1.78	
Potassium (mmol/l)	3.5–5.0	Neonates often higher; poor-quality samples
Pyruvate (μmol/l)	50–100	
Total protein (g/l)	Neonates: 46–77; 1–12 months: 56–73	
Sodium (mmol/l)	135–145	
Free thyroxine (pmol/l)	Up to 1 year: 7.5–30	
Thyroid-stimulating hormone (mU/l)	0–48 h: 2.5–66; 3 days–1 month: 0.5–10; 1 month–5 years: 0.7–8.5	Ranges vary with method
Urate (μmol/l)	1–12 months: 80–390; neonates: 120–340	
Urea (mmol/l)	1.0–5.0	
Blood volume (ml/kg)	At birth: 61–100 (mean 78); then gradual fall to adult values: 53–87 (mean 71)	May be higher in preterm neonates
Plasma volume (ml/kg)	Term neonates: 39–72; infants: 40–50; older children: 30–54	

blood–brain barrier. Causes of intracranial AFP synthesis include primary or metastatic germ-cell tumours.

β2-Microglobulin is synthesized by all nucleated cells, and in high concentrations by activated T-lymphocytes. Measurement of the CSF/albumin index corrects for increases in blood–CSF barrier permeability. Causes of increased intracranial synthesis include CNS lymphoma and leukaemias. An increase may predict relapse (note: this is non-specific: CNS infection may also increase levels).

INORGANIC IONS
Measurement in CSF has little practical value. CSF potassium and total and ionized calcium are lower than in plasma, and magnesium is higher. Their concentrations are regulated largely by choroid plexus transport mechanisms and do not vary with plasma levels. CSF sodium reflects plasma levels.

HAEMOGLOBIN AND BILIRUBIN
After the first month of life, normal CSF is crystal clear, with no red cells or detectable bilirubin. In normal preterm and some term neonates without evidence of intracranial bleeding, CSF bilirubin (mostly unconjugated) is increased and the fluid appears yellow (xanthochromic). This is correlated with serum bilirubin levels and largely explained by hyperbilirubinaemia and increased permeability of the blood–CSF barrier to proteins.

Following haemorrhaging into the subarachnoid space, red blood cells undergo lysis and phagocytosis. Liberated oxyhaemoglobin is converted *in vivo* into bilirubin in a time-dependent manner. Negative brain computed tomography does not exclude *subarachnoid haemorrhage*. Visual inspection of the CSF supernatant fluid for xanthochromia is insensitive and should not be used. Examination of CSF for blood cannot distinguish between an *in vivo* haemorrhage and a traumatic tap. In these cases, the most appropriate investigation is analysis by spectrophotometry to look for oxyhaemoglobin and its product bilirubin in CSF collected more than 12 h after the acute event. For interpretation, results are also required for serum bilirubin and serum and CSF protein levels. Most positive cases have increases in both oxyhaemoglobin and bilirubin, but increased bilirubin alone is more likely after a lapse of several days. Subarachnoid haemorrhage is unlikely if results are negative and further investigation (for example cerebral angiography) is not indicated. Results from patients with hyperbilirubinaemia or CSF protein of more than 1000 mg/l must be interpreted cautiously.

CSF rhinorrhoea
Fluid leaking into the nasal passages after trauma can be confirmed to be CSF by demonstrating β2-transferrin (desialated transferrin) by electrophoresis. β2-Transferrin is not normally present in serum, nasal or aural fluid. Analysis of paired serum controls for genetic variants of transferrin. If this test is not available, the presence of glucose will differentiate CSF from nasal mucus.

Specimens for biochemistry tests

Results of biochemical tests from inappropriate samples may provide misleading information and lead to incorrect management. Special requirements are needed for the tests listed below. Refer to the clinical sections of this book for investigation protocols. Analysis of samples for DNA and collection of skin and tissue biopsies requires informed written parental consent.

Blood

- *Acylcarnitines and carnitine*: these may be analysed from blood spotted onto filter paper, or separated plasma or serum.

- *Amino acids (plasma)*: if possible, collect at least 4 h after food or from infants just before a feed. Plasma should be separated within 4 h and stored at −20°C. Causes of spurious abnormalities: delayed separation.

- *Ammonia*: plasma concentrations rise rapidly after venesection. Free-flowing blood should be collected into Ethylenediaminetetraacetic acid (EDTA) or lithium-heparin (check with local laboratory) in an ammonia-free tube, transported to the laboratory within 15 min, preferably on water ice, and separated on receipt. If not analysed immediately, plasma may be stored for up to 4 h at 4°C. Causes of spurious increases: delayed separation, haemolysis, struggling during venesection.

- *Lactate*: plasma concentrations rise rapidly after venesection. If not measured on a blood gas analyser, samples must be separated within 15 min. Causes of spurious increases: delayed separation, haemolysis, venous obstruction with a tourniquet, struggling and crying during venesection, breath-holding.

- *Lead*: more than 95% of blood lead is in red blood cells; hence whole blood and not plasma is analysed. Samples must be collected into EDTA or heparin and *not* centrifuged.

- *Pyruvate*: pyruvic acid is very unstable and blood must be collected into perchloric acid at the bedside following strict protocols and centrifuged under refrigeration. Analysis is required only exceptionally.

- *Red cell enzymes*: samples should not be collected until 3 months after blood transfusion.

- *White cell enzymes* (e.g., for lysosomal storage disorders): at least 7 ml of blood (absolute minimum 5 ml) is required, even from very small infants, to extract and wash enough cells for analysis. Whole-blood samples must be delivered to a specialist laboratory within 24 h at room temperature and hence should not be collected before weekends or public holidays.

Urine

- *Amino acids and organic acids (random samples)*: faecal contamination alters the profiles and should be avoided. A bag urine sample is preferred. If this proves difficult, unsoiled urine collected into a cotton wool ball may be the only option; it is essential to obtain urine for analysis at presentation of an acutely ill child, even if the sample is of poor quality. If transport to the laboratory is delayed, samples should be refrigerated (4°C if overnight; −20°C if longer).

- *Other metabolites*, for example creatine, glycosaminoglycans (mucopolysaccharides), purines, orotic acid and other pyrimidines, are analysed on random urine samples, not faecally contaminated, collected into a sterile container and stored at −20°C until analysed. Fluids should not be increased to induce a diuresis. Causes of spurious results: bacterial contamination, very dilute samples.

- *Sulphite*: there is a dip-stick test (Merckoquant Sulfi-Test®). Because sulphite is unstable, urine must be tested within minutes of voiding or frozen immediately if this is not possible. False negatives occur even with fresh samples.

CSF
- *Bilirubin and oxyhaemoglobin spectrophotometry* to investigate for subarachnoid haemorrhage with negative brain scan: CSF samples are collected 12 h or more after the acute event in sequence for (1) glucose and protein, (2) microbiology and lastly (3) spectrophotometry (around 20 drops). The third sample must be protected from light and sent immediately for analysis. Blood is collected simultaneously for bilirubin and protein analysis. Causes of spurious results: samples collected too early, delayed analysis, interpretive difficulties if there is hyperbilirubinaemia or CSF protein exceeds 1000 mg/l.

- *Glycine analysis* for suspected nonketotic hyperglycinaemia: CSF must be clear since blood contamination makes the result uninterpretable (glycine in plasma is normally 10–20 times higher than in CSF). A paired blood sample must be taken for glycine analysis to calculate the CSF/plasma ratio. Causes of spurious results: blood contamination, treatment with valproate.

- *Glucose analysis*: paired blood and CSF samples are needed for interpretation. If the test is to exclude inherited deficiency of the GLUT1 glucose transporter, samples should be collected after a 4–6 h fast when non-ictal, and blood collected first to minimize stress-induced increase in plasma glucose.

- *Lactate*: samples must either be analysed immediately at the bedside, using, for example, a blood gas analyser), or reach the laboratory within 15 min of collection. Causes of spurious results: delayed analysis especially if blood contamination, an increase in white blood cells or if tumour cells are present.

- *Neurotransmitters*: because there is a lumbosacral gradient, samples must be collected in a standardized volume fraction following protocols provided by the referral laboratories. The samples must be frozen immediately after collection (at the bedside) in solid carbon dioxide or liquid nitrogen.

- *Serine analysis* for 3-phosphoglycerate dehydrogenase deficiency: paired plasma and CSF samples are needed and analysed for amino acids.

Tissue biopsies
- *Skin*: local anaesthetic is injected or applied to the skin of the forearm, upper leg or armpit and the skin cleaned carefully. A 3 mm full-thickness punch biopsy is taken with full aseptic technique and placed in tissue culture fluid for fibroblast

culture. If culture medium is not available, the biopsy may be stored overnight at 4°C (*not* frozen) either in an empty sterile container or in sterile saline, according to instructions from the local tissue culture laboratory. Fibroblasts can often be cultured from skin taken 2 or 3 days after death and autopsy biopsies should be taken if indicated (with prior consent).

- *Muscle*: biopsies should be undertaken in collaboration with the muscle histopathologist so that samples are collected and processed appropriately for histology, histochemistry, electron microscopy and biochemical analyses. The tissue for biochemistry must be frozen at the bedside in solid carbon dioxide or liquid nitrogen.

- *Liver*: a biopsy should be obtained if possible when nonketotic hyperglycinaemia is diagnosed, and in a very small number of inborn errors involving enzymes expressed only in liver when mutation analysis is not an option, or if mitochondrial depletion is likely. One or two good needle biopsy cores are transferred to sterile containers and frozen immediately at the bedside in solid carbon dioxide or liquid nitrogen. An additional core is needed for histology and electron microscopy if required, and should be stored as directed by the histopathologist. If open biopsy is undertaken, 1 cm^3 of tissue should suffice.

Reference ranges

Good reference range data for neonates and young children are sparse. The ranges shown in Tables 9.1 and 9.2 are relevant for neurological investigations. They were compiled from ranges used in Southampton, UK, and from a number of published sources, including Belton (2003) and Soldin et al. (2007) which provide comprehensive lists. Referral laboratories supply their own ranges for specialist tests such as white cell enzymes and CSF neurotransmitters.

Haematology investigations

Full blood count

Fully automated cell counters provide a result for haemoglobin, total leukocyte count with differential and platelet count. Normal age-related reference ranges need to be applied as these are different from adult values. Spurious results may arise due to blood sampling (often difficult in small children with poor venous access), hence it is essential to correlate the clinical findings with the laboratory result.

In thrombocytopenia, the blood film should be reviewed to confirm the low platelet count, as clumping of platelets will give rise to a spuriously low count.

The full blood count (FBC) result includes a value for the red cell indices, mean cell volume (MCV) reflecting the size of the red cells and mean corpuscular haemoglobin (MCH) indicating the haemoglobin content. These values, in addition to a reticulocyte count, are also helpful in assessing the *cause* of anaemia.

Laboratory investigations for iron deficiency

- haemoglobin may be low.

- reduced mean cell volume, mean corpuscular haemoglobin.

- blood film shows hypochromic, microcytic red cells.

- reduced serum ferritin (ferritin is an acute-phase protein which increases in infection and inflammation); whereas a low serum ferritin reflects iron deficiency, a normal level does not necessarily confirm iron sufficiency; and

- reduced serum iron with raised total iron-binding capacity (transferrin); however, both can fall with inflammation.

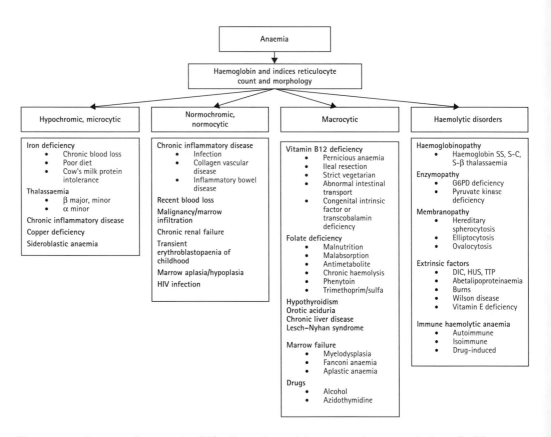

Figure 9.1 Causes of anaemia. DIC, disseminated intravascular coagulation; G6PD, glucose-6-phosphate dehydrogenase; HUS, haemolytic uraemic syndrome; TTP, thrombotic thrombocytopaenic purpura.

CAUSES OF IRON DEFICIENCY
See Figure 9.1

Most common:

- inadequate intake:
  - prolonged breast feeding
  - formula milk without iron fortification
  - undernourishment
- blood loss.

CLINICAL FEATURES OF IRON DEFICIENCY
- Tiredness
- Pallor if anaemic
- Angular stomatitis.

INVESTIGATIONS FOR HAEMOLYSIS
- Full blood count and film examination (red cell morphology), reticulocytes
- Direct antiglobulin test
- Elevated lactate dehydrogenase
- Elevated unconjugated bilirubin.

In haemolytic anaemia, the child may be jaundiced (usually not clinically apparent until 40 µmol/l) and have splenomegaly, but not always.

LEUKOCYTE ABNORMALITIES
Causes of neutrophilia (see Table 9.4) include

- infection
- inflammation
- metabolic disturbance
- neoplasia
- steroid therapy
- myeloproliferative disorders.

Causes of lymphocytosis include

- viral infections
- tuberculosis
- brucellosis
- thyrotoxicosis.

Table 9.3 Normal haematological values in children

Age	Haemoglobin (g/dl)		Mean cell volume (fl)		Mean corpuscular haemoglobin (pg)	
	Mean	−2 SD	Mean	−2 SD	Mean	−2 SD
Birth (cord blood)	16.5	13.5	108	98	34	31
1–3 days (capillary)	18.5	14.5	108	95	34	31
1 week	17.5	13.5	107	88	34	28
2 weeks	16.5	12.5	105	86	34	28
1 month	14.0	10.0	104	85	34	28
2 months	11.5	9.0	96	77	30	26
3–6 months	11.5	9.5	91	74	30	25
0.5–2 years	12.0	10.5	78	70	27	23
2–6 years	12.5	11.5	81	75	27	24
6–12 years	13.5	11.5	86	77	29	25
12–18 years						
Female	14.0	12.0	90	78	30	25
Male	14.5	13.0	88	78	30	25

Haemostasis

The coagulation system is immature at birth and even more so in the preterm infant. Plasma concentrations of coagulation proteins may vary from the adult normal range. Managle (2006) provides comprehensive age-related normal values for the coagulation proteins in preterm and term infants. Blood for coagulation tests is taken into tubes containing a measured amount of citrate which is used as the anticoagulant. The correct amount of blood should be added. Under- or overfilled tubes will cause abnormal results. The laboratory should reject these samples.

Table 9.4 Reference ranges for leukocyte counts in children

Age	Total leukocytes		Neutrophils			Lymphocytes			Monocytes	
	Mean	Range	Mean	Range	%	Mean	Range	%	Mean	%
Birth	18.1	9.0–30.0	11.0	6.0–26.0	61	5.5	2.0–11.0	31	1.1	6
12 h	22.8	13.0–38.0	15.5	6.0–28.0	68	5.5	2.0–11.0	24	1.2	5
24 h	18.9	9.4–34.0	11.5	5.0–21.0	61	5.8	2.0–11.5	31	1.1	6
1 week	12.2	5.0–21.0	5.5	1.5–10.0	45	5.0	2.0–17.0	41	1.1	9
2 weeks	11.4	5.0–20.0	4.5	1.0–9.5	40	5.5	2.0–17.0	48	1.0	9
1 month	10.8	5.0–19.5	3.8	1.0–9.0	35	6.0	2.5–16.5	56	0.7	7
6 months	11.9	6.0–17.5	3.8	1.0–8.5	32	7.3	4.0–13.5	61	0.6	5
1 year	11.4	6.0–17.5	3.5	1.5–8.5	31	7.0	4.0–10.5	61	0.6	5
2 years	10.6	6.0–17.0	3.5	1.5–8.5	33	6.3	3.0–9.5	59	0.5	5
4 years	9.1	5.5–15.5	3.8	1.5–8.5	42	4.5	2.0–8.0	50	0.5	5
6 years	8.5	5.0–14.5	4.3	1.5–8.0	51	3.5	1.5–7.0	42	0.4	5
8 years	8.3	4.5–13.5	4.4	1.5–8.0	53	3.3	1.5–6.8	39	0.4	4
10 years	8.1	4.5–13.5	4.4	1.8–8.0	54	3.1	1.5–6.5	38	0.4	4

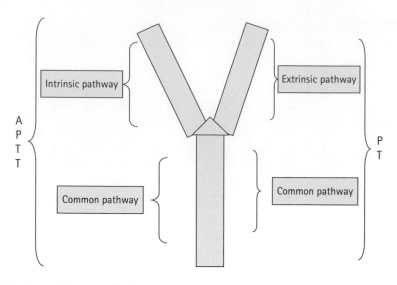

Figure 9.2 Prothrombin time (PT) and activated partial thromboplastin time (APTT).

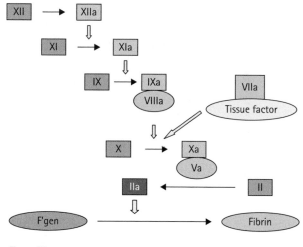

F'gen, Fibrogen.

Figure 9.3 The coagulation cascade.

LABORATORY INVESTIGATIONS

Prothrombin time (PT) is a measure of the 'extrinsic system' (Figure 9.2), whereas activated partial thromboplastin time (APTT) is a measure of the 'intrinsic system'. Also measured are: thrombin clotting time (or TCT), fibrin degradation products (or D-dimers) and fibrinogen.

COAGULATION CASCADE

PT measures the vitamin K-dependent coagulation factors (Factors II, VII, IX and X; see Figure 9.3). PT is prolonged because of:

- sampling error
- vitamin K deficiency
- deranged liver function
- factor deficiency
- warfarin (the therapeutic effect is achieved by a reduction in the vitamin K-dependent factors synthesized in the liver).

Vitamin K deficiency may cause haemorrhagic disease of the newborn, which can be classified into three patterns depending on the time of onset (see list below). Intracranial haemorrhaging may occur as well as from other sites and into vital organs (see Table 9.5):

- early: within 24 h, serious haemorrhaging including intracranial haemorrhage;
- classic: days 1–7, breast-fed infants;
- late: beyond the first week up to 6 months, breast-fed infants, usually associated with underlying disorders that compromise the supply of vitamin K.

Table 9.5 Vitamin K deficiency

	Early	Classic	Late
Age at onset	<24 h	Day 1–7	Week 2 – 6 months
Etiology	Drugs administered in pregnancy	Inadequate milk intake, low vitamin K in breast milk	Low vitamin K in breast milk, malabsorption of vitamin K (liver and bowel disease)
Frequency without prophylaxis	<5% in high-risk groups	0.01–1.5%	4–10 in 100 000 births
Precautions	Stop or substitute offending drugs	Adequate vitamin K supply by early breast feeding, prophylaxis	Vitamin K prophylaxis recognition of predisposing factors

APTT measures Factors VIII, IX, XI and XII, and the kallikrein–kinin system. It is prolonged for the following reasons:

- sampling error
- factor deficiency

- inhibitor: lupus anticoagulant
- heparin.

Caution: even small amounts of heparin in the blood taken from central lines will prolong the APTT. Deficiencies of factor XII, high-molecular-weight kininogen and pre-kallikrein result in a prolonged APTT, but do not cause haemorrhaging.

Thrombin clotting time measures the amount and quality of fibrinogen and the rate of conversion of fibrinogen to fibrin. A prolonged thrombin clotting time may indicate a deficiency of fibrinogen (<1 g/l) as seen in congenital hypofibrinogenaemia or afibrinogenaemia. It is markedly prolonged in the presence of heparin.

A fibrinogen assay should be included in the basic coagulation screening tests. It is reduced in acquired (disseminated intravascular coagulation, liver dysfunction, increased fibrinolysis) and hereditary (afibrinogenaemia, hypofibrinogenaemia and dysfibrinogenaemia) coagulopathies. Haemorrhaging does not usually occur until the level is less than 1.0 g/l, *unless it is a dysfunctional protein.*

DISSEMINATED INTRAVASCULAR COAGULATION – LABORATORY ABNORMALITIES
- Prolonged PT and APTT
- Thrombocytopenia
- Reduced fibrinogen
- Raised fibrin-degradation products.

ACQUIRED DISORDERS OF COAGULATION
- Vitamin K deficiency
- Liver disease
- Disseminated intravascular coagulation
- Associated with malignancy
- Acquired inhibitors: lupus anticoagulant
- Massive blood transfusion.

CONGENITAL COAGULATION DISORDERS
- Haemophilia A: deficiency of Factor VIII
- Haemophilia B: deficiency of Factor IX (Christmas disease)
- Von Willebrand disease Type 1, 2, 3
- Deficiency of Factors II, V, VII, X, XI, XII and XIII
- Dys-/hypo-fibrinogenaemia.

FACTOR XIII DEFICIENCY
Severe Factor XIII deficiency can result in intracranial haemorrhage. The PT and APTT are normal and a specific factor assay is necessary to make the diagnosis.

Haemoglobinopathy

Haemoglobinopathies are disorders of haemoglobin arising as a result of a disturbance of globin chain production or a mutation resulting in an abnormal haemoglobin (Hb variant). Thalassaemia syndromes are characterized by diminished or absent production of alpha or beta globin chain synthesis. Alpha-thalassaemia occurs in people of African, Mediterranean, South and South-east Asian origin. Beta-thalassaemia is found in the Mediterranean, India, Pakistan and Africa.

Haemoglobin variants arise as a result of a single amino acid substitution in the alpha or beta globin chains. This results in alteration in the structure of the normal adult haemoglobin. The most common of these are S, C, E, D^{Punjab}. HbS and HbC are found in the Afro-Caribbean population, HbE in the South-east Asian population and HbD^{Punjab} in the Indian population. The most important of these is sickle haemoglobin found in Africa, the Near East, Mediterranean and parts of India, which in the homozygous or double heterozygous state can result in a condition characterized by chronic haemolysis and sickle cell crises.

Haemoglobinopathy could be suspected for the following reasons:

- family history
- hypochromic, microcytic indices not due to iron deficiency
- target cells on blood film
- red cell fragments or sickle cells.

LABORATORY DIAGNOSIS
- Examination of a blood film
- Cellulose acetate electrophoresis to identify an abnormal Hb band
- High-pressure liquid chromatography (HPLC) to identify the various haemoglobins
- Sickle solubility test which detects the presence of HbS, but does not distinguish the hetero- from the homozygous state.

Caution: the majority of haemoglobin at birth is fetal Hb F before the switch to adult HbA. Children with a haemoglobinopathy should be referred to a haematologist.

References

Belton NR. Biochemical & physiological tables & reference ranges for laboratory tests. In: McIntosh N, Helms P, Smyth R, eds. *Forfar and Arneil's textbook of pediatrics*, 6th ed. Edinburgh, Churchill Livingstone, 2003:1879–1916.

Monagle P et al. *Paediatric thromboembolism and stroke*, 3rd ed. Hamilton, ON, BC Decker, 2006.

Nathan D et al. *Nathan and Oski's haematology of infancy and childhood*, 6th ed. Philadelphia, Saunders, 2003.

Soldin SS, Brugnara C, Wong EC, eds. *Pediatric reference intervals*, 6th ed. Washington DC, AACC Press, 2007.

Chapter 10
Drug treatments: drugs, vitamins and minerals

Imti Choonara and Peter Baxter

Key messages

Neonatal drugs

- Use drug doses adjusted for age-specific metabolism (e.g. reduced doses in preterm infants).
- Administer drugs less frequently (for drugs that are renally excreted).
- Avoid highly protein-bound drugs.

Medication errors

- Tenfold errors occur more frequently in neonates and infants.
- Errors involving aminoglycosides and morphine are particularly dangerous.
- Errors with intravenous drugs are more likely to result in harm.

Anti-infective drugs

- Ceftriaxone is contraindicated in neonates.

General principles

- Avoid polypharmacy.
- Avoid intramuscular administration of medicines.
- Be aware that all medicines have side effects.
- Use the lowest effective dose of a medicine for the shortest duration.

Common errors

- Using drug treatments without a clear diagnosis.
- Using drug treatments for which there is no justification.
- Using oral preparations of phenytoin under the age of 6 months.

When to worry

- Unexplained adverse clinical change associated with addition of a drug.

Introduction

Medicines are extremely useful in the treatment of diseases. It is important, however, to recognize that medicines can also be harmful, especially if used inappropriately. It is important to try to use as few medicines as possible and ideally to use the medicine in the lowest dosage that is effective and for the shortest duration of time. This will hopefully reduce the risk of drug toxicity while ensuring that the child receives appropriate treatment.

Is the treatment evidence-based?

Medicines are licensed by regulatory agencies if they are shown to be more effective than placebo. Unfortunately, medicines may be licensed even if they are less effective than existing treatment. Therefore, one always needs to critically evaluate licensed medicines. An additional problem for infants is that many medicines are not licensed for use in young children because clinical trials have not been performed. This does not automatically mean we should not use any medicine that is not licensed, but that we should always try and evaluate the existing evidence to see whether the medicine is likely to be of benefit or not. The most supportive evidence for efficacy of a medicine is a clinical trial and this is ideally performed as a randomized clinical trial. Clinical trials, however, are not that effective in detecting uncommon side effects. One needs to recognize that new medicines may be associated with side effects that have not been detected in a small randomized clinical trial.

Drug metabolism

Drugs are excreted either by metabolism in the liver or through the kidneys. Drug metabolism is usually decreased in the neonatal period and renal function is also impaired, especially in the sick preterm infant. The most important metabolic pathway for the elimination of drugs in the liver is the CYP3A4 pathway. This is reduced at birth but then increases during the first year of life. Midazolam is an example of a medicine that is eliminated by this pathway and it is important that one therefore uses lower doses of midazolam in the first year of life and especially in neonates. Another major metabolic pathway in the liver is the CYP1A2 pathway, which again is reduced at birth and then gradually increases during infancy. The CYP3A4 and CYP1A2 pathways both involve oxidation.

Other pathways include conjugation into a glucuronide or a sulphate. Morphine undergoes conjugation to both morphine 3-glucuronide and morphine 6-glucuronide. The latter is an important metabolite as it has considerable analgesic activity. Glucuronidation of morphine is decreased in the neonatal period and then increases in activity during the first year of life. As the metabolism of morphine is decreased in the neonatal period, one needs to use lower doses of morphine. Paracetamol undergoes metabolism by both glucuronidation and sulphation. Glucuronidation of paracetamol is reduced in neonates and infants, but sulphation is increased. The overall metabolism of paracetamol is reduced in the neonatal period but from the age of 1 month onwards it is similar to that in older children because of the increased sulphation. Paracetamol is the exception in that for all the other drugs mentioned in this section drug metabolism is decreased in the first year of life.

Many drugs, such as aminoglycosides and cephalosporins are eliminated by renal excretion. Renal function is impaired in the first few days of life, especially in the preterm neonate. The dosing interval for these drugs is therefore increased in sick preterm neonates. After the neonatal period renal function is usually normal.

Drug toxicity

The effect of reduced drug metabolism in the neonatal period is illustrated by the grey baby syndrome that was reported in association with chloramphenicol. When chloramphenicol was first used in infants, individuals were unaware that drug metabolism in the early stages of life was reduced. Unfortunately, several infants developed catastrophic cardiovascular collapse and died because they had received too high a dose of chloramphenicol.

Sulphonamides were noted to result in an increased mortality in neonates. This was due to the displacement of bilirubin from albumin and the subsequent development of kernicterus. It is essential therefore that one does not use a medicine that is highly protein-bound in sick neonates.

There are cases of drug toxicity that have affected infants where the mechanism is not fully understood. An example is the use of sodium valproate in children under the age of 3 years, especially if on more than one medicine. These children are at greater risk of liver toxicity. This is thought to be due to the activation of different metabolic pathways in young children. These different metabolic pathways can also be enhanced in children with developmental delay or by the use of polypharmacy.

We know that one in 10 children in hospital will experience an adverse drug reaction. One in eight of these adverse drug reactions will be severe and 2% of children admitted to hospital will be admitted directly as a result of an adverse drug reaction. We cannot prevent adverse drug reactions entirely but we can do our best to reduce the incidence.

Medication errors and route of administration

Medication errors occur in adults and children. The most frequent type of medication error in children is the wrong dose of the medicine being given. A particular problem in infants is tenfold errors whereby the decimal point is placed incorrectly. Tenfold errors occur more frequently in neonates and infants as one can administer 10 times the dose of a drug from a single ampoule. The clinical impact of a medication error is greater with certain medications, in particular morphine, phenytoin and aminoglycosides. Medication errors associated with intravenous formulations are more likely to result in significant harm. One therefore needs to be especially careful with intravenous medicines.

Medicines are usually given orally. This is the preferred route for children who are able to take medicines orally and who are not critically ill. Intravenous administration of medicines should be reserved for children with severe acute infections or if they are critically ill; that is, in status epilepticus. Intramuscular medicines are not routinely recommended in neonates or infants. Oral medicines should be given as a suspension/liquid to infants in the first year of life as they are unable to take tablets. Unfortunately, many medicines are not available in a suitable format for infants and extemporaneous preparations are frequently required.

Essential drug lists

In order to ensure children receive the medicines that are essential, the WHO has developed an Essential List of Medicines. These were originally designed for adults. More recently an Essential List of Medicines for Children has been developed. This is available on the WHO website (www.who.int/medicines/publications/essentialmedicines/en/index.html). One needs to question the routine use of medicines that are not on the WHO Essential List of Medicines for Children.

Antiepileptic drugs

In the neonatal period, intravenous phenobarbital has been shown to be effective and is the first-line drug of choice. Outside the neonatal period, buccal midazolam has been shown to be more effective than rectal diazepam for acute seizures. If intravenous medication is required, then lorazepam is the drug of choice. A particular problem in the first year of life is infantile spasms and oral corticosteroids (prednisolone) are the preferred treatment for these. Infants requiring oral medication for epilepsy should ideally be given carbamazepine in preference to sodium valproate which is more likely to be associated with hepatotoxicity in children under the age of 3 years. Hepatotoxicity is rare, and exactly how rare is not precisely known, but unfortunately is usually fatal and therefore valproate should only be used if carbamazepine or phenobarbital has been ineffective. Exceptions to this rule apply to certain specific epilepsy syndromes with certain types of epileptic seizure becoming more severe when carbamazepine, phenytoin or lamotrigine are added to treatment (see Chapter 16). Nevertheless, valproic acid should not *routinely* be used in infants with developmental delay or in those receiving more than one anticonvulsant, as hepatotoxicity is significantly increased in this group of infants.

Anti-infective drugs

In the neonatal period, intravenous benzylpenicillin and gentamicin are the usual first-line choice of antibiotics. Ceftriaxone is contraindicated in neonates for two reasons. First, it is highly protein-bound and may displace bilirubin and second it has been associated with death in several neonates and infants who have also received calcium supplements. Cefotaxime is the cephalosporin of choice in the neonatal period. The first-line choice of intravenous antibiotic for meningitis in infants will depend upon local resistance. Benzylpenicillin remains the drug of choice for meningococcus and pneumococcus if local strains are penicillin-sensitive. In areas of high resistance, intravenous cephalosporins such as cefotaxime or ceftriaxone (except in neonates) can be given. If herpes encephalitis/meningitis is suspected, then aciclovir is recommended. For tetanus, intravenous benzylpenicillin is the drug of choice.

Analgesia and antipyretics
A fever is not usually a problem in the neonatal period and antipyretics are not routinely recommended. In the first year of life it is more important to try to determine the cause of the fever than simply to reduce the temperature. If an antipyretic is required, paracetamol is the drug of choice as it is safer than ibuprofen which, as a nonsteroidal anti-inflammatory drug, may cause gastrointestinal symptoms and rarely may cause gastrointestinal bleeding. Paracetamol is also the initial drug of choice for mild pain. If more potent analgesia is required, then one should consider the use of morphine either intravenously or orally.

Sedative agents
For critically ill children or neonates who require sedation, intravenous midazolam is the drug of choice. For infants who are able to tolerate oral or nasogastric medication then chloral hydrate and promethazine are alternatives to midazolam. Sedation should only be used to benefit the infant. It should never be used to make life easier for health professionals.

Antispasmodics
Children with cerebral palsy may have hypertonicity/spasticity of their voluntary muscles. If this is chronic then oral baclofen may be beneficial. Skeletal muscle relaxants are, however, usually of benefit in children only after the first year of life and baclofen and other muscle relaxants should not routinely be used in infancy.

Gastro-oesophageal reflux
Gastro-oesophageal reflux is a physiological event which is self-limiting and is common in infants in the first 6 months of life. Not all infants with gastro-oesophageal reflux require medication. If the reflux is causing significant medical problems, such as failure to thrive or excessive vomiting, then one should consider using thickeners such as Carobel or alternatively alginates such as Gaviscon. The efficacy of motility stimulants such as domperidone and metoclopramide has not been established in gastro-oesophageal reflux and therefore they should not be used. Histamine H2 receptor antagonists, such as ranitidine, again should not routinely be used for gastro-oesophageal reflux. Proton-pump inhibitors, such as omeprazole, should not routinely be used for reflux as they have been shown to be ineffective in infants.

Diuretics for hydrocephalus

Historically, acetazolamide has been used to try and prevent hydrocephalus. Systematic literature reviews including Cochrane Reviews have shown that acetazolamide and furosemide are ineffective in reducing the the need for surgical intervention and cause significant harm in increasing the risk of subsequent motor disability and of nephrocalcinosis (Whitelaw et al., 2001). It is best to therefore avoid the use of diuretics for post-haemorrhagic hydrocephalus in the neonatal period.

Vitamins and minerals

Neurological conditions that respond to treatment with vitamins, minerals or other substances such as amino acids are rare. However, if in doubt it is always worth considering a trial of treatment since a response can be dramatic and can, at times, save a child from further damage. As a general principle, deficiencies occur when there is an inadequate diet, malabsorption, disorders of transport or with some metabolic disorders. In addition, maternal deficiency can affect newborn infants.

Vitamins and minerals can have possible therapeutic benefits in a wide range of conditions presenting with seizures, encephalopathy, reflex anoxic syncope, extrapyramidal movement disorders, early developmental impairment, weakness/myopathy, deafness, oculomotor disorders and retinopathy.

Possible indications and dose ranges are given in Table 10.1. Please refer to later chapters in this volume for more details on the relevant conditions, as well as appropriate doses for specific disorders.

Various vitamin and mineral treatments have also been tried in conditions such as Down syndrome, autism, Fragile X syndrome and Duchenne muscular dystrophy. Formal trials have shown that they are ineffective and should not be used.

Drugs to avoid

It is important that one only uses medicines that have been shown to be effective. This does not mean that we need a large multinational randomized clinical trial before medicines are used in neonates or in infants. It is, however, important to recognize that there needs to be some evidence to justify the use of the medication in an infant. Doctors throughout the world are very quick to copy colleagues who will start to use a medication with no scientific evidence to justify its use in a particular clinical situation. An example of this is the widespread use of domperidone in infants with mild gastro-oesophageal reflux in the UK. Similarly, there does not appear to be any scientific rationale for the use of medicines such as Actovegin and Citicoline. It is not possible to list all the medicines that are used inappropriately but each doctor who writes out a prescription for a medication should be able to justify the use of such a medication and this justification needs to be based on articles published in the scientific literature rather than copying the practice of other individuals.

Table 10.1 Possible indications, dose ranges and some adverse effects of vitamins and minerals

Vitamins	Specific conditions	Dose range	Route	Adverse effects
A (retinol)	Vitamin A deficiency ?Retinitis pigmentosa	Neonate: 100 mg/kg/day; older child: 5000–15000 IU/day	Oral	Raised intracranial pressure
B1 (thiamine)	Maple syrup urine disease Leigh syndrome Mitochondrial cytopathies Pyruvate dehydrogenase deficiency (girls) Wernicke encephalopathy	Neonate 5 mg/kg/day 10–1000 mg/day	Oral or IV	Anaphylactic shock may follow injection
B2 (riboflavin)	Fazio-Londe or Brown Vialetto van Laere Syndrome Multiple acyl-CoA dehydrogenase deficiency Mitochondrial cytopathies MTHFR deficiency	5–300 mg/day	Oral	

B3 (nicotinamide)	Pellagra Hartnup disease	50–300 mg/day	Oral	
B6 (pyridoxine)	Pyridoxine dependency Hypophosphatasia Epilepsy including West syndrome Homocystinuria ?Tetanus	Initial: 30–50 mg/kg/day; Maintenance: 5–50 mg/kg/day; 12–24 hourly	Oral/IV	Immediate: apnoea Long term: sensory neuropathy
B6 (pyridoxal-5-phosphate)	Pyridoxal phosphate dependency (or PNPO deficiency) Pyridoxine dependency Hypophosphatasia Epilepsy including West syndrome	30–50 mg/kg/day; 4–6 hourly	Oral	Immediate: apnoea Long term: sensory neuropathy
B12 (hydroxocobalamin)	B12 deficiency Methylmalonic aciduria	1–2 mg/day initially, later 1 mg 1–8 times monthly	IM	

Table 10.1 *Continued*

	Specific conditions	Dose range	Route	Adverse effects
C (ascorbic acid)	Mitochondrial cytopathies Prolidase deficiency	50–60 mg/kg/day or 1–4 g/day	Oral	
D (cholecalciferol)	Rickets (all forms) Hypocalcaemia	Cholecalciferol or ergocalciferol: 400–6000 units/day; or 1α-cholecalciferol: 0.015–0.05 µg/kg/day	Oral	Nephrocalcinosis, hypercalcaemia
E (aloha-tocopherol)	Vitamin E deficiency Ataxia with vitamin E deficiency Hypobetalipoproteinaemia	10–300 mg/kg/day	Oral	

			Oral/IM/IV	
K (phytomenadione)	Haemorrhagic disease of the newborn Mitochondrial cytopathies	10 mg/day K3 Menadione 1.1–1.5 mg/kg/day	Oral/IM/IV	Risk of hyperbilirubinemia in neonates
Biotin	Biotinidase deficiency Leigh syndrome Biotin responsive encephalopathy Holocarboxylase synthetase deficiency	5–30 mg/day	Oral	
Folinic acid	Folinic acid-responsive seizures (≈Pyridoxine dependency) Remethylation defects	3–5 mg/kg/day 12 hourly; 10–20 mg/day	Oral	Immediate: apnoea

Table 10.1 *Continued*

	Specific conditions	Dose range	Route	Adverse effects
Folic acid	Remethylation defects	1–5 mg/day Up to 100 mg/day	Oral	
Minerals				
Calcium	Hypocalcaemia Rickets		Oral/IV	Nephrocalcinosis
Iron	Iron deficiency		Oral	Hepatopathy
Magnesium glycerophosphate	Magnesium deficiency	0.6 mmol/kg/day	Oral	Constipation

Other			
Serine	Serine deficiency, e.g. due to 3-phosphoglycerate dehydrogenase deficiency	400–650 mg/kg/day, 8 hourly	Oral
Carnitine	Primary or secondary carnitine deficiency Reye syndrome Mitochondrial cytopathies	1–3 g/d or 100 mg/kg/day	Oral or IV	Vomiting/diarrhoea
Ubiquinone (coenzyme Q)	Ubiquinone deficiency	4–5 mg/kg/day or 30–300 mg/day	Oral
Idebenone	Mitochondrial cytopathy ?Friedreich's ataxia*	5–15 mg/kg/day or 90 mg/day	Oral

Table 10.1 *Continued*

Specific conditions	Dose range	Route	Adverse effects
Creatine	Creatine-deficiency syndromes	100–2000 mg/kg/day	Oral	
Dicloroacetate	Pyruvate dehydrogenase deficiency	15–200 mg/kg/day	Oral	Renal tubulopathy, pericardial effusion, neuropathy
Betaine	5,10-MTHFR reductase deficiency; other disorders of folate and cobalamin metabolism	500 mg/kg/day, or 2–3 g/day in young children and 6–9 g/day in older children	Oral	If powder inhaled, severe pneumonia

IM, intramuscularly; IV, intravenously; MTHFR, 5,10-methylenetetrahydrofolate reductase.
*The suggested benefit of idebenone in Friedreich ataxia is currently uncertain.

Reference

Whitelaw A, Kennedy C, Brion L. Diuretic therapy for newborn infants with posthemorrhagic ventricular dilatation. *Cochrane Library*, 2001, Issue 2.

Resources

Blau N et al., eds. *Physician's guide to the treatment and follow-up of metabolic diseases*. Berlin, Springer-Verlag, 2006.

Scriver CR et al. *The metabolic and molecular bases of inherited disease*, 8th ed. New York, McGraw-Hill, 2001.

Chapter 11
Nonpharmacological treatment

Ilona Autti-Rämö

Key messages

- Learn the spectrum of normality.
- High-risk groups need structured follow-up.
- Teaching parents to handle and be in contact with their child is the first step.
- Start individually planned interventions when abnormalities persist or increase.
- Establish a quality-control system for the follow-up of at-risk children.

Common errors

- Not involving parents in early intervention.
- Treating a symptom without proper clinical and developmental evaluation.

When to worry

- Regression in development (suspect progressive disease).
- Poor response to visual or/and acoustic stimulation (suspect visual or auditory problems).
- Poor social interaction.
- Abnormalities in posture and/or movement that do not respond to adequate handling.

During the first year of life the infant learns more than in any subsequent year. However, the pace of learning is individual. Individual properties like basal tone, genetic predisposition to normal developmental variants (e.g. age at first independent steps in crawlers versus bottom shufflers; age at first expressed words with meaning), relationships within the family and between the parents and the child and the challenges the child is faced with when learning to take his or her body and the environment under control all have an effect on the developmental trajectories of the individual child. Acute or chronic diseases and physical disabilities, whether hidden or obvious, can lead to developmental trajectories being either delayed or deviant – that is, qualitatively different to the normal trajectory with abnormal postures, movements or social behaviour – or even progressively disordered with stasis then loss of previously acquired developmental skills. Early developmental concerns do not necessarily mean long-term difficulties, but more severe early developmental impairments do tend to mean that there will be long-term disabilities. Identification and early intervention will decrease the longer-term disability.

Protocol for follow-up

In infants born with a risk factor for later developmental difficulties it is not possible to predict the developmental outcome without follow-up. It is important that there is a structured protocol for follow-up and the parents are aware of why and how the child is being followed and what kind of interventions may possibly be instituted. If any abnormality is observed, the parents should first be given advice on how to handle their child in daily life. Often this active contact (tactile, visual and auditory) and daily 'training' shows, within a matter of a few weeks, how the infant can benefit from such handling. If the developmental trajectory doesn't normalize, individual treatment may need to be started. The intensity, content and length of individual treatment are based on the severity and complexity of the developmental disorder. Usually it is best to start with only one therapist (usually the physiotherapist) and other members of the multiprofessional team (e.g. occupational therapist for visual and play activities, speech therapist for oral motor and feeding functions, psychologist for social interaction and psychological support) are consulted. It is important that the bonding between parents and the child is not disturbed but the parents are supported in their growth as parents: they are the best for their child and the use of their capacity should be encouraged and supported.

What to do when development is not normal

When there are obvious abnormalities in development – either failure to reach developmental milestones or abnormality in posture, movement or performance of any specific task – one has to decide on the treatment strategy. A strategy requires goals – specific, measurable, achievable, relevant and timed – in order to be effective and transformed into therapeutic actions. Skilled therapists are important for identifying the optimal ways to challenge the child and realistic goals. The most important part of early intervention, however, is confirmation that the parents have learned what they were encouraged to learn and have changed their daily practice of handling their child accordingly. The infant cannot be helped with individual therapies only.

Delay in early motor development may be due to hypotonia that normalizes with age. Basal tone affects the way the child needs to be treated and handled. *Hypotonia* is often associated with inactivity and poor muscle strength. *Hypertonia* can lead to abnormal motor development in either posture or movement patterns. The more severe the hypertonia, the more difficult it is for the child to move smoothly and to balance. Hypertonia can also co-occur with hypotonia as a compensation (hypertonia in neck extensors and shoulder girdle in hypotonic infants). Hypotonia, inactivity and hypertonia are characteristics that can be overcome with specific handling techniques: they need follow-up and parental coaching but only rarely intensive treatment.

Asymmetry of posture or movement is sometimes a red-flag feature of an evolving hemiplegic (unilateral) type of cerebral palsy and the asymmetric patterns become more evident as the child initiates active movement.

Delay in motor development is often combined with other variations of normal development like dissociated movement in which fine motor development proceeds normally but early gross motor development is delayed. Some motor developmental patterns are idiosyncratic. For example, bottom shuffling is a developmental variation in which the child doesn't crawl but moves in a sitting position by pushing with the feet. Age of independent walking is delayed in both these movement variations but most of these children perform normally by preschool age. Indications for individual therapies need to be decided on a case-by-case basis. Counselling and specific home training guides are often all that is required. These developmental variations are often familial; for example, one of the parents may have had the same pattern of motor development.

Delay in overall development may be due to difficulties in vision, hearing, social skills or cognition. Vision – especially the ability to accommodate – needs always to be checked in case of delayed development and if there is any kind of suspicion of delayed or impaired vision an ophthalmological assessment should be undertaken. The toys used should have strong contrasts in colour (black/white is best) and the figures and shapes must be easy to perceive. Hearing impairment also affects overall development and hearing should be checked with age-appropriate means. A disorder of social development can be due to neuropsychiatric disorders, impaired attachment, maternal depression or cognitive delay. All these etiologies need to be considered to identify the best treatment strategy. Cognitive delay nearly always also causes delay of motor development as this is led by curiosity and the intrinsic need to learn to use one's body and search the environment. Children with delayed cognitive development need much repetition in order to remember causal relationships and learn to use their body in meaningful way.

Clearly abnormal development: several disorders – described elsewhere – can lead to clearly abnormal development (motor and/or cognitive) and the level of functional disability can vary from minor to severe. A definite abnormality in an infant is, however, for the parents always a severe disability and it is important that the parents are supported in their parenthood so that the child is always accepted as he or she is.

Individual therapies, technical equipment and orthosis should be planned according to individual needs by a multiprofessional team.

The role of technical equipment

Many parents believe that the various types of technical equipment currently being marketed to enhance the child's development are good for the infant. This is not necessarily so and it is important to check what kind of technical equipment the parents have bought as they may sometimes intensify abnormal movement patterns. For example, bouncing swings and infant walking aids may enhance toe walking, increasing hypertonia and spasticity. Or a child placed for too long in a sitting position will spend a reduced amount of the time on the tummy (prone), which is necessary for developing active control of extensors. For hypertonic infants a supportive baby seat may, however, be helpful in feeding situations as they help the child to remain in a flexed and symmetrical position. Children with any kind of visual problem see better toys and pictures that have clear contrasts and are not crowded (a simple pattern of black and white is often best).

Novel treatment methods without evidence should not be recommended

Having a child with a definite developmental impairment is always a shock for the parents and they want to do everything in their power to help their child to reach normal development. Some centres provide very intensive, time-consuming and often expensive treatment programmes with strict treatment protocols including manipulation and various alternative treatment methods. There is, however, no evidence so far that such very intensive and complex treatment programmes offer any advantage over standard care. Early intervention with a local multidisciplinary team working in partnership with the family is always important but some intensive, expensive treatment programmes can lead to a stressful life without joy and weaken or otherwise damage the relationship between the child and the main carers with negative consequences in the longer term. In addition, to date there is no evidence that stem cell transplantation or various pharmaceutical injections (e.g. extracts) will cure a child with damage to the central nervous system.

Resources

Anttila H et al. Effectiveness of physical therapy interventions for children with cerebral palsy: a systematic review. *BMC Pediatrics*, 2008, 8:14.

Azari MF et al. Mesenchymal stem cells for treatment of CNS injury. *Current Neuropharmacology*, 2010, 8(4):316–323.

Cioni G, D'Acunto G, Guzzetta A. Perinatal brain damage in children: neuroplasticity, early intervention, and molecular mechanisms of recovery. *Progress in Brain Research*, 2011, 189:139–154.

Drotar D et al. A randomized, controlled evaluation of early intervention: the Born to Learn curriculum. *Child: Care, Health and Development*, 2009, 35(5):643–649.

Guzzetta A et al. Plasticity of the visual system after early brain damage. *Developmental Medicine and Child Neurology*, 2010, 52(10):891–900.

Nordhov SM et al. Early intervention improves cognitive outcomes for preterm infants: randomized controlled trial. *Pediatrics*, 2010, 126(5):e1088–e1094.

Orton J et al. Do early intervention programmes improve cognitive and motor outcomes for preterm infants after discharge? A systematic review. *Developmental Medicine and Child Neurology*, 2009, 51(11):851–859.

Shapiro BK et al. Precursors of reading delay: neurodevelopmental milestones. *Pediatrics*, 1990, 85:416–420.

Shevell M et al. Developmental and functional outcomes in children with global developmental delay or developmental language impairment. *Developmental Medicine and Child Neurology*, 2005, 47(10):678–83.

Spittle AJ et al. Preventive care at home for very preterm infants improves infant and caregiver outcomes at 2 years. *Pediatrics*, 2010, 126(1):e171–e178.

Whittingham K, Wee D, Boyd R. Systematic review of the efficacy of parenting interventions for children with cerebral palsy. *Child: Care, Health and Development*, 2011, 37(4):475–483.

Ziviani J, Feeney R, Rodger S, Watter P. Systematic review of early intervention programmes for children from birth to nine years who have a physical disability. *Australian Occupational Therapy Journal*, 2010, 57(4):210–223.

Chapter 12
Neonatal encephalopathy

Gian Paolo Chiaffoni and Daniele Trevisanuto

Key messages

- It is estimated that each year 814 000 neonatal deaths result from intrapartum related causes; of which, almost all (99%) occur in low–middle-income countries.
- Antenatal care, availability of skilled health professionals and equipment significantly reduce still births and improve perinatal outcome.
- Effective neonatal resuscitation is a cornerstone in the management of the asphyxiated newborn.
- The clinical assessment remains central to all investigations for the first evaluation, day-to-day medical care and follow-up of the newborn infant with acute encephalopathy.
- Prolonged moderate hypothermia reduces mortality and increases survival with normal outcome in asphyxiated neonates.
- Although perinatal asphyxia represents the main reason for neonatal encephalophathy, other causes have to be considered.

Common errors

- Low Apgar scores misunderstood as signs of perinatal brain damage.
- Clinical evaluation not standardized and considered to be difficult.
- Neurophysiological/neuroimaging investigations considered the only means to recognize neonatal brain damage.
- Hyperoxygenation of an asphyxiated term newborn misunderstood as a way to protect the brain.
- Multiple drug treatment believed to be have a role in 'protecting' brain against post-asphyxial damage.

When to worry

- When a term newborn is unable to initiate or sustain autonomous breathing.
- When a term newborn shows decreased alertness, seizures and apneas.
- When a newborn still presents seizures and multiple signs of central nervous system depression after the first week.

Definition

Neonatal encephalopathy (NE) is a clinical – not etiological – term that describes an *altered level of consciousness* of the neonate at the time of the examination. NE is a clinical syndrome characterized by a combination of findings including altered level of consciousness, seizures, abnormalities of muscle tone, movements and reflexes, with or without poor respiratory control and poor feeding. Although NE may be caused by hypoxic ischaemic encephalopathy (HIE), it does not necessarily imply HIE; NE is the preferred term to describe a newborn depressed at birth, as it may be produced by causes different from HIE, mainly metabolic disorders, infections, drug exposure, stroke and malformations. The definition of NE is very frequently confused with other different etiological and/or clinical conditions. For this reason it is very important to understand the exact definition of NE and related terms.

Other frequently used and potentially confusing terms are listed below.

HIE

This term describes encephalopathy as defined above with, in addition, evidence that the mechanism is hypoxic/ischemic in nature. HIE can be defined as mild, moderate or severe according to combination of signs and symptoms

Perinatal hypoxia, anoxia and hypoxaemia

These terms describe partial or total lack of oxygen supply to the brain or blood.

Ischaemia

Reduction (partial) or cessation (total) of blood flow to an organ, such as the brain, which impairs both oxygen and substrate delivery to the tissue.

Perinatal asphyxia

This is an insult to the fetus or newborn due to a lack of respiratory gas exchange, causing hypoxia and hypercapnia, and may be associated with ischaemia. This problem can involve several organs and be of sufficient magnitude and duration to produce functional and/or biochemical changes (e.g. lactic acidosis). Asphyxia leads to increased acidity (decreased pH) in the blood resulting both from the lack of oxygen, referred to as metabolic acidosis, and from hypercapnia (i.e. the build-up of carbon dioxide), referred to as respiratory acidosis. The base deficit is an index of the balance between respiratory and metabolic components of acidosis with a larger metabolic (or smaller respiratory) component leading to a more negative base deficit.

Perinatal asphyxia is defined by the presence of all of the following criteria (according to the American Academy of Pediatrics, 1997):

- umbilical arterial cord pH <7.0 and absolute base excess <−12 mmEq/l
- Apgar score 0–3 at 5 min
- seizures
- signs of multiorgan (renal, cardiovascular, pulmonary, gastrointestinal) dysfunction/failure.

Table 12.1 The timing of hypoxic ischaemic insult and related causes

Timing of the insult	Approximate percentage of total	Possible related causes
Antepartum	20	Maternal hypotension with uterine haemorrhage, abdominal trauma, IUGR, multiples
Intrapartum	35	Malpresentation, forceps extraction, abruptio placentae, cord prolapse, maternal pyrexia
Intrapartum±antepartum	35	Stress during labour and delivery in pre-existing antepartum difficult conditions (maternal diabetes, pre-eclampsia, IUGR)
Postnatal	10	Severe apneic spells, congenital heart disease, iatrogenic reasons

IUGR, intrauterine growth retardation. Modified from Volpe (1995).

The timing of hypoxic ischaemic insult is not easy to establish. Table 12.1 provides approximate percentages occurring at different times relative to birth with likely causes.

Hypoxic ischaemic brain injury
This describes brain injury due to exposure to hypoxia and/or ischaemia, as evidenced by biochemical, electroencephalography (EEG), neuroimaging (magnetic resonance imaging (MRI), computed tomography) or pathological (post-mortem examination) findings.

Neonatal depression
This is a general term that describes the condition of the infant in the immediate postnatal period (approximately the first hour of life) without implying any specific association with prenatal condition or postnatal investigations.

Incidence
Incidence of birth asphyxia is about 1–1.5 cases in every 1000 births, and 0.5 cases in every 1000 births with gestational age ≥36 weeks. Birth asphyxia is the cause of 23% of all neonatal deaths worldwide. It is estimated that each year 814 000 neonatal deaths result from intrapartum-related causes; of these, almost all (99%) occur in low–middle-income countries. Furthermore, the WHO *World Health Report* (WHO, 2005) estimated

that as many as 1 million survivors of birth asphyxia may develop cerebral palsy, intellectual disability, learning difficulties and other disabilities each year.

Clinical neurobehavioural assessment of the newborn

The clinical assessment remains central to all investigations for the first evaluation, day-to-day medical care and follow-up of the newborn infant. The clinical neurobehavioural assessment of the newborn is aimed at

- evaluating gestational age, which may be related to specific clinical conditions;
- identifying signs of neural damage and planning for short- and long-term management; and
- making a tentative and preliminary evaluation of the prognosis.

The core questions to be answered are listed below.

- What has happened? Is the neural damage structural or functional?
- Where is it located in the central/peripheral nervous system?
- When did it happen? Was it pre-, peri- or postnatal?
- Why and how did it happen?

The clinical neurobehavioural assessment has to be considered an ongoing process, which needs to be followed-up over time, to be adapted to the age and clinical status of the newborn and to be compared with reference values. The essential components are history; general assessment; neurobehavioural assessment conducted in a standardized way; evaluation of environment and quality of care; and follow-up.

The *history* has to investigate which specific conditions may be related to NE: health problems within the family (in particular unexplained and/or recurrent infant/child deaths, stillbirths, abortions, genetic and/or neurological diseases, seizures, cerebral palsy, intellectual disability), maternal illnesses, drug treatments or unhealthy behaviours (alcohol, smoking, drug addiction), before and during pregnancy, fetal, perinatal and postnatal problems. When investigating for perinatal and postnatal problems, specific attention has to be paid to the following:

- clinical status of the newborn at birth and Apgar score at 1 and 5 min;
- need for – and response to – resuscitation at birth;
- clinical status of the newborn after birth: alertness, cry, social contact, posture, tone and movements, reaction to stimulation, patterns of breathing, feeding and sleeping, consolability with breastfeeding, skin-to-skin contact and nesting;
- presence of 'unusual' signs, such as purposeless sucking, unusual movements/postures such as boxing, cycling, fisting, unusual behaviours such as frequent yawning and sneezing; and
- how the newborn looks day-by-day: stable, improved or worsened.

When taking history, mother, father and nurses are to be trusted as best sources, as they care for the newborn day and night. Therefore, specific recommendations have to be made to caregivers to record what they observe when caring for the newborn, remembering that any non-recorded observation is a missed one.

The *assessment* of the newborn has to be conducted, if possible, when the newborn is awake, in a quiet, warm place and without interruptions; it is recommended to encourage the mother to attend and to inform and reassure her while performing the assessment. When assessing a newborn for suspected NE or other neural damage, a single evaluation is rarely sufficient and usually needs to be repeated twice daily or even more frequently.

With specific reference to excellent reviews for a detailed description (Volpe, 2008; Amiel-Tison and Gosselin, 2009), the main steps of evaluation are summarized as follows:

- gestational age: this is estimated through history, morphological and neurobehavioural criteria (e.g. the Dubowitz and New Ballard standardized examination scores);
- general condition: aimed at assessing patterns and/or abnormalities of breathing, circulation, thermal control, feeding and nutrition, level of alertness and at recognizing malformations and dysmorphic signs;
- head: size (frontal-occipital head circumference with centiles), shape, fontanelles and sutures, murmurs (heard through stethoscope over anterior fontanelle), traumas, craniosynostosis, rate of growth;
- signs of trauma: if present, specifying whether they are birth-related and/or involving head, trunk, spine, limbs, impaired function or pain;
- alertness and sleep: highly informative with regard to neurological status, they are recognizable from the 28th week, normally variable during the day, best evaluated through integrated assessment of eye-opening, breathing, spontaneous movements and crying pattern;
- visual and auditory communication: visual fixation and tracking, response to sound and consolability, defined by the response of the crying infant to voice or soothing;
- posture and tone–best evaluated from 24 h after birth:
  - the spontaneous posture for a term newborn delivered with a cephalic presentation is of full flexion of all four limbs,
  - passive tone: defined as muscular tonus at rest; that is, minimal contraction of the resting muscle, best evaluated through posture and range of movement with standard manoeuvres (e.g. forward traction, ventral suspension),
  - active tone: observed during spontaneous movements, best evaluated through motor performance,
  - spontaneous movements: assessed as spontaneous and/or in response to stimulation, they are normally smooth, symmetrical and varied; abnormal

movements may be slow and stereotyped, or paroxysmal and purposeless, or chewing and repetitive tongue-thrusting movements;

- reflexes: both deep tendon and primitive reflexes may be present, absent, decreased, increased or asymmetrical. The primitive (or inborn automatic) reflexes are automatic responses that appear during the second half of pregnancy, are present at birth and gradually disappear by 6 months of age. Abnormal findings are reflexes not elicited at birth (CNS depression), or reflexes persisting beyond a specific age limit (CNS damage); the following are used in routine evaluation:
  - ○ Moro reflex,
  - ○ finger grasp and response to traction,
  - ○ automatic walking,
  - ○ crossed extension,
  - ○ sucking,
  - ○ asymmetric tonic neck reflex,
- cranial nerves, evaluated through their specific sensory and/or motor functions including response to light, visual behaviour, eyelid elevation (II, III), extra-ocular movements (III, IV, VI), facial sensibility, biting (V), facial motility, taste (VII), hearing, vestibular responses (VIII), sucking, swallowing, vocalization, taste, gag reflex (IX and X), head and neck movements (XI), movements of the tongue (XII);
- peripheral nerves: look for injuries at the level of brachial plexus (immobile floppy upper limb), phrenic nerve (dyspnea), facial nerve (facial asymmetry), laryngeal nerve (stridor, dyspnea), median nerve, radial nerve (loss of normal hand posture and movement), lumbosacral plexus, sciatic nerve, peroneal nerve; look also for generalized neuropathy: congenital or chronic sensory or sensorimotor neuropathy, acute polyneuropathy;
- autonomic function: respiratory, cardiovascular, bowel and bladder functions; and
- higher cognitive functions: social contact and interaction, behavioural responses to tactile, thermal, painful, visual and auditory stimulation, specifically investigating for latency, habituation, modulated/stereotyped responses.

Abnormal findings leading to suspicion of neonatal CNS damage occur in the following common clinical presentations:

- *CNS depression*, seen in NE, trauma, other encephalopathies, drug intoxications: characterized by decreased alertness, tone, movements and reflexes, poor feeding;
- *hyperalertness/seizures*: seen in mild NE caused by HIE, infection, acute dysmetabolism (hypoglycaemia, hypocalcaemia), drug withdrawal (opioids, cocaine, other psychotropes); seizures are clinically differentiated from tremors by abnormal eye movements, unresponsiveness to passive flexion of limbs, possible associated apnoea, bradycardia and cyanosis, abnormal EEG, if available; be aware that neonatal

seizures may be subtle, that is, only characterized by abnormal gaze, eyelid blinking, sucking and other oral-lingual movements, swimming, boxing, cycling;

- *intracranial hypertension*, seen in acute severe infection, intracranial haemorrhage, intracranial mass: signs may include enlarged head and sutures, full/bulging fontanelles, decreased alertness, forced downgaze (sunsetting), bradycardia, apnea, vomiting, yawning, hypertonia, extensor posturing, opisthotonus;

- *generalized muscular hypotonia*, seen in HIE (early stages), intracranial haemorrhage, infection, kernicterus, drugs: decreased passive and active tone.

- *upper body hypotonia*, involving head/upper limbs: seen in NE from HIE (mild or recovery from): with or without associated to impaired alertness, sucking/swallowing, fix and track; and

- *axial (i.e. muscles of neck and torso) extensor hypertonia*: rare and severe, seen in HIE, massive intracranial haemorrhage, infection, hyperekplexia (stiff baby syndrome; see Chapter 17 and Gastaut & Villeneuve, 1967), associated with an exaggerated startle response and apnea.

Once the diagnosis of NE is suspected, the following clinical considerations may be useful in orienting towards possible timing and etiologies:

- the infant was normal at birth and abnormal thereafter: consider the following perinatal/postnatal causes:
  - intraventricular haemorrhage,
  - HIE,
  - acute/congenital dysmetabolism,
  - infection,
  - degenerative disease,
  - drug withdrawal;
- the neonate was abnormal at birth, then improved/worsened thereafter: consider the following causes:
  - HIE,
  - trauma,
  - intracranial haemorrhage,
  - degenerative/metabolic disease;
- The neonate was abnormal at birth and stable thereafter: consider the following prenatal causes:
  - CNS malformations and developmental disorders,
  - infections (TORCH; TO, toxoplasmosis; R, rubella; C, cytomegalovirus; H, herpes simplex virus. See also Chapter 19.),
  - prenatal hypoxic ischaemic brain damage,
  - degenerative/metabolic disease.

Clinical presentations of HIE with/without multiorgan failure

The Sarnat and Sarnat 1976 classification is the most widely used instrument to identify the prognostic risk of a term neonate with HIE. This classification is based on a clinical and EEG findings and enables patients with HIE to be divided into three prognostic groups within the first 24–48 h after birth (see Table 12.2). The stages in Table 12.2 are a continuum reflecting the spectrum of clinical states of infants over 36 weeks' gestational age.

Perinatal asphyxia may involve several organs other than the brain, to different degrees. Vulnerability, clinical presentation and recoverability are tabulated in Table 12.3.

Diagnosis and differential diagnosis of HIE

When assessing a newborn with suspected HIE, the differential diagnosis has to be considered including the following conditions which can mimic neonatal HIE:

- inborn errors of metabolism e.g. nonketotic hyperglycinaemia, disorders of pyruvate metabolism, urea-cycle defects, Zellweger syndrome and mitochondrial disorders;
- drug exposure, abstinence syndrome, drug withdrawal;
- stroke;
- neuromuscular disorders including neonatal myopathies;
- brain tumours;
- developmental defects;
- infections.

Many new technologies aimed at documenting early CNS damage can support, when available and reliable, the already mentioned central role of clinical assessment in recognizing and evaluating NE.

Laboratory studies in HIE

HIE is a *clinical* diagnosis because the diagnosis is made based on the history, physical and neurological examination with *supporting* biochemical, imaging and/or EEG investigation. Many of the tests are performed to assess the severity of brain injury and to monitor the functional status of systemic organs. Laboratory studies should include those listed below.

- *Arterial blood gas-analysis*: blood gas monitoring is used to assess acid-base status and to avoid hyperoxia and hypoxia as well as hypercapnia and hypocapnia.
- *Serum electrolyte levels:* in severe cases, daily assessment of serum electrolytes are valuable until the infant's status improves. Markedly low serum sodium, potassium and chloride levels in the presence of reduced urine flow and excessive weight gain may indicate acute tubular damage or syndrome of inappropriate antidiuretic hormone (SIADH), particularly during the initial 2–3 days of life.

Table 12.2 Sarnat and Sarnat (1976) classification

	Stage 1 (mild)	Stage 2 (moderate)	Stage 3 (severe)
Level of consciousness	Hyperalert, irritable	Lethargic or obtunded	Stuporous, comatose
Neuromuscular control	Uninhibited, overreactive	Diminished spontaneous movement	Diminished or absent spontaneous movement
Muscle tone	Normal	Mild hypotonia	Flaccid
Posture	Mild distal flexion	Strong distal flexion	Intermittent decerebration
Stretch reflexes	Overactive	Overactive, disinhibited	Decreased or absent
Segmental myoclonus	Present or absent	Present	Absent
Complex reflexes	Normal	Suppressed	Absent
Suck	Weak	Weak or absent	Absent
Moro	Strong, low threshold	Weak, incomplete; high threshold	Absent
Oculovestibular	Normal	Overactive	Weak or absent
Tonic neck	Slight	Strong	Absent
Autonomic function	Generalized sympathetic	Generalized parasympathetic	Both systems depressed
Pupils	Mydriasis	Miosis	Variable, often unequal, poor light reflex
Respirations	Spontaneous	Spontaneous, occasional apnea	Periodic, apnea

Table 12.2 *Continued*

	Stage 1 (mild)	Stage 2 (moderate)	Stage 3 (severe)
Heart rate	Tachycardia	Bradycardia	Variable
Bronchial and salivary secretions	Sparse	Profuse	Variable
Gastrointestinal motility	Normal or decreased	Increased, diarrhoea	Variable
Seizures	None	Common, focal or multifocal	Uncommon (excluding decerebration)
EEG findings	Normal (awake)	Early: low-voltage showing continuous delta and theta Later: periodic pattern (awake); seizures focal or multifocal; 1.0–1.5 Hz spike-and-wave	Early: periodic pattern with isoelectric phases Later: totally isoelectric
Duration	<24 h	2–14 days	Hours to weeks
Outcome	About 100% normal	80% normal; abnormal if symptoms more than 5–7 days	About 50% die; remainder with severe sequelae

Similar changes may be seen during recovery; increased urine flow may indicate ongoing tubular damage and excessive sodium loss relative to water loss.

- *Renal function:* serum urea and creatinine levels and creatinine clearance suffice in most cases.
- *Cardiac and liver enzymes:* these values are an adjunct to assess the degree of hypoxic ischaemic injury to these other organs. These findings may also provide some insight into injuries to other organs, such as the bowel.
- *Haematological and coagulation system evaluation:* increased nucleated red blood cells, neutropenia or neutrophilia and thrombocytopenia have been reported. Coagulopathy includes alteration of prothrombin time, partial thromboplastin time and fibrinogen levels.

Table 12.3 Multi-system organ injuries

Organ/system	Vulnerability	Clinical presentation	Recoverability
Brain	++++	Apnea, hypoxia, encephalopathy, coma, seizures	+
Kidneys	+++	Acute renal failure	+++
Lungs	+++	PPHN, ARDS, pulmonary haemorrhage	++++
Liver	++	Transaminase derangement, coagulopathy	++++
Heart	++	Cardiogenic shock, valvular regurgitation	++++
Blood	++	Thrombocytopenia, DIC	++++
Vascular	++	Capillary leak, sclerema	++++
Gastrointestinal tract	++	Feeding intolerance, necrotizing enterocolitis	++++

ARDS, acute respiratory distress syndrome; DIC, disseminated intravascular couagulation; PPHN, persistent pulmonary hypertension of the newborn. Vulnerability: +, less likely to occur; ++++, most likely to occur. Recoverability: +, likelihood of complete recovery without impairments is very scarce; ++++, likelihood of complete recovery without impairments is very likely.

Neuroimaging and neurophysiological investigations in HIE

We can consider three phases of perinatal asphyxia management: antenatal, delivery room and postnatal management (see Table 12.4. See also Chapters 7 and 8).

Prevention of HIE

Preventing fetal asphyxia through effective obstetric care is greatly preferable to managing an asphyxiated newborn. When asphyxia has occurred, the key to effective resuscitation is to restore adequate blood and oxygen supply to vital organs, particularly the brain. This can be achieved through anticipating neonatal resuscitation by knowing in advance the presence of maternal, uteroplacental and intrapartum risk factors for birth asphyxia, and knowledge and skill among nurses, midwives and doctors in neonatal resuscitation at birth. Once an asphyxiated neonate is born, optimal management has to be systematic (see Table 12.4) and brain-centred.

Table 12.4 The three phases of perinatal asphyxia management: antenatal, delivery room and postnatal management

Problem	Recommendations	
(a) Antenatal phase		
Clinical environment	Clean and warm (26 °C) delivery suite; availability of equipment including radiant warmer (37 °C), suction system (max. pressure 100 mmHg), oxygen (flow rate: 5 l/min), self-inflating bag, facial mask, set for neonatal tracheal intubation, medications (epinephrine [adrenaline], volume expanders, sodium bicarbonate)	
Fetal heart rate and rhythm abnormalities and/or presence of thick meconium. Scarce fetal movements	Consider emergency caesarean section	
(b) Delivery room phase		
Apnea and/or heart rate <100 beats/min; cyanosis, hypotonia	Neonatal resuscitation including positive pressure ventilation, chest compressions, drugs (see Perlman et al., 2010)	
Aspect	**Objective**	**Things to avoid (and why)**
(c) Postnatal management		
Ventilation	To maintain CO_2 in normal ranges (35–45 mmHg)	Hypercapnia (causes cerebral vasodilation) Hypocapnia, CO_2 <25 mmHg (decreases cerebral blood flow)
Oxygenation	To maintain O_2 in normal range (SaO_2, 85–95%)	Hyperoxia (may increase free radical damage and decrease cerebral blood flow)
Temperature	To maintain core temperature in normal range (36.5–37.5° C). Consider moderate therapeutic hypothermia (33–34° C for 72 h)	Hyperthermia (may increase brain damage)

Table 12.4 *Continued*

Aspect	Objective	Things to avoid (and why)
(c) Postnatal management		
Blood circulation	To maintain blood pressure and haemoglobin in normal range (consider blood transfusion) Judicious fluid management (60 ml/kg/day) To consider inotropes (dopamine)	Hypotension and anaemia (may decrease cerebral and body perfusion) Fluid overload (may cause cerebral oedema and generalized oedema due to SIADH)
Metabolic state	To maintain blood glucose levels in normal range (2.2-6.6 mmol/l)	Hypoglycaemia (may potentiate excitotoxic amino acid) Hyperglycaemia (may increase oedema, brain lactate)
	To maintain calcium levels in normal range (1.98-2.65 mmol/l)	Hypocalcaemia (may cause seizures and compromise cardiac contractility) Hypercalcaemia (may cause cardiac arrest)
Neurological problems	To control seizures with anticonvulsants (phenobarbital, phenytoin, lorazepam) and correction of metabolic perturbations (hypoglycaemia, hypocalcaemia, hyponatremia)	
Renal problems	To monitor urine output	Avoid fluid overload
Haematologic problems	Based on coagulation profile (INR >1.5) and platelet count, consider fresh frozen plasma and platelet transfusion, respectively	

Table 12.4 *Continued*

Aspect	Objective	Things to avoid (and why)
(c) Postnatal management		
Gastrointestinal problems	Start feeding with caution	Avoid large amount of feeding during the acute phase (necrotizing enterocolitis)
Liver function	To evaluate transaminases (alanine transferase, aspartate transferase), clotting (prothrombin time, PTT, fibrinogen), glucose, albumin, bilirubin, ammonia To monitor levels of drugs metabolized and/or eliminated through the liver	

INR, International Normalized Ratio; PTT, partial thromboplastin time; SIADH, syndrome of inappropriate antidiuretic hormone. For reference ranges, see Chapter 9.

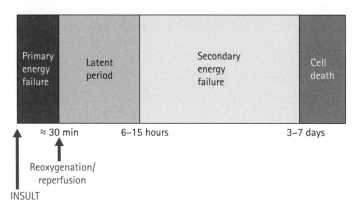

Figure 12.1 Phases of perinatal asphyxia.

Neuroprotective strategy

Perinatal asphyxia occurs in two phases: primary and secondary energy failure (Figure 12.1). During secondary energy failure, there are four main mechanisms determining neuronal cell death. They are: (1) excitotoxic, in which adenosine triphosphate (ATP) and glutamate are abundant in the synaptic spaces; (2) accumulation of intracellular calcium; (3) formation of free radicals; and (4) production of pro-inflammatory cytokines.

Table 12.5 Effects of moderate hypothermia (33–34°C) for 72 h

	Risk ratio (95% CI)	Number needed to treat (95% CI)
Death or severe disability	0.81 (0.71–0.93)	9 (5–25)
Survival with normal outcome	1.53 (1.22–1.93)	8 (5–17)
Mortality	0.78 (0.66–0.93)	14 (8–47)
Severe disability in survivors	0.71 (0.56–0.91)	9 (5–30)
Cerebral palsy in survivors	0.69 (0.54–0.89)	8 (5–24)
Adapted from Edwards et al. (2010).		

Experimental studies show that therapeutic hypothermia can be used as a treatment to limit the damage caused by all these processes. A recent meta-analysis of 10 randomized clinical trials including 1320 neonates (gestational age ≥36 weeks) demonstrated the positive effects of moderate hypothermia (33–34°C) for 72 h on the outcomes listed in Table 12.5. The results of this meta-analysis provide evidence for the benefit of prolonged moderate hypothermia in asphyxiated neonates (Edwards et al., 2010) (see Figure 12.2).

Follow-up and outcome after NE
Once the diagnosis of NE has been made and management has been started, one of the major concerns for both family and caregivers is the expected/suspected short- and long-term outcome, which will influence the child's and family future life and, if not favourable, will challenge the family's ability to cope with the child's problems and society's adequacy to meet the child's special needs. The prognosis of NE is highly unpredictable because of different etiologies, timing of occurrence and diagnosis, management options and environmental factors.

Outcome after neonatal HIE
It is well known that NE caused by cerebral hypoxia/ischaemia due to perinatal asphyxia is an important cause of neonatal mortality and morbidity. The outcome is influenced by the combination of duration and severity of the insult to the brain, gestational age, presence and duration of seizures, associated problems from infection, trauma and metabolic alterations.

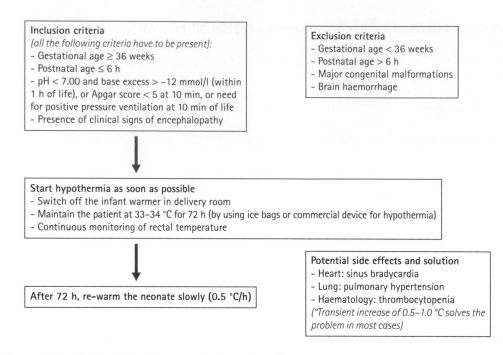

Figure 12.2 Protocol for therapeutic hypothermia.

Several predictors of mortality and neurological morbidity after perinatal hypoxia/ischaemia have been reported (Levene and de Vries, 2011):

- extended period (up to 20 min) of very low (3 or less) Apgar scores,
- prolonged delay in establishing spontaneous respirations after birth,
- severity and duration of intrapartum metabolic acidosis (umbilical artery pH less than 7.00),
- neonatal neurological examination findings,
- brain imaging (ultrasound, MRI) findings,
- EEG or amplitude-integrated EEG findings, and
- visual, brainstem auditory, somatosensory evoked potentials findings.

With specific attention to neonatal neurological examination, follow-up studies (Sarnat and Sarnat, 1976; Finer et al., 1981; Robertson and Finer, 1985; Low et al., 1985; Levene et al., 1986) have shown that mild HIE has virtually no risk of adverse outcome (death or major neurodevelopmental disability); moderate HIE is associated with few deaths and 75% survival without major neurological deficits; and severe HIE had a very poor outcome, with 50–100% mortality rate and severe disability (cerebral palsy, intellectual disability, sensory-neural impairment, epilepsy) in up to 75% of survivors.

Other studies (Thompson et al., 1997, Miller et al., 2004) have correlated outcome to early neurological signs through numerical scoring systems. In summary, the prognosis for children with HIE depends on the severity and duration of the neurological abnormalities, with a significant risk of death after severe HIE and major developmental problems after moderate or severe HIE.

The neurological findings present by the end of the first week of life may provide a preliminary estimate of the likely severity of neonatal brain damage:

- Mild, if the newborn at 7 days presents
  - hyperalertness,
  - abnormal muscular tone,
  - no seizures, and
  - no signs of CNS depression;
- Moderate, if the newborn at 7 days presents
  - abnormal muscular tone,
  - no more than two isolated seizures, and
  - signs of CNS depression;
- Severe, if the newborn at 7 days presents
  - repeated seizures, and
  - multiple important signs of CNS depression.

Clinical predictors of poor outcome are the following:

- isolated persistent abnormal neurological signs,
- combination of neurological signs persistent over time at serial evaluations,
- abnormal neurological signs still present at 40 weeks of corrected age,
- poor head growth leading to head size more than at least two standard deviations below and away from the mean level (microcephaly),
- hypertonus of neck and upper limbs; palmar grasp beyond 3 months of corrected age,
- abnormal findings in tracking motor development
  - poor repertoire of strategies,
  - stereotyped movements and lack of initiative in performance;
- no head control, no social smile at 3 months of corrected age, other milestones not reached by the following age limits:
  - visual fixing and following by 3 months,
  - reaching out for objects by 5 months,
  - sitting unsupported by 10 months,
  - walking unsupported by 18 months,

○ using words with meaning by 18 months, and

○ putting words together by 30 months.

Ellis et al. (1999) reported that there are very few studies in developing countries of outcome in HIE survivors and that only 36% of survivors with any grade of HIE were normal at 1 year. Growing attention is being paid to less severe forms of disability in older children surviving neonatal HIE, such as minor motor impairments, attention-deficit–hyperactivity disorders, significant perceptual-motor or cognitive difficulties and abnormalities in brain MRI (Barnett, 2002; Moster et al., 2002; Marlow et al., 2005).

Regular clinical follow-up over time enables prognosis to be estimated appropriately. This follows from evaluating performance according to postnatal age (corrected, up to 2 years, for gestational age) against the limits of normality for age (see above), recognizing retarded/disrupted developmental trends, considering parental and professional quality of care. Any estimate of long-term prognosis made before 8–12 months of corrected age has a wide margin of error.

References

American Academy of Pediatrics, American College of Obstetrics and Gynecologists. *Guideines for Perinatal Care,* Fourth edition, 1997.

Amiel-Tison C, Gosselin J. Clinical assessment of the infant nervous system. In: Levene MI and Chervenak FA. *Fetal and neonatal neurology and neurosurgery,* 4th ed. Philadelphia, Churchill Livingstone Elsevier, 2009:128–154.

Barnett A et al. Neurological and perceptual-motor outcome at 5–6 years of age in children with neonatal encephalopathy:relationship with neonatal brain MRI. *Neuropediatrics,* 2002, 33(5):242–248.

Edwards AD et al. Neurological outcomes at 18 months of age after moderate hypothermia for perinatal hypoxic ischaemic encephalopathy: synthesis and meta-analysis of trial data. *British Medical Journal,* 2010, 340:1–7.

Ellis M et al. Outcome at 1 year of neonatal encephalopathy in Kathmandu, Nepal. *Developmental Medicine and Child Neurology,* 1999, 41:689.

Finer NN et al. Hypoxic-ischaemic encephalopathy in term neonates:perinatal factors and outcome. *Journal of Pediatrics,* 1981, 98:112.

Gastaut H, Villeneuve A. The startle disease or hyperekplexia: pathological surprise reaction. *Journal of the Neurological Sciences,* 1967, 5:523–542.

Levene MI et al. Comparison of two methods of predicting outcome in perinatal asphyxia. *Lancet,* 1986, 1:67.

Levene MI and de Vries LS. Hypoxic-ischaemic encephalopathy. In: Martin RJ, Fanaroff AA, Walsh MC, eds. *Neonatal-perinatal medicine: diseases of the fetus and infant,* 9th ed. St Louis, Elsevier Mosby, 2011:952–976.

Low JA et al. The relationship between perinatal hypoxia and newborn encephalopathy. *American Journal of Obstetrics and Gynecology,* 1985, 152:256.

Marlow N et al. Neuropsycological and educational problems at school age associated with neonatal encephalopathy. *Archives of Disease in Childhood. Fetal and Neonatal Edition,* 2005, 90:F380.

Miller SP et al. Clinical signs predict 30-month neurodevelopmental outcome after neonatal encephalopathy. *American Journal of Obstetrics and Gynecology,* 2004, 190:93.

Moster D et al. Joint association of APGAR scores and early neonatal symptoms with minor disabilities at school age. *Archives of Disease in Childhood. Fetal and Neonatal Edition,* 2002, 86:F16.

Perlman JM et al. Neonatal resuscitation: 2010 International consensus on cardiopulmonary resuscitation and emergency cardiovascular care science with treatment recommendations. *Pediatrics*, 2010, 126:e1319–e1344.

Robertson C and Finer NN. Term infants with hypoxic-ischaemic encephalopathy: outcome at 3.5 years. *Developmental Medicine and Child Neurology*, 1985, 27:473.

Sarnat HB, Sarnat MS. Neonatal encephalopathy following fetal distress: a clinical and electroencephalographic study. *Archives of Neurology*, 1976, 33:696–705.

Thompson CM et al. The value of a scoring system for hypoxic-ischaemic encephalopathy in predicting neuro-developmental outcome. *Acta Paediatrica*, 1997, 86:757.

Volpe JJ. *Neurology of the newborn*, 3rd ed. Philadelphia, WB Saunders, 1995.

Volpe JJ. *Neurology of the newborn*, 5th ed. Philadelphia, Saunders Elsevier, 2008.

WHO. *The World Health Report 2005: Make every mother and child count*. Geneva, World Health Organization, 2005. www.who.int/whr/2005/whr2005_en.pdf.

Resources

American Academy of Pediatrics and American College of Obstetricians and Gynecologists. *Guidelines for Perinatal Care*. 1997.

Ballard JL et al. New Ballard score, expanded to include extremely premature infants. *Journal of Pediatrics*, 1991, 119(3):417–423.

Carlo WA et al., First Breath Study Group. Newborn-care training and perinatal mortality in developing countries. *New England Journal of Medicine*, 2010, 362:614–623.

Cowan F et al. Origin and timing of brain lesions in term infants with neonatal encephalopathy. *Lancet*, 2003, 361(9359):736–742.

de Vries LS, Toet MC. Amplitude integrated electroencephalography in the full-term newborn. *Clinics in Perinatology*, 2006, 33:619–632.

Murray DM et al. The predictive value of early neurological examination in neonatal ischaemic encephalopathy and neurodevelopmental outcome at 24 months, *Developmental Medicine and Child Neurology*, 2010, 52(2):e55–e59.

Perlman JM et al. Neonatal resuscitation: 2010 International Consensus on Cardiopulmonary Resuscitation and Emergency Cardiovascular Care Science with Treatment Recommendations. *Pediatrics*, 2010, 126:e1319–e1344.

Spitzmiller RE et al. Amplitude-integrated EEG is useful in predicting neurodevelopmental outcome in full-term infants with hypoxic-ischemic encephalopathy: a meta-analysis. *Journal of Child Neurology*, 2007, 22:1069–1078.

Wall SN et al. Reducing intrapartum-related neonatal deaths in low- and middle- income countries – what works? *Seminars in Perinatology*, 2010, 34:395–407.

Chapter 13

Neonatal seizures, including metabolic epileptic encephalopathies

Barbara Plecko

Key messages

- Electroencephalography is mandatory to diagnose neonatal seizures.
- Neonates with recurrent seizures need to be admitted to an intensive care unit.

Common errors

- Subtle seizures are often unrecognized.
- Physiological episodic phenomena may be overdiagnosed as seizures.

When to worry

- Therapy-resistance.
- Affected siblings with neonatal seizures and poor prognosis.

Definitions

The newborn period is defined as the first 4 weeks of life and comprises the time of birth, postpartum adaptation and first weeks of infantile development. The estimated incidence of neonatal clinically recognized seizures is around 2% in term infants, and around 5–13% in newborns with a birth weight below 1500 g. According to the clinical setting one can distinguish three seizure patterns: (1) clinical seizures diagnosed by observation only, (2) electroclinical seizures with documented ictal electroencephalography (EEG) patterns and (3) electrographic-only pattern with an ictal EEG pattern in the absence of any temporally related clinical symptoms or signs.

It is a common problem that neonatal seizures may be very subtle, and that non-convulsive seizures remain largely unrecognized by pure clinical observation. On the other hand there is an overestimate of physiological episodic clinical phenomena as being epileptic in nature. Therefore the clinical diagnosis of neonatal seizures is unreliable and EEG investigations are mandatory in every newborn with unclear, episodic phenomena. If the newborn shows signs of neurological functional impairment in between seizures the diagnosis of epileptic encephalopathy is met. A newborn with recurrent seizures needs to be admitted to a neonatal intensive care unit for continuous monitoring of vital parameters (heart rate, oxygenation, blood pressure).

Clinical approach

Recognition of neonatal seizures can be difficult and needs a high degree of suspicion whenever there are episodic or repetitive patterns observed. Neonatal seizures are usually focal, brief and subtle with motor automatism and eye blinking or eye opening. As the newborn brain is largely unmyelinated and synapses are still immature, generalized seizures are not seen in this young patient group. Involvement of all four extremities at that age rather represents bilateral epileptic discharges with some degree of synchrony. While clonic seizures are easily recognized clinically and electrographically, myoclonic, tonic or subtle seizures, as listed in Table 13.1, may need repeated EEG tracing to prove their epileptogenic nature. In term infants, subtle seizures are by far the most common seizure type (Table 13.1). In preterm infants the prevalence of seizure types differ, with about 50% clonic, 33% tonic, 26% subtle and 10% myoclonic seizures. Autonomic signs (increase or decrease in heart rate, blood pressure, etc.) along with seizures are more frequent in preterm (37%) than in term infants (6%).

The occurrence of combined episodic symptoms is more likely to represent seizure events than isolated symptoms. On the other hand some non-epileptic episodic phenomena may be distinguished from seizures by clinical criteria. Jitteriness is distinguished from clonic seizures by preceding stimuli, interruption by changes in position, suppression by holding the affected limb and lack of abnormal eye movements. Sleep myoclonus is distinguished from seizures by its strict occurrence during rapid eye movement (REM)-sleep phase I, the non-stereotyped clonic jerks mainly in upper limbs, but also legs and face and normal muscle tone in between

Table 13.1 Different seizure patterns according to their typical clinical and ictal electrographic patterns

Semiology	Ictal EEG correlate	Etiology
Clonic (25–30%) (focal, segmentary or bilateral)	+++ Repetitive spikes	Various, frequent in stroke
Myoclonic (15–20%) erratic, fragmentary or more generalized	– to +++	Various, frequent in metabolic disorders
Tonic (5%) (resembling decerebrate rigidity)	– to +++ Rhythmic delta activity	Most often structural brain anomalies
Subtle seizures 50–70% (nystagmus, tonic eye deviation, blinking, limb posturing, pedalling movements, repetitive sucking/chewing, recurrent apnea, vasomotor change)	– to ++ flattening of EEG (more than one EEG tracing may be needed to show epileptic discharges)	Various, frequent in hypoxic ischaemic encephalopathy

Numbers in parentheses are estimates of relative frequencies in term neonates (Pitt and Pressler, 2005). ++, frequent feature; –, absent; +++, prominent feature.

myoclonus. In recurrent isolated apnea, normal EEG tracing during apnea excludes an epileptic nature.

According to the International League Against Epilepsy (ILAE) there are three epilepsy syndromes, that manifest within the first 4 weeks of life.

- Benign familial neonatal convulsions (BFNCs) have their onset between day 2 and 15 of life with very frequent focal tonic and bilateral clonic seizures. Neurological status is normal and seizures remit spontaneously. EEG shows frontal spikes propagating to temporal. Family history is positive and in line with autosomal dominant inheritance. The prognosis is favourable in most cases. BFNCs are caused by mutations in either of two genes (*KCNQ2* or *KCNQ3*), both of which encode voltage-gated potassium-channel subunits.

- Early myoclonic encephalopathy (EME): seizures consist of fragmentary myoclonic jerks. EEG shows a burst-suppression pattern. The etiology is variable and comprises cortical dysgenesis, but also metabolic disorders, for example pyridoxine-dependent epilepsy (PDE) and nonketotic hyperglycinaemia (NKH).

- Early infantile encephalopathy with epilepsy (EIEE) is also named Ohtahara syndrome. Patients have tonic spasms and bilateral seizures, indistinguishable from West syndrome. EEG shows a burst suppression pattern and from age 4–6 months may develop into typical hypsarrhythmia and West syndrome. The causal background is heterogeneous (brain malformations, Aicardi syndrome, dentate-olivary dysplasia) and prognosis is usually poor.

EEG

Video EEG over 40–60 minutes including a sleep phase is standard for investigating seizures in the neonate using the protocol described in Chapter 8 in this volume. Knowledge and experience of normal EEG patterns in term and preterm neonates is necessary, as pathological paroxysmal features are not as readily differentiated in this young age group.

In the neonatal period discharges are frequently focal, with decreasing prevalence from temporal to occipital and to central and frontal. Usually there is abnormal background activity in inter-ictal periods. Term infants produce sharp waves, spikes, sharp and slow waves at onset of seizures, while in preterms rhythmic delta activity is the most common ictal pattern. In both groups ictal patterns may vary in frequency, morphology, duration or propagation during a single event or from one seizure to another. Seizures tend to be longer (about 10 min) in term than in preterm neonates (2–3 min). There is no correlation of EEG patterns, onset of seizures or frequency to the underlying etiology. Status epilepticus is diagnosed in newborns if there is over 50% spike-wave activity in a 30 min EEG tracing, and is more frequent in term infants. Severely abnormal background activity usually indicates poor prognosis, if side effects of drugs are excluded (e.g. phenobarbitone, morphine, surfactant, etc.).

Correlation of EEG and clinical seizures

It is a common problem, that mainly clonic seizures are clinically recognized, while subtle seizures easily escape clinical detection (Murray et al., 2008; Malone et al., 2009). When matching EEG data to clinical video observation only 27% of seizure events were diagnosed correctly. As newborns have spikes and waves as physiological EEG patterns, rhythmic activity over 10 seconds plus clinical symptoms have to be present to diagnose an electroclinical seizure. Therefore an ictal EEG tracing is of utmost importance. Conventional EEG is able to detect about 90% of seizure events correctly as most seizures propagate to the surface in neonates. In certain circumstances conventional EEG may show ictal events without clinical seizures. These so-called electrographic-only events are mostly seen after the administration of antiepileptic drugs (electroclinical uncoupling) or with very high seizure activity, for example status epilepticus.

Amplitude-integrated EEG (aEEG) is increasingly used for long-term monitoring of neonates at risk or under treatment for repeated seizures (see Chapter 8). One-channel aEEG (see Figure 8.4, p. 103) will pick up about 25%, while two-channel aEEG will pick up about 50% of seizures. This gross limitation is due to restriction to the central area and to the fact that low-amplitude spike-wave discharges escape detection by aEEG.

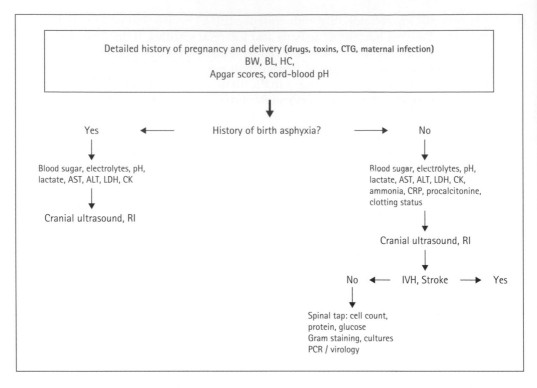

Figure 13.1 First-line investigations in neonatal seizures. ALT, alanine transferase; AST, aspartate transferase; BL, birth length; BW, birthweight; CK, creatine kinase; CRP, C-reactive protein; CTG, cardiotocography; HC, head circumference; IVH, intraventricular haemorrhage; LDH, lactate dehydrogenase; PCR, polymerase chain reaction; RI, resistance index.

Common etiologies of neonatal seizures

Neonatal seizures are rarely idiopathic and therefore need a standardized first- and second-line diagnostic work up (Figures 13.1 and 13.2). The most common causes are (1) birth asphyxia, (2) intracranial haemorrhage (in preterm infants) and (3) central nervous system (CNS) infection. As seizures have the potential to induce apoptosis they represent an independent and often additional threat to the developing brain. When seizures are observed in a newborn, easily treatable causes have to be considered first. Immediate assessment of blood sugar and electrolytes will help to detect hypoglycaemia, hypo- or hypernatremia, hypocalcaemia or hypomagnesaemia as underlying conditions. Most often imbalance of glucose or electrolytes are part of a more complex derangement such as marked preterm birth, infection, anoxia or intracranial haemorrhage and should not be considered as isolated conditions unless proven otherwise. For the following section it is recommended to consider locally accepted normal laboratory values with recognition of term and preterm birth as well as strict dependency on postnatal age in days.

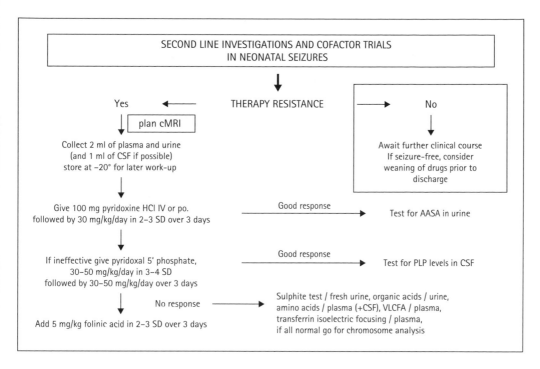

Figure 13.2 Second-line investigations and cofactor trials in neonatal seizures. AASA, alpha-aminoadipic semialdehyde; cMRI, cranial magnetic resonance imaging; CSF, ccrebrospinal fluid; IV, intravenous; PLP, pyridoxal 5'-phosphate; po, per os; SD, single dosages; VLCFA, very-long-chain fatty acids.

Hypoglycaemia is frequently seen in preterm infants and is associated with seizures in about 50% of cases. Correction and maintenance of normal blood glucose levels is mandatory in every newborn. Hyponatremia may occur along with intracranial haemorrhages or CNS infections, most likely due to inappropriate secretion of antidiuretic hormone. Hypernatremia may occur along with excessive administration of sodium bicarbonate, given to buffer acidosis or in the instance of dehydration. Hypocalcaemia can nowadays be largely prevented by adequate calcium and phosphate supply in parenteral or enteral nutrition. While early hypocalcaemia within the first days of life is difficult to treat, later occurrence around day 7 has a favourable response. Hypomagnesaemia can present with focal or multifocal convulsions along with restlessness as an isolated finding in the occasional patient and responds well to intravenous or oral correction.

Around 50–75% of neonatal seizures are caused by birth asphyxia and about 64% of asphyxiated newborns will experience seizures. Asphyxiated neonates usually start having seizures before day 2, when acute cell death and damage by secondary cytotoxins has reached its maximum impact. Seizure semiology is variable and ictal

EEG is necessary to assess the epileptic character of the clinical manifestations and to detect subtle seizures or even status epilepticus. Inter-ictal background activity is a helpful prognostic marker in children who experienced perinatal asphyxia. Seizures in asphyxiated newborns are often accompanied by other signs such as apathy, hypotonia or hypertonia, absence of Moro reflex and bulbar signs, especially difficulty with sucking and swallowing, that may indicate hypoxic-ischaemic encephalopathy (HIE). Caution should be used before ascribing seizures to hypoxia/asphyxia as this may prevent patients from receiving a correct diagnosis of an eventually treatable condition such as meningitis or genetic conditions such as pyridoxine dependent epilepsy (PDE). To relate (or not) seizures to an anoxic event, a careful history of peripartum risk factors has to be taken (dips on cardiotocogram, meconium staining, abruption of placenta, cord prolapse, slow or fixed fetal heart rate, prolonged labour, prolonged low Apgar scores, or low cord-blood pH). Usually asphyxiated newborns suffer from other organ involvement beside the CNS and show transient renal failure or cardiac insufficiency. High plasma lactate is a sign of anaerobic glycolysis, and high lactate dehydrogenase and creatine kinase may reflect tissue damage and, though non-specific, serve as laboratory indicators of birth asphyxia. Cranial imaging may show changes supporting a diagnosis of HIE (see Chapter 7). Cranial ultrasound, as a bedside method, allows serial investigation with minor burden for the patient, while for computed tomography and magnetic resonance imaging (MRI) the burden of transport and sedation has to be weighed against the higher diagnostic yield of these imaging techniques. Doppler sonography may be used to measure cerebral blood flow and vascular resistance with high resistance associated with poor cerebral perfusion.

Around 15–30% of neonatal seizures are due to intracranial haemorrhage or ischaemic infarction, especially in preterm infants. These events usually occur between day 1 and 5 of life. Seizures are usually focal, clonic, unilateral and more stereotyped and rarely lead to status epilepticus. The ictal EEG may show spikes in the Rolandic region and the inter-ictal EEG is asymmetrical with unilateral or focal continuous or discontinuous abnormal patterns. In contrast to asphyxiated newborns, patients with haemorrhage or ischaemic stroke do not show signs of encephalopathy and focal neurological deficits, if they are to appear, usually do not become evident before 3–4 months of corrected age. Nevertheless intraventricular haemorrhage associated with repeated convulsions in a preterm infant indicates a rather poor prognosis. Cranial ultrasound is a suitable method to detect most intracerebral haemorrhages and infarctions, with less sensitivity for events of the posterior fossa or pathology close to cortical areas.

Besides asphyxia and stroke as the two major causes of neonatal seizures, meningitis or encephalitis have to be considered. Intracranial infections account for about 12% of neonatal seizures. CNS infections usually occur during the first week of life, especially after day 2–3. Meningitis may be part of systemic septicaemia (most frequently caused by Group B *Streptococcus* (GBS) and *Escherichia coli*), but may occur as isolated late-onset (i.e. after the first week of life) meningitis (especially Group B *Streptococcus*, *E. coli* and other Gram-negative bacteria such as *Citrobacter* or *Proteus mirabilis*). Other infections in the newborn are caused by parasites such as *Toxoplasma gondii*, and viruses such as rubella, herpes simplex I and II, cytomegalovirus or coxsackie B. In the absence of a suggestive history of birth asphyxia and after having obtained normal imaging on cranial ultrasound, every newborn with unexplained seizures should undergo a lumbar puncture.

Rare etiologies of neonatal seizures

In newborns with repeated seizures but a normal birth history and normal first-line investigations, rare aetiologies have to be considered, especially if seizures are resistant to therapy. In this situation, consider second-line investigations (Figure 13.2) for (1) metabolic disorders, (2) chromosomal/genetic disorders and (3) cerebral dysgenesis. Metabolic disorders are genetically determined inborn errors of metabolism that usually have a biomarker to be measured in urine, plasma or cerebrospinal fluid (CSF). As some metabolic conditions manifesting with neonatal epilepsy are amenable to causal treatment of the underlying cause, they have to be considered in every newborn with therapy-resistant seizures of unknown etiology. The following entities have been selected because of either availability of treatment options or high relative frequency of the disorder.

Pyridoxine dependent epilepsy (PDE)

PDE is one of the more common vitamin-responsive encephalopathies. Patients usually present with refractory seizures soon after birth. In therapy-resistant neonatal seizures or status epilepticus, 100 mg or, if ineffective, up to 500 mg of pyridoxine HCl should be given intravenously during EEG monitoring. Pyridoxine HCl should be continued intravenously or by mouth with 30 mg/kg/day divided into two or three single dosages over three consecutive days. Apnea and comatose state following the initial administration of pyridoxine have been observed in patients with PDE, but not in non-responders. Thus resuscitation equipment should be at hand. PDE patients would also respond to pyridoxal 5'-phosphate (PLP), but this substance is unfortunately unlicensed, except in Japan. In some patients the addition of folinic acid 3–5 mg/kg/day has an additional positive effect. About 30% of PDE patients have a history of complicated delivery, leading the clinician incorrectly to think that their seizures are symptomatic of HIE. Therapy-resistance, sleeplessness and erratic myoclonus, resembling drug-withdrawal, should alert the clinician to test for pyridoxine dependency.

Most pyridoxine-dependent seizures are caused by an autosomal recessive defect of the antiquitin gene. Pipecolic acid and alpha-aminoadipic semialdehyde (AASA) in plasma, urine and CSF serve as reliable diagnostic biomarkers of PDE, even when on pyridoxine. If genetically proven, patients with PDE need lifelong pyridoxine therapy.

Pyridoxal phosphate-dependent epilepsy (PLP)

This autosomal recessive disorder (MIM#610090) has to be differentiated from PDE in that seizures are resistant to pyridoxine and only respond to the administration of PLP. About 25 patients have been reported so far and presented with therapy-resistant neonatal, mainly myoclonic seizures and burst-suppression pattern on EEG. Preterm birth and fetal distress are common. Oral administration of PLP 30–50 mg/kg/day, divided into three or four single dosages, leads to prompt cessation of seizures and can be followed by apnea and comatous state. Thus resuscitation equipment should be at hand. PLP is not licensed outside of Japan and usually only available as a purified, chemical powder. Despite early treatment outcome seems to be poor in most patients. Patients with PLP-dependent epilepsy have a genetic defect of the pyridox(am)ine 5'-phosphate oxidase (*PNPO*) gene, essential for the formation of PLP (the active form of vitamin B_6) in liver. Very low PLP concentrations in CSF are the only reliable biomarker and would need collection and deep-freeze preservation before treatment.

Biotinidase deficiency
This disorder affects the recycling of biotin (vitamin H), an essential cofactor of many carboxylases in glucose, protein and lipid metabolism. As it is easily treatable, biotinidase deficiency is included in the neonatal screening programme of many countries. Seizures have been recognized as the presenting symptom in 38% of 78 patients and are accompanied by other symptoms such as muscular hypotonia or breathing problems. Seizures are mainly myoclonic and therapy-resistant to anticonvulsants in about 50% of cases. Analysis of urinary organic acids by gas chromatography will reveal elevated lactate, 3-OH isovaleric acid, methylcitrate and methylcrononylglycine, but as these metabolic findings vary, measurement of biotinidase in serum is used to establish the diagnosis. Oral treatment with biotin 5–10 mg/day leads to complete resolution of symptoms if started early.

Molybdenum cofactor and sulphite oxidase deficiency
Molybdenum acts as a cofactor of three different enzymes involved in cysteine degradation, and it has been shown to be impaired sulphite oxidation that gives the typical phenotype. Patients present with neonatal tonic-clonic seizures and high risk of status epilepticus. MRI shows toxic brain oedema followed by cystic white matter changes and global brain atrophy. Low urinary uric acid and plasma homocysteine as well as a positive sulphite test in fresh urine serve as diagnostic markers and can be accomplished by determination of elevated xanthine and hypoxanthine in urine. Diagnosis has to be established in fibroblasts by enzyme analysis and two complementation groups have been identified. Patients lacking Molybdenum cofactor (Moco) precursor Z can be treated with purified cyclic pyranopterin monophosphate (cPMP), but this has to be started before irreversible brain damage has occurred.

Non-Ketotic Hyperglycinaemia (NKH)
This is one of the more frequent metabolic epilepsies but is unfortunately untreatable. The autosomal recessive defect leading to NKH is located in one of the four subunits of the glycine-cleavage system. Patients with NKH usually present at birth with severe epileptic encephalopathy, profound hypotonia, chronic hiccups and myoclonic jerks accompanied by prolonged apnea. In the surviving patients, the initial burst suppression pattern evolves into hypsarrhythmia and infantile spasms by around 3 months of age. Elevated plasma and CSF glycine as well as an increased CSF/plasma ratio of more than 0.08 in the classical and more than 0.04 in atypical forms are diagnostic of NKH. Diagnosis needs to be confirmed by enzyme assay in lymphoblasts or by molecular analysis. Protein-restricted diet, administration of sodium benzoate for

alternate glycine elimination and dextromethorphan, an *N*-methyl d̲-aspartate (NMDA) receptor antagonist, have been tried without convincing results in typical NKH cases, but seem to be promising in atypical cases if implemented early.

Beyond these listed entities where neonatal seizures are the hallmark of the disease, seizures can be part of the clinical spectrum in other treatable or untreatable metabolic disorders such as urea-cycle defects, propionic or methylmalonic acidaemia, peroxisomal disorders or congenital disorders of glycosylation (or CDG) syndromes. These disorders have to be considered in the presence of hyperammonaemia or metabolic acidosis. Measurement of ammonia needs rapid processing and cooling to avoid false elevation caused by storage at room temperature.

Chromosomal anomalies with neonatal seizures

Chromosomal lesions leading to epilepsy can be divided into three major subgroups: duplication syndromes where additional genetic material is present, deletions where a segment of genetic material is lost and disruption where only one or few genes are affected. If dysmorphic features are present along with epilepsy, the likelihood of chromosomal anomalies is about 50%. Some of those chromosomal disorders are associated with brain malformation.

Disorders of cerebral dysgenesis

Several disorders of cerebral dysgenesis can manifest with neonatal seizures with a broad spectrum ranging from focal cortical dysplasia to more generalized syndromes such as lissencephaly or double cortex. MRI is superior to computed tomography in detecting areas of cortical dysplasia and should be the investigation of choice in this selection of patients. As subcortical U-fibres are largely unmyelinated until the end of the second year of life, detectability of cortical dysplasia may change with age and MRI may need to be repeated at that age if no other explanation has been identified. Complex brain malformation is often caused by chromosomal or monogenetic defects and parents need genetic counselling for further family planning. Table 13.2 lists some chromosomal abnormalities associated with brain malformation.

Treatment of neonatal seizures

Every newborn, if mature or preterm, that suffers from recurrent seizures should be admitted to a neonatal intensive care unit for monitoring of vital signs. The drug most commonly used in the treatment of neonatal seizures is phenobarbitone, although studies on its effect have been disappointing and animal studies have shown apoptosis in the presence of high concentrations. In many countries it remains a first-line drug and a loading dose of 40 mg/kg will lead to cessation of seizures in about 50% of patients with neonatal seizures. Maintenance dosage should keep phenobarbitone plasma levels at around 25 mg/ml. Electroclinical uncoupling is frequent and aEEG or daily EEG studies should be performed to detect electrographic-only events. There is no guideline supporting the use of phenobarbitone for the prevention of seizures in at risk

Table 13.2 Chromosomal anomalies associated with cortical malformations

Condition	Chromosomal anomaly
Lissencephaly	Miller–Dieker syndrome (del17p13.3)
Polymicrogyria	1p36 deletion
	Monosomy 1q44
	Duplication 11q12–11q13
	Monosomy 3p
	Trisomy 5p
	Partial monosomy 18p
	Partial monosomy 21q
	22q deletion
	Duplication 3q
Double cortex	Trisomy 9p
Heterotopia	Deletion 4q
	Ring 17
	Trisomy 13
	Trisomy 19
	69XXX

neonates. Intravenous phenytoin will stop neonatal seizures in around 45% of patients. The usual loading dose is 15–20 mg/kg with a maximum rate of administration of 1 mg/kg/min and ECG monitoring to test for cardiac arrhythmia. Owing to its non-linear pharmacokinetics and variable protein binding in sick neonates, phenytoin is more difficult to handle, requiring monitoring of blood concentrations, and its impact on cerebellar growth is a potential serious side effect. Unlike phenobarbitone, enteral absorption of phenytoin is erratic in infants aged less than 6 months after term.

Although irritant to veins, it needs to be used intravenously at this age. A Cochrane review in 2004 showed poor effect with a combination therapy of phenobarbitone plus phenytoin.

This unsatisfactory situation has lead to the use of benzodiazepines, especially clonazepam or midazolam, as a second-line drug in many European countries. Clonazepam at a dosage of 0.1 mg/kg (i.e. 100 micrograms/kg) has been effective in *newborn* patients unresponsive to phenobarbitone. One dose per 24 hours is recommended. Midazolam with an initial bolus of 0.15 mg/kg followed by dosages up to 0.1 mg/kg/h by continuous infusion has been highly effective in a non-randomized study. Continuous administration of benzodiazepines can lead to apathy, poor feeding and apnea and may aggravate sleep myoclonus.

In the presence of neonatal seizures resistant to therapy with two conventional drugs, it is strongly recommended to have a standardized procedure for a therapeutic trial of therapy with vitamins: pyridoxine and/or pyridoxal 5'-phosphate and folinic acid. To prevent irreversible brain damage in children with potentially treatable disorders, such as PDE, this trial has to be performed early in the course of disease (Figure 13.2).

There are recent reports on the successful off-label use of newer antiepileptic drugs, such as levetiracetam (10 mg/kg on day 1, 20 mg/kg on day 2 and 30 mg/kg on day 3) or topiramate (1 mg/kg with stepwise increase to 4 mg/kg/day) in newborns with refractory seizures, but no formal studies have been performed. Valproate is associated with hepatotoxicity with that association being stronger in infants. Undiagnosed metabolic disease contributes to this risk, and valproate is therefore not recommended for the treatment of neonatal seizures.

About 48% of preterm but only 30% of term infants with neonatal seizures will develop epilepsy in later life. No antiepileptic therapy has as yet proven to be effective in the prevention of later-onset epilepsy. Thus newer concepts discuss weaning of the anticonvulsant therapy before discharge in patients who are seizure-free and have a normal EEG record.

References

Malone A et al. Interobserver agreement in neonatal seizure identification. *Epilepsia*, 2009, 50(9):2097–2101.

Murray DM et al. Defining the gap between electrographic seizure burden, clinical expression and staff recognition of neonatal seizures. *Archives of Disease in Childhood. Fetal and Neonatal Edition*, 2008, 93(3):F187–F191.

Pitt M, Pressler R. Neurophysiological testing in the newborn infant. *Early Human Development*, 2005, 81:939–946.

Resources

Bassan H et al. Neonatal seizures: dilemmas in workup and management. *Pediatric Neurology*, 2008, 38(6):415–421.

Plecko B, Stöckler S. Vitamin B$_6$ dependent seizures. *Canadian Journal of Neurological Sciences*, 2009, 36 Suppl 2:S73–S77.

Roberton NRC, Rennie JM. *Textbook of neonatology*, 3rd ed. Edinburgh, Churchill Livingston, 1999.

Stöckler-Ipsiroglu S, Plecko B. Metabolic epilepsies: approaches to a
diagnostic challenge. *Canadian Journal of Neurological Sciences*, 2009, 36 Suppl 2:S67–S72.

Vento M et al. Approach to seizures in the neonatal period: a European perspective. *Acta Paediatrica*, 2010, 99(4):497–501.

Volpe JJ. *Neurology of the newborn*, 5th edition. Philadelphia, Saunders Elsevier, 2008.

Wheless J, Willimore J, Brumback RA, eds. *Advanced therapy in epilepsy*. New York, McGraw Hill, 2009.

Chapter 14

Acute non-febrile encephalopathy

Tiina Talvik, Fenella Kirkham, Tuuli Metsvaht and Inga Talvik

Key messages

Acute encephalopathy

- Altered level of consciousness is the clinical hallmark of acute encephalopathy.
- In infants, look for disturbed behaviour, poor feeding, irritability and high-pitched cry.
- Recognise extraocular palsies, facial weakness, hemiparesis and seizures.
- Recognize decorticate or decerebrate (extensor) posturing, loss of pupillary reflexes.
- Always measure true blood glucose and ammonia in acute encephalopathy.
- Provide supportive intensive care, whatever the cause.
- Consult a specialist in suspected inherited errors of metabolism.

Stroke

- Seizures, as well as hemiparesis, are a common presentation of stroke.
- Neuroimaging, including the venous sinuses, should be performed as early as possible.
- Intracerebral haemorrhage may require urgent neurosurgery.
- In children without prior cardiac disease, echocardiography is rarely abnormal.
- Electroencephalography may help distinguish stroke from epilepsy and migraine.
- Consider aspirin (5 mg/kg acutely, 1–3 mg/kg longer term) if stroke recurrence risk is high.
- Consider anticoagulation for cerebral venous sinus thrombosis or extracranial dissection.
- Surgical decompression for unconscious children with brain swelling following stroke may occasionally be life-saving in neurosurgical units with appropriate experience.

Traumatic and inflicted traumatic brain injury
- Distinguish inflicted head injury from accidental traumatic head injury.
- Multidisciplinary management of inflicted injury is required.

Common errors
- Missing meningitis/meningo-encephalitis, the most common diagnosis in paediatric emergency malpractice claims: always be alert to the possibility.
- Withholding antimicrobial treatment if infection is a possibility: if in doubt, treat.
- Performing lumbar puncture on a child with Glasgow Coma Scale score of less than 9 without neuroimaging.

Stroke
- Delay in recognizing that a child has had a stroke.
- Misdiagnosing Todd's paresis after focal seizure as stroke or vice-versa.
- Delay in recognizing depressed consciousness level and risk of raised intracranial pressure.
- Difficulty in distinguishing between hemiplegic migraine and stroke.
- Mistaking parieto-occipital infarction due to venous sinus thrombosis as arterial stroke.
- Reducing instead of supporting blood pressure when cerebral perfusion pressure is low.

Traumatic and inflicted traumatic brain injury
- Misinterpreting history given by caretakers.
- Failing to diagnose fractures caused by previous abuse.
- Failing to identify retinal haemorrhages.

When to worry
- Lethargy, coma, progressive decrease in level of consciousness.
- Hypotension; bradycardia with hypertension.
- Persistent seizures or status epilepticus, not controlled with medication.
- Persistent vomiting; recurrent apnoeas, forced downgaze (sunsetting).
- Emergence of focal neurological symptoms or extensor posturing.

Stroke
- Acute hemiplegia.
- Acute focal or generalized seizures.
- Lethargy, coma, vomiting.
- Focal neurological signs.

> *Traumatic and inflicted traumatic brain injury*
> – Any progressive decrease in level of consciousness.
> – Decreased consciousness level in a previously alert child after trauma.
> – Emerging restlessness in an infant with depressed level of consciousness.
> – Acute acquired encephalopathy/injury without reasonable explanation.
> – Inconsistent history from caregivers following trauma.

Definition

Acute encephalopathy refers to a state of rapid deterioration of brain function, usually presenting as an alteration in state of consciousness which may or may not be accompanied by focal neurological signs.

Causes

There are many possible causes of acute encephalopathy. In this chapter, traumatic, metabolic, toxic and cerebrovascular causes are considered. Infection and post-infective causes are considered in Chapter 15 but non-infectious causes that may mimic infection are considered in this chapter. It is important to note, however, that cases of acute infective encephalopathy with rapid deterioration, and even death, may occur without fever (e.g. recent reports of this due to shigellosis and salmonellosis with only mild diarrhoea). Other possible causes not considered in further detail include neoplastic and systemic conditions.

The initial differential diagnosis of acute encephalopathy may be based on the presence or absence of fever and neuroimaging findings (see Figure 14.1). However, remember that in infancy sepsis may present with temperature instability rather than fever.

General principles of management

The key to rational assessment of the clinical state of the infant is systematic and repeated recording of level of consciousness, pupillary responses, pulse and respiratory rate and blood pressure. The assessment of consciousness is based on observable behavioural responses to stimulation: eye opening, verbal response, motor response that in combination make up the Glasgow Coma Scale (GCS). In infants the scoring is modified to be age-appropriate (Table 14.1). A total score is obtained by summing the scores on the eye opening, verbal and motor subscales but stating the three clinical observations that constitute the subscale scores is more informative than the total score.

Clinical assessment of a child with acute encephalopathy

History of the present illness and previous medical and family history, medication and access to medication in the household that may have been accidentally ingested, and

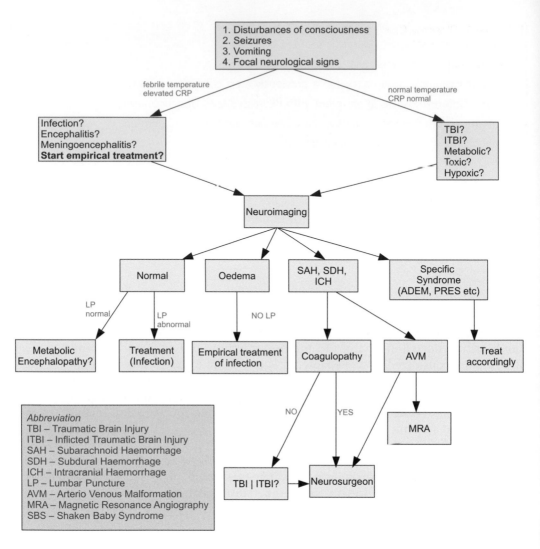

Figure 14.1 Algorithm in acute infantile encephalopathy. PRES, posterior reversible leukoencephalopathy syndrome

history of illness in contacts are all potentially relevant. In the youngest children the symptoms and signs may be subtle, like poor feeding or poor social cognition, and easily missed by caregivers.

On examination, assess level of consciousness using the GCS. Assess airway, breathing and circulation. Measure the blood pressure. In addition, look for a rash (purpuric in meningococcal infection or bleeding disorders, variable in viral infection), signs of inflicted injury or neglect; cardiac murmurs; signs of lower respiratory tract infection

Table 14.1 Glasgow Coma Scale modified for infants

Eye opening	Spontaneous	4
	To verbal stimuli	3
	To pain only	2
	No response	1
Verbal response	Coos and babbles	5
	Irritable cries	4
	Cries to pain	3
	Moans to pain	2
	No response	1
Motor response	Moves spontaneously and purposefully	6
	Withdraws to touch	5
	Withdraws in response to pain	4
	Decorticate posturing in response to pain	3
	Decerebrate posturing in response to pain	2
	No response	1

(tuberculosis, mycoplasma, pneumococcus); hepatosplenomegaly; any other diagnostic clue on general examination. Measure the occipitofrontal head circumference (or OFC) with a disposable paper measuring tape and plot on the centile chart appropriate for age and sex: macro- or microcephaly are potentially relevant. Note any separation of the cranial sutures which may signify intracranial hypertension. Fullness and firmness of the anterior fontanelle, if possible with the infant supported in a sitting position, can be a useful additional sign.

Raised intracranial pressure (ICP) may accompany both traumatic and non-traumatic acute encephalopathies. It impairs cerebral perfusion pressure (CPP), which is arterial blood pressure minus ICP. Low CPP leads to cerebral ischaemia and has consistently been shown to be an important determinant of outcome following central nervous system (CNS) traumatic brain injury (TBI) and non-traumatic brain injury in children. Cerebral ischaemia itself causes cerebral oedema which compounds the rise in ICP from other causes (e.g. trauma, metabolic derangement). Progressive uncontrolled increase in ICP ultimately causes death by brainstem compression.

Persistent unexplained vomiting, loss of upgaze or forced downgaze (sunsetting) may indicate increasing pressure on the tegmentum, caused, for example, by hydrocephalus. If the infant is awake but sleepy, try to assess eye movements. Depressed level of consciousness may be associated with focal neurological signs or with abnormal posturing to noxious stimulation. This may be decorticate (flexion of the upper limbs and extension of the lower limbs) or decerebrate with extension of all four limbs. The emergence of such signs and/or abnormal respiratory patterns may indicate life-threatening deterioration.

Laboratory and radiological assessment of a child with acute encephalopathy
Remember the value of simple laboratory tests: white cell count (and increase in immature cells or 'shift to the left'); may be seen in infection or prolonged seizure; acute-phase proteins such as C-reactive protein; cell count in the cerebrospinal fluid (CSF); CSF protein; paired plasma and CSF glucose (you cannot interpret one without the other); lumbar CSF pressure measured with a manometer or, more easily in an infant, with a tape measure held next to a vertically orientated sterile thin-bore flexible plastic tube (e.g. IV giving set), attached via a three way tap to the lumbar puncture needle.

Test for non-infective causes of meningitis/meningo-encephalitis should include consideration of antibody-mediated illness and haemophagocytic lymphohistiocytosis (HLH). In practice, investigation for a possible infective cause (see Chapter 15) may also be required.

Ultrasound is good for defining the size of the cerebral ventricles but less informative in describing extra cerebral and subdural spaces or abnormalities of the cerebral parenchyma. Therefore computed tomography (CT) or magnetic resonance imaging (MRI; the method of choice) is needed to confirm ultrasound findings.

Clinical management of a child with acute encephalopathy
The GCS score (Table 14.1) and vital signs should be systematically monitored over time. If seizures are a feature, does the infant return to his or her usual self between seizures? Identify seizure type, duration, any localizing features, and conscious level and responsiveness between seizures. If GCS is less than 8 or there is declining level of consciousness, admit to the intensive care unit and manage airway. Restore normal circulating blood volume and manage seizures and CPP.

A child with encephalopathy needs empirical treatment at presentation often several days before a definitive diagnosis is available. When an infective cause is suspected an

Table 14.2 Anticonvulsants used for seizures with acute encephalopathy

Drug	Route of administration	Paediatric dose
Drugs used as first line treatment of status epilepticus		
Diazepam	IV bolus Rectal	0.25–0.5 mg/kg 0.5–0.75 mg/kg*
Lorazepam	IV bolus	0.1 mg/kg
Midazolam	Buccal, nasal	0.15–0.3 mg/kg*
Drugs in established status epilepticus or acute encephalopathy with seizures		
Phenytoin	IV bolus/infusion	20 mg/kg at 25 mg/min
Phenobarbital	IV bolus	15–20 mg/kg
Valproate (beware in suspected metabolic encephalopathy)	IV bolus	20–40 mg/kg
*May be repeated. IV, intravenous.		

antimicrobial, such as a cephalosporin, and aciclovir as an antiviral should be commenced. Better outcome is associated with the starting of appropriate therapy before the conscious level deteriorates (see Chapter 15).

Status epilepticus is less likely to be refractory to medical therapy if treated early with appropriate medication (Table 14.2). If status epilepticus continues in spite of use of the drugs in Table 14.2, continuous intravenous infusion of diazepam, midazolam (in high care) or of thiopentone (in intensive care) may be required.

Management of intracranial hypertension
Consideration of surgical placement of an ICP monitor is desirable but not possible in some clinical settings. Management aims to optimize CPP and reduce ICP. Methods include positioning (head straight, trunk and head at 30° to horizontal); temperature regulation to avoid fever (and, in post-hypoxic brain injury, mild hypothermia to 33–34 °C; see also discussion of hypothermia in Chapter 12); sedation; external ventricular drainage of CSF; operative decompression; osmotherapy with hypertonic saline or, for acute short-term management of an emergency, mannitol.

Hyperventilation is no longer recommended as the resulting vasoconstriction can exercerbate cerebral ischaemia. Early consultation with neurosurgical colleagues is important for early discussion of ICP monitoring and/or surgical removal of space occupying causes of ICP (e.g. extradural haematoma).

Boluses of glycerol or mannitol achieve transient reduction in ICP; however, there is a risk of a significant rebound with subsequent rise in ICP. The role of this treatment is therefore confined to acute severe deterioration due to raised ICP to buy time to institute other measures to reduce ICP. Hypertonic saline has achieved greater reduction in ICP and, in non-traumatic acute encephalopathy, is associated with a lower mortality when compared to mannitol or normal saline. The benefit is sustained for longer when given as a continuous infusion.

Specific non-infectious acute encephalopathies that may mimic infection
Infection and post-infective causes are considered in Chapter 15.

Haemophagocytic lymphohistiocytosis (HLH) may cause meningoencephalitis and significant neurological sequelae. The term HLH encompasses the recessively inherited primary form, familial haemophagocytic lymphohistiocytosis (or FHL)-mostly affecting young children, and secondary HLH – predominantly associated with infections or malignancies. Common features are fever, pancytopenia, hypertriglyceridaemia, hypofibrinogenaemia and hepatosplenomegaly. The majority have a pronounced inflammatory response with hypercytokinaemia and hyperferritinaemia, in association with deficient lymphocyte cytotoxic activity. Importantly, they also develop a meningoencephalitis that may be severe. About 66% will have neurological symptoms – with seizures, meningismus and irritability being the three most common – and/or abnormal CSF findings at the time of diagnosis. CT and MRI findings of HLH are ring-enhancing parenchymal lesions (at times calcified) which are nonspecific and mimic abscess. In the immunosuppressed child increased diffusion at the centre on diffusion-weighted imaging may help differentiate these lesions from an abscess, which has restricted diffusion at their centre. Prompt treatment (etoposide and marrow transplantation) of active HLH at onset or relapse may reduce neurological sequelae and this is therefore important to consider in undiagnosed encephalopathy.

In long-term survivors, neurological sequelae – usually neurodevelopmental impairment and epilepsy – are reported in approximately 15% of cases. Late sequelae affect approximately 25% of those with an abnormal CSF at onset and are about three times as common as in those with normal CSF. Approximately 75% of children aged less than 12 months at time of diagnosis have abnormal CSF without any neurological symptoms.

Aicardi–Goutieres syndrome is a rare genetically determined disorder with a phenotype classically characterized by episodic acute irritability with or without fever. It is associated with elevated levels of interferon in the CSF and often with increased CSF white cell count. Chilblains and other skin manifestations may be seen (see also pp 208 and 265).

Acute necrotizing encephalopathy (ANE) is predominantly a disease of infants and young children. It is characterized by fever, acute encephalopathy, seizures and rapid progression to coma within days of onset of a viral illness; more frequently influenza A, but also influenza B, parainfluenza, human herpesvirus 6 and others. Brain T2-weighted MRI classically shows multiple symmetrical lesions affecting primarily the thalami but also the upper brainstem tegmentum, periventricular white matter, putamina and cerebellum. A genetic form of the disease, ANE1, is recognized with mutations in the gene *RANBP2* (OMIM 601181).

Acute disseminated encephalomyelitis (ADEM) is monophasic inflammatory multifocal demyelinating disorder of the CNS usually appearing after an infection and by definition including a degree of encephalopathy (i.e. depression of consciousness level). It is a rare disorder and very unlikely to present in the first year of life. There may also be focal neurological signs. MRI typically shows multifocal large areas of demyelination in white matter but grey matter involvement (e.g. lesions in thalamus and basal ganglia) also occurs. Diagnosis is based on the combination of clinical and radiological features and exclusion of diseases that mimic ADEM. Treatment is with intravenous methylprednisolone 30 mg/kg, up to a maximum dose of 1 g/day, for 3–5 days (level of evidence, class III). Higher doses have been used in severe forms of steroid-resistant post-infectious encephalomyelitis. This is usually followed by oral steroid (prednisone 1 mg/kg per day) tapered over 4–6 weeks, but might be unnecessary if symptoms improve. Monitor for hyperglycemia, hypokalemia, high blood pressure and mood disorders. Outcome is usually favourable, with good functional recovery and mortality rates less than 5%.

Posterior reversible leukoencephalopathy syndrome (PRES) is a condition also recognized on the basis of encephalopathy associated with high signal change on MRI in parieto-occipital areas. Risk factors include hypertension, hypotension, treatment with tacrolimus, cyclosporin, cyclophosphamide, methotrexate and some of the newer immunosuppressive agents. It is very rare in the first year of life.

Vaccinations and acute encephalopathy
Recent reviews of cases of long-term neurological impairment with onset of acute epileptic encephalopathy immediately following diphtheria-tetanus-pertussis (DTP) vaccination have found that the majority of these had a *SCN1A* gene deletion. They were, in fact, cases of Dravet syndrome (see Chapter 16) and their neurological outcome was no different from those with the same gene deletion and onset of seizures unrelated to vaccination. There are isolated reports of aseptic meningitis, without any known long-term sequelae, following measles, mumps and rubella (MMR) vaccination. The risk is less than 1 in 534 000 vaccinees. Research in the 1990s suggesting a link between vaccination and autism has now been discredited and the publications retracted. The resulting debate on this issue led to large amounts of high-quality epidemiological research that has provided reassurance that there is no such link. There is no evidence of increased risk of encephalopathy after DTP/*Haemophilus influenzae* B (Hib) or MenC vaccines 15–35 days after MMR vaccine.

TBI and inflicted TBI

Definitions

TBI results from external forces being absorbed by cranial and intracranial structures. It may be closed or penetrating. It is a major cause of death and disability worldwide, especially in infancy and childhood. TBI is characterized by extra- or subdural haemorrhages, often accompanied by cerebral contusion.

TBI including inflicted TBI

Causes in infancy include falls, or being a passenger in a road traffic accident, but the focus should always be on safe-guarding and whether the infant before you is the victim of deliberate inflicted TBI (ITBI). ITBI may be caused by direct impact or shaking often accompanied by areas of hypoxia ischaemia. Pathological data indicate that ITBI is probably a better term than the previously used shaken-baby syndrome (or SBS) as no one mechanism is implied. The level of violence used is recognized by others as excessive, dangerous and likely to harm the child.

Caregivers at risk for abusive behaviour generally have unrealistic expectations for their children and may exhibit a role reversal whereby caregivers expect their needs to be met by the child. Professionals should be aware that a crying infant is at higher risk of ITBI, especially when parents are complaining of excessive crying and are in a social position that could put pressure on the family situation. The actual duration of crying at a given moment seems to be less relevant than the parents' perception of the crying over the long term.

Epidemiology of TBI

The incidence of TBI in childhood is high and higher if measured prospectively rather than retrospectively (Table 14.3).

Clinical approach

Take a careful and exact history. Look for consistency in accounts given by the different people involved. Does their version of events stay constant? Assess the injury: open, closed or penetrating? Focal or diffuse? Associated soft-tissue trauma; damage to internal organs? Focal neurological signs? Are subtle seizures contributing to apparent depression of consciousness? ITBI is often seen in association with bruising, a torn frenulum, retinal haemorrhages and fractures of long bones or ribs.

Investigation of TBI
- Blood clotting screen
- Imaging:
  - CT to verify the possibility of intracranial haemorrhage (see Table 14.4),
  - MRI,
  - cranial ultrasound in young infants (screening),
  - ophthalmoscopy (retinal haemorrhage in ITBI,

Table 14.3 Incidence of traumatic brain injury by region

Location	What is measured	Rate	
South West England and Wales	SDH under 1 year of age	21 per 100 000	Jayawant et al. (1998)
Scotland	SDH under 1 year of age (retrospective)	11.2 per 100 000	Barlow et al. (1998)
Scotland	SDH under 1 year of age (prospective)	24.6 per 100 000	Barlow et al. (2000)
North Carolina, USA	Hospital surveillance (prospective)	29.7 per 100 000	Keenan et al. (2003)
Canada	Hospital surveillance (retrospective)	40 cases/year	King et al. (2003)
Germany	Estimation	100–200 per year	Matchke et al. (2009)
Switzerland	Nationwide	14 per 100 000 live births	Fanconi et al. (2010)
New Zealand		14.7–19.6 per 100 000	Kelly et al. (2008)
Estonia	Retrospective	13.5 per 100 000	Talvik et al. (2006)
Estonia	Prospective	40.5 per 100 000	Talvik et al. (2006)

SDH, subdural haemorrhage.

○ skeletal survey in traffic trauma or suspected ITBI including repeat chest X-ray at 7 days for, initially radiologically inapparent, rib factures; in 30–40% of children with inflicted injuries, signs of previous inflicted injury are present: old fractures, chronic subdural haemorrhage,

○ ultrasound and/or CT of abdomen.

Management
Assess level of consciousness with GCS score (Table 14.1). If GCS is less than 8 or there is declining consciousness, admit to the intensive care unit and manage airway. Restore

Table 14.4 Causes of subdural haemorrhage in infancy

Cause	Clinical or imaging feature	Possible other features	Comment/ management
Inflicted	SDH	External signs of abuse, inconsistent history, discrepancy between history and injury severity	Abdominal trauma, skeletal survey CT, MRI, surgery if necessary
Trauma	SDH	External signs of trauma	CT, surgery if necessary
Haemorrhage	SDH, ICH	Signs of haemorrhaging outside the CNS (e.g. nosebleed) and/or bruising, CNS parenchymal haemorrhage; bruises	Coagulation profile
Stroke including AVM	SDH, ICH	Focal neurological signs	MRI, MRA
Infection	SDH	Fever; differentiate focal infection from meningitis (see Chapter 15)	Enhancement with contrast, lumbar puncture if not contraindicated
Metabolic disorder	SDH	Previous developmental impairment or arrest	MRI, metabolic screening

AVM, arteriovenous malformation; ICH, intracranial haemorrhage; MRA, magnetic resonance angiography; SDH, subdural haemorrhage.

normal circulating blood volume and manage seizures and CPP. In possible ITBI, involve the inter-disciplinary safe-guarding team, typically including hospital doctor and nurse, a family doctor that knows the family, social worker and specialist police officer.

Outcome of TBI and inflicted brain injury
The majority of children with ITBI have poor outcomes. About 20% die and only 20% survive without impairment. The remainder have impairments in their motor and cognitive abilities, language, vision and behaviour. These impairments affect future

educational and social attainment. The reasons for the poor outcomes in infants and children who sustain ITBI are not known but are probably attributable to associated ischaemia and hypoxia.

Acute metabolic encephalopathies

The clinical presentation in children with a metabolic encephalopathy is non-specific. In newborn infants it usually occurs after a symptom-free period following delivery. Poor feeding, vomiting, central hypotonia with limb hypertonia, abnormal movements followed by seizures and coma may occur (see Chapter 12). In older infants, it may be associated with periods of metabolic stress (e.g. fasting, intercurrent infection). Inborn errors of metabolism should always be considered in children – and especially infants – with unexplained changes in their consciousness, alongside CNS infections (bacterial or viral), haemorrhage, hypoxia and/or ischaemia or poisoning.

Management

Supportive management is as for any child with an encephalopathy. Specific therapy depends upon the underlying disorder and the biochemical abnormalities. The three main biochemical disturbances associated with an encephalopathy due to inherited errors of metabolism are hypoglycaemia, hyperammonaemia and metabolic acidosis. Therefore the important investigations are ammonia, glucose, pH, serum lactate and organic acids.

The most common causes of severe hyperammonaemic encephalopathy in children are enzyme deficiencies of the urea cycle (see Figure 14.2), which functions to convert ammonia (highly toxic) arising from the catabolism of amino acids to urea (non-toxic). Hyperammonaemia may also occur in children with organic acidaemias and less commonly in fat oxidation disorders The outcome for children with hyperammonaemic encephalopathy is generally poor. However, permanent CNS damage can be limited by a rapid reduction in blood ammonia.

Figure 14.2 The urea cycle. AL, argininosuccinate lyase; AS, argininosuccinate synthetase; CPS, carbamoyl phosphate synthetase; NAGS, N–acetylglutamate synthase; OTC, ornithine transcarbamoylase.

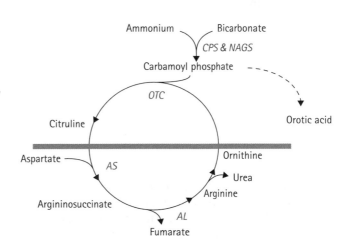

191

Although hypoglycaemia is a common non-specific feature of many sick infants, it may arise as a result of the following disorders:

- fat oxidation (most common),
- glycogen metabolism,
- gluconeogenesis,
- glucose transport,
- galactose and fructose conversion to glucose, or
- ketone metabolism.

True blood sugar must be measured in any encephalopathic child with the following essential investigations:

- true blood glucose,
- lactate,
- free fatty acids, 3-hydroxybutarate, acyl carnitines,
- insulin, urinary cortisol,
- organic acids,
- later: growth hormone.

Figure 14.3 shows the principles of glucose metabolism. Once identified the principles of management are

- glycogen storage disorders: maintain glucose with nocturnal enteral feeding;
- fatty oxidation defects: regular feeding, carnitine supplements;

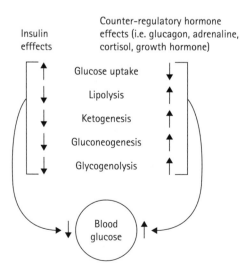

Figure 14.3 The principles of glucose metabolism.

- gluconeogenesis defects: avoid fasting (tolerance increases with age);
- growth hormone/cortisol: replace as appropriate;
- organic acids/amino acids: may be vitamin-responsive, protein restriction;
- galactos-/fructos-aemia (HFI): avoid galactose/fructose respectively; and
- insulin excess: central venous line, hypotonic glucose, give somatostatin with or without diazoxide.

Metabolic acidosis is very common in sick infants and children and is most often caused by sepsis, poor tissue perfusion and/or hypoxia. Severe metabolic acidosis is most often associated with the organic acidaemias (mainly propionic and methylmalonic acidaemia) and disorders of ketone body utilization. The absence of acidosis does not exclude these disorders. In contrast to secondary causes of metabolic acidosis, sodium bicarbonate is usually a necessary part of therapy.

Some inborn errors of metabolism present with an acute encephalopathy without prominent biochemical abnormalities of blood glucose, ammonia or acid/base balance and should still be considered in a child with an unexplained encephalopathy even if initial biochemical investigations are normal. These include, for example, pyridoxine-dependent seizures, maple syrup urine disease, sulphite oxidase deficiency and glutaric aciduria type 1.

Acute toxic encephalopathies
The most common cause of acute toxic encephalopathy is sepsis, but remember that the crawling infant may be able to access drugs or poisons in the home. Deliberate poisoning will also rarely occur.

Acute necrotizing encephalopathy
Mentioned in the section on encephalopathy with fever (Non-infectious acute encephalopathies that may mimic infection), remember this may present without fever.

Stroke
Stroke is one of the most common causes of death and disability in childhood. There have been controversies about the optimal timing for investigation and emergency management strategies but a consensus is now emerging. This section suggests an evidence-based pathway for investigation and management. More details can be found in the UK Royal College of Physicians and American Heart Association Stroke Council and the American College of Chest Physicians guidelines (see Resources).

Epidemiology
Stroke affects between 130 000 and 1.3 million children per year; at least a third are haemorrhagic while a similar proportion have ischaemic stroke. Other conditions may mimic stroke (important to exclude before treatment is considered). Fatalities are highest in haemorrhagic stroke (mainly due to the ICP from space-occupying lesions

such as intracranial haematomata), but some children with arterial ischaemic stroke also die with widespread cerebral oedema. Mortality and morbidity are higher with an underlying condition such as cardiac malformation or haematological disease. Neuroimaging will increase diagnostic yield in acutely ill children, for example in intensive care, especially where there are focal signs. There is a wide differential diagnosis (Table 14.5).

Pathology and causation
Half the incident cases of stroke in infancy or childhood are seen in association with congenital heart disease or sickle-cell anaemia. Of the remainder, a post-varicella (within the last 12 months) arteriopathy is the most common cause, with rarer causes of arteritis also contributing. Traumatic dissection of the carotid artery in the neck is to be considered in the older, more robust and mobile child. There are no reports of cerebral autosomal dominant arteriopathy with subcortical infarcts and leukoencephalopathy (CADASIL) in infancy. In a report of post-mortem findings, more than half of the children had venous sinus thrombosis. Antenatal events will cause a hemiparesis that, in many cases, presents later in infancy. Causes include neuronal migration disorders, schizencephaly and intra-uterine stroke causing porencephaly.

Neonatal stroke occurs in about 1 in 4000 term neonates. Risk factors for neonatal stroke include congenital heart disease; blood, homocysteine and lipid disorders; infection; maternal disorders (autoimmune disorders, coagulation disorders, anticardiolipin antibodies, twin-to-twin transfusion syndrome, *in utero* cocaine exposure, infection); placental disorders (thrombosis, abruption or infection); fetomaternal haemorrhage; vasculopathy including maldevelopment such as arteriovenous malformations; trauma and catheterization; hypoxia ischaemia at birth; dehydration; and extracorporeal membrane oxygenation. Commonly the source of the embolism is undetermined but a placental origin is suspected in many.

There is a high prior probability that the stroke will be embolic and there is currently no evidence to support thrombolysis. Cerebral abscess should be considered especially when cyanotic heart disease and/or endocarditis is present (infarcts, haemorrhages and mycotic aneurysms may be seen).

In congenital heart disease neuroimaging may show focal infarcts pre-operatively (40% in transposition of the great arteries). This may be due to prior atrial septostomy, hypotension at presentation or perinatal events. Post-operatively infarcts and haemorrhages are seen in 15% of cases. These arise from micro-emboli as bypass clamps or device closures are released. Extracorporal membrane oxygenation and anticoagulation may predispose to haemorrhage. Low-flow cardiac conditions, for example a hypoplastic left heart, predispose to thrombus and embolic stroke and require anticoagulation and/or antiplatelet treatment. Paradoxical emboli with right-to-left shunting from the right side of the circulation in children may be seen with cyanotic heart disease.

Cerebral vein thrombosis may lead to central venous hypertension that may provoke multifocal infarcts and haemorrhages.

Table 14.5 Differential diagnosis, investigation and management in the child with suspected stroke

Etiology	Clinical/laboratory/neuroradiological features	Specific treatments to be considered
Space-occupying mass	Focal signs, seizures, deteriorating level of consciousness	Surgical opinion
Spontaneous intracerebral haemorrhage	Sudden onset, obvious on plain CT, may be secondary to VST so CTV/MRV, distinction between aneurysm and AVM may require MR and conventional arteriography	Surgical opinion ?decompression, exclude haemorrhaging diastheses, polycystic kidneys and other genetic causes of AVM or aneurysm
Ischaemic stroke, anterior circulation e.g. large hemispheric Ischaemic stroke or posterior circulation e.g. cerebellar (with hydrocephalus) or brainstem	Preceding transient ischaemic attacks in some cases, at <24 h may be subtle changes on CT but MRI often required Preceding transient ischaemic attacks in some cases, at <24 h may be subtle changes on CT but MRI often required	Unusual to present <4.5 h so *not thrombolysis*. ?Surgical decompression Consider thrombolysis adolescents at <12 h Surgical opinion:? decompression or drainage
Tumour	Preceding headache and other symptoms and signs, CT with or without MRI	Surgical opinion
Cerebral abscess	Fever, obvious on contrast CT	Antibiotics including cover for anaerobes
Venous sinus thrombosis	Focal signs, seizures, deteriorating level of consciousness, haemorrhage or ischaemia or normal CT; needs CTV or MRV	Anticoagulation, exclude prothrombotic disorders especially prothrombin 20210

Table 14.5 *Continued*

Etiology	Clinical/laboratory/neuroradiological features	Specific treatments to be considered
Accidental head injury	History of head injury	
Extradural or intracerebral hematoma	Obvious on plain CT	Surgical opinion
Extracranial dissection	Fat-saturated T1 MRI of neck shows blood in vessel wall	Consider anticoagulation; may be suitable for interventional neuroradiology
Intracranial dissection	Double lumen may be demonstrated on MR arteriography or conventional arteriography	Anticoagulation contraindicated; may be suitable for interventional neuroradiology if haemorrhage in view of recurrence risk
Diffuse brain oedema	Exclude venous sinus thrombosis on CTV or MRV	Surgical opinion ?decompression
Non-accidental injury	Retinal haemorrhages on funduscopy, bruises, fractures	Child protection
Subdural or intracerebral haemorrhage/effusion Intracerebral haemorrhage		Neurosurgery opinion Surgical opinion
Hemispheric ischaemia, diffuse brain oedema	Exclude secondary VST	Surgical opinion ?decompression

Etiology	Clinical/laboratory/neuroradiological features	Specific treatments to be considered
Acute disseminated encephalomyelitis (ADEM)	Demyelination on MRI, may have had infection	?Corticosteroids, intravenous immunoglobulin
Congenital heart disease	Exclude VST, dissection, moyamoya, aneurysm, embolus	Discuss with cardiologists
Sickle cell disease	Exclude VST, PRES, focal cerebral arteriopathy of childhood, dissection, moyamoya, aneurysm, embolus through PFO	Exchange transfusion, very slowly Appropriate management of stroke syndrome
Other anaemias including iron deficiency	Exclude VST, PRES, focal cerebral arteriopathy of childhood, dissection, moyamoya, aneurysm, embolus through PFO	Appropriate management of anaemia and stroke syndrome; care with transfusion
Haemolytic–uraemic syndrome	Anaemia, jaundice, Burr cells on blood film, AIS, VST or PRES	Dialysis; appropriate management of anaemia and stroke syndrome
Nephrotic syndrome	Typically VST	?Anticoagulate acutely and in relapse
Inflammatory bowel disease	VST, PRES, focal cerebral arteriopathy of childhood	VST ?anticoagulate acutely and in relapse
Leukaemia	VST, PRES, focal cerebral arteriopathy of childhood	VST ?anticoagulate acutely and in relapse
Hypoglycaemia	Encephalopathic, hemiparesis, seizures	Glucose
Epilepsy	Subtle seizures, EEG may show, e.g. Rolandic spikes	Consider anticonvulsants

Table 14.5 *Continued*

Etiology	Clinical/laboratory/neuroradiological features	Specific treatments to be considered
Hypertensive encephalopathy	Preceded by visual symptoms and seizures, macular star, CT may show subtle changes but MRI (DWI) shows PRES	Slow reduction blood pressure
Migraine e.g. hemiplegic	Family history, headache, EEG shows unilateral slowing	May respond to calcium-channel blockers, phenytoin or acetazolamide
Metabolic conditions		
Ornithine transcarbamylase deficiency	Unilateral cerebral oedema; High ammonia	
Mitochondrial	MRI: parieto-occipital lesions not typical of AIS; high lactate	?Arginine
Moyamoya	Preceding transient ischaemic attacks in some cases, may be a family history or clues to an underlying diagnosis	Revascularization
Lacunar stroke with no obvious precipitant and normal vascular imaging	Exclude PFO using transoesophageal ECHO; role of bubble TCD not established	Long-term aspirin; consider closure of PFO after randomized controlled trials have evaluated

AIS, arterial ischaemic stroke; AVM, arteriovenous malformation; CTV, computed tomographic venography; DWI, diffusion-weighted imaging; ECHO, echocardiography; EEG, electroencephalography; MRV, magnetic resonance venography; PFO, persistent foramen ovale; PRES, posterior reversible encephalopathy syndrome; TCD, transcranial Doppler ultrasonography; VST, venous sinus thrombosis.

Clinical clues to the diagnosis
Neonatal stroke may present as cardiorespiratory instability, seizures, abnormal posturing or limb weakness. Clinical assessment is often hampered by the fact that the infant is ventilated. In post-neonatal infants take a history for underlying conditions and recent trauma or infections, including chicken pox within the previous year and apparently minor upper respiratory tract infections. Family history may reveal a prothrombotic tendency (note any history of early stroke, coronary heart disease or venous thrombosis).

Clinical examination should note the pattern of motor impairment and features of vasculitis or hypertension; also include a careful heart examination and a search for neurocutaneous stigmata (linear sebaceous naevus may be associated with cerebrovascular disease).

Most perinatal strokes occur in the territory of the middle cerebral artery. There is a left-sided predominance of lesions, which may be related to the haemodynamics of a patent ductus arteriosus, or easier transfer from the left common carotid. Preterm infants tend to have multifocal lesions involving the cortical or lenticulostriate branches of the middle cerebral artery, but term infants tend to have occlusions of the main middle cerebral artery.

Investigations
See also Table 14.5.

Neuroimaging: Cranial ultrasound is a sensitive method of detecting hemorrhage but two thirds of ischaemic strokes seen on MRI are missed. CT does not show parenchymal infarction reliably within 24 h of an ischaemic stroke, but may be required urgently to exclude haemorrhage (Figure 14.4a). Although ischaemic infarction (Figures 14.4b) may not be obvious within the first 24 h on CT, MRI is more sensitive (Figure 14.4c) and other abnormalities, for example collaterals associated with moyamoya, may be seen (Figure 14.4d) and CT may reveal venous sinus thrombosis (Figures 14.4e and f), particularly post-contrast. Occasionally other vascular abnormalities may be revealed (Figures 14.4g and h). CT venography and arteriography may be the appropriate modality for making the diagnosis quickly in a sick child, although the radiation dose is relatively high.

MRI will exclude haemorrhage, reveal venous sinus thrombosis and may be useful for documenting vascular abnormalities in more detail; in addition include MR venography and extra- and intracranial arteriography (MR arteriography) and sequences for fat-saturated T1 MRI of the neck (FS-T1). If there is no obvious arterial disorder involving the intracranial vessels on MR arteriography, venous sinus thrombosis should be investigated either with CT venography or MR venography and dissection in the neck vessels should be excluded using Doppler sonography, or if necessary conventional arteriography. MRI is also the modality of choice for diagnosing conditions mimicking stroke.

Electroencephalography can be useful in demonstrating that focal signs are epileptic or migrainous in origin (Figure 14.5).

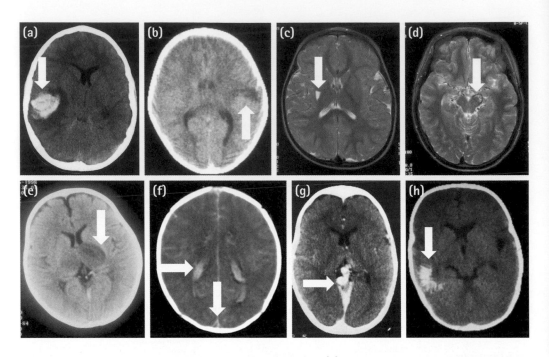

Figure 14.4 Emergency imaging in unilateral stroke. (a) CT showing acute intracerebral haemorrhage with surrounding focal oedema in a child presenting in coma after a focal seizure, (b) CT scan showing infarction in a child with a hemiparesis after minor trauma, (c) MRI showing a small infarct in a child with arteriopathy of the middle cerebral artery after chickenpox, (d) abnormal collateral arteries seen as filling defects on MRI in moyamoya, (e) CT scan showing thalamic infarction in a child with iron-deficiency anaemia and venous sinus thrombosis, (f) venous thrombosis in the sagittal sinus: empty delta sign on contrast CT scan, (g) contrast CT scan showing a vein of Galen malformation in a child with proptosis and (h) 'tramline' calcification on CT in a child with Sturge–Weber syndrome.

Echocardiography, ideally with bubble contrast during a Valsalva manouevre to detect a significant right to left shunt at the atrial level, should be undertaken in all children with stroke, whether or not they have another underlying condition. It is, however, rare for a previously undiagnosed cardiac lesion to be revealed and poor ventricular function is at least as common as patent foramen ovale on echocardiography. The role of bubble-contrast transcranial Doppler ultrasonography in detecting minor degrees of shunting has not yet been established and the need to close any patent foramen ovale found is currently very controversial.

Laboratory investigation: examination of red-blood-cell indices is important, since a substantial proportion of young children with cerebrovascular disease (particularly venous sinus thrombosis) have iron deficiency (ferritin levels or, if necessary, more detailed iron studies). There is now substantial evidence linking prothrombotic

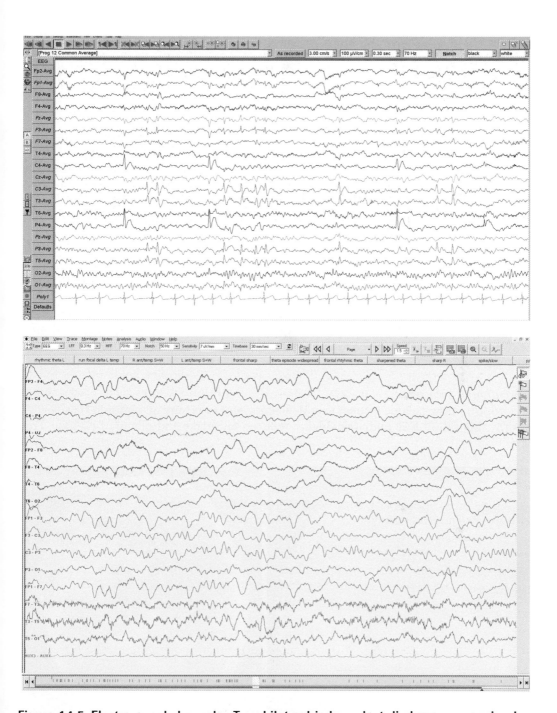

Figure 14.5 Electroencephalography. Top: bilateral independent discharges, occurring in typical doublets (and a quadruplet) on the left, typical of benign Rolandic epilepsy, in a child presenting with a persistent, but ultimately reversible, hemiparesis. Bottom: unilateral slowing on electroencephalography in a child with familial hemiplegic migraine and a calcium-channel gene mutation. (See colour plate 1)

disorders to childhood stroke, but extensive investigation is expensive. In some circumstances it may be appropriate to limit the investigation to the tests which will make a difference to management, for example excluding prothrombin 20210, which appears to increase the risk of recurrence of venous sinus thrombosis.

Acute management
If there is any reduction in level of consciousness the child requires emergency transfer to a centre in which emergency intervention can be undertaken; imaging such as CT can be performed while transportation is organized but neuroimaging should not delay transfer. It is very important that principles of good emergency management of a sick child are followed, with attention to management of the airway, circulation and any seizures.

There are no randomized controlled trials of emergency management of stroke in childhood and thrombolysis is not recommended for children in view of the risk of haemorrhaging. Very occasionally, children with a high risk of recurrent stroke may be suitable for interventional neuroradiological procedures, such as coils or stents but, in many settings, access to these skills will not be available. This also applies to vascular neurosurgery, such as clipping of an aneurysm, or stereotactic radiotherapy to obliterate an arteriovenous malformation. Surgical decompression (Figure 14.6) may be life-saving if the patient is deeply unconscious.

Prevention of recurrence
It is important to exclude or treat iron deficiency and to ensure all children have a healthy diet full of fruit and vegetables, a reduced fat intake and plenty of exercise. For

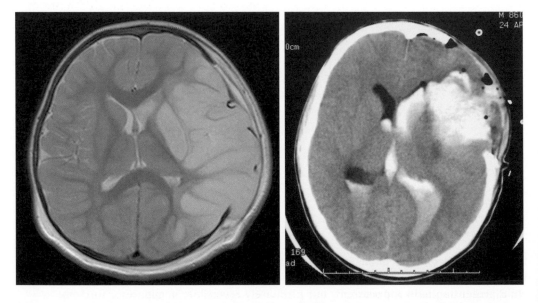

Figure 14.6 Surgical decompression in ischaemic (left) and haemorrhagic (right) stroke.

arterial ischaemic stroke, in view of the data from adults and, in spite of the very low risk of complication by haemorrhage or Reye syndrome, most physicians give aspirin at a dose of 5 mg/kg per day in the acute situation and continue this at the same dose or a reduced dose of 1 mg/kg per day. Recent cohort studies suggest that aspirin prophylaxis may have been associated with reduction in the risk of recurrence, at least for anterior stroke, but there have been no randomized controlled trials.

Many physicians would consider anticoagulation in older children with venous sinus thrombosis, as the adult randomized controlled trials showed benefit in terms of mortality and morbidity and the risk of haemorrhage is low. In such cases, anticoagulation is usually continued for 3–6 months and then discontinued except in high-risk situations such as recurrence of nephrotic syndrome or exacerbation of inflammatory bowel disease. Some physicians would also consider anticoagulation in children with proven dissection of the extracranial portion of the carotid or vestibular arteries but not in those with intracranial dissection because of the risk of subarachnoid haemorrhage.

Although prothrombotic disorders do appear to be associated with stroke risk and perhaps with the risk of recurrence, investigation of individual risk factors has not yet led to secondary prevention. The exception to this rule is the observation that children with the prothrombin 20210 mutation are at high risk of recurrence. It is therefore reasonable to undertake this test, if available, and to consider long-term anticoagulation these children following venous sinus thrombosis without any other triggers.

Rehabilitation and reintegration into school
Some children make a very rapid recovery from stroke while others have considerable residual disability. Early rehabilitation by a skilled team can make a big difference to the long-term outcome. Children may need an educational statement on return to school, and they and their families need considerable support.

References

Barlow KM, Milne S, Minns RA. A retrospective epidemiological analysis of non-accidental head injury in children in Scotland over the last 15 years. *Scottish Medical Journal*, 1998, 43:112–114.

Barlow KM, Minns RA. Annual incidence of shaken impact syndrome in young children. *Lancet*, 2000, 356(9241):1571–1572.

Fanconi M, Lips U. Shaken baby syndrome in Switzerland: results of a prospective follow-up study, 2002-2007. *European Journal of Pediatrics*, 2010, 169(8):1023–1028.

Jayawant S et al. Subdural hemorrhages in infants: population based study. *British Medical Journal*, 1998, 317:1558–1561.

Keenan HT et al. A population based study of inflicted traumatic brain injury in young children. *Journal of the American Medical Association*, 2003, 290:621–626.

Kelly P, Farrant B. Shaken baby syndrome in New Zealand, 2000-2002. *Journal of Paediatrics and Child Health*, 2008, 44:99–107.

King WJ, MacKay M, Sirnick A, Canadian Shaken Baby Study Group. Shaken baby syndrome in Canada: clinical characteristics and outcomes of hospital cases. *Canadian Medical Association Journal*, 2003, 168(2):155–159.

Matschke J et al. Nonaccidental head injury is the most common cause of subdural bleeding in infants <1 year of age. *Pediatrics*, 2009, 124(6):1587–1594.

Talvik I et al. Inflicted traumatic brain injury (ITBI) or shaken baby syndrome (SBS) in Estonia. *Acta Paediatrica*, 2006, 95(7):799–804.

Resources

Monagle P et al, and American College of Chest Physicians. Antithrombotic therapy in neonates and children: American College of Chest Physicians Evidence-Based Clinical Practice Guidelines (8th Edition). *Chest*, 2008, 133(6 Suppl):887S–968S.

Paediatric Accident and Emergency Research Group. *The management of a child (aged 0-18 years) with a decreased conscious level. An evidence-based guideline for health professionals based in the hospital setting.* Royal College of Paediatrics and Child Health and British Association for Emergency Medicine, 2008 (www.nottingham.ac.uk/paediatric-guideline/home2.htm).

Paediatric Stroke Working Group. *Stroke in childhood. Clinical guidelines for diagnosis, management and rehabilitation.* London, Royal College of Physicians. 2004 (www.rcpch.ac.uk/child-health/standards-care/child-health-guidelines-and-standards/guidelines-endorsed-rcpch-subsp-14#RCP_stroke).

Roach ES et al, and American Heart Association Stroke Council, Council on Cardiovascular Disease in the Young. Management of stroke in infants and children: a scientific statement from a Special Writing Group of the American Heart Association Stroke Council and the Council on Cardiovascular Disease in the Young. *Stroke*, 2008, 39:2644–2691. Erratum in: *Stroke*, 2009, 40:e8–e10.

Talvik I, Alexander R, Talvik T. Shaken baby syndrome and baby's cry. *Acta Paediatrica*, 2008, 97(6):782–785.

Chapter 15

Acute neurological illness with fever: meningitis, encephalitis and infective space-occupying lesions

Rachel Kneen and Charles Newton

Key messages

- Central nervous system (CNS) infections are neurological emergencies. The outcome is improved by early recognition and appropriate management.
- Clinical features are useful but cannot be used to predict the risk of CNS infections. Therefore appropriate investigations are needed, especially a lumbar puncture (LP) if no contraindications exist.
- The findings of cerebrospinal fluid (CSF) analysis are very useful for children with suspected CNS infections. All children should have a LP unless an established contraindication exists (Table 15.1).
- CSF analysis in both meningitis and encephalitis usually shows a pleocytosis but it can be normal, especially if the LP was done early in the illness (see Table 15.2).
- An LP, postponed because of previous contraindication, still adds important diagnostic information.
- In encephalitis, brain imaging findings are useful, but computed tomography (CT) can be normal especially in the early stages of the illness. Magnetic resonance imaging is more sensitive, but may not be available in many settings.
- The list of pathogens causing CNS infections is extensive, but careful history taking and examination can help establish the correct diagnosis.
- The causes of CNS infections vary geographically. Local knowledge is important to understand the individual risks of particular pathogens.
- An immunocompromised child with a CNS infection may have a subtle presentation. Clinical suspicion needs to be high in these patients. Different pathogenic organisms also need to be considered.

Common errors

- Failing to investigate a child with a prolonged 'post-ictal phase' after an assumed febrile convulsion (see Chapter 16).
- Diagnosing febrile convulsion in epilepsy (e.g. Dravet syndrome; see Chapter 16).
- Failing to properly investigate a child with symptoms suggestive of a CNS infection (in particular, not doing a LP when no contraindications exist).
- Failing to appreciate that a child may have a CNS infection for other reasons including: discounting the parents' history that their child is excessively irritable, a bit confused or subdued, has a change in personality or is 'not quite right'. It is usually a mistake to ignore parents' opinions.
- Relying on cranial imaging (especially CT) to rule out raised intracranial pressure: CT may be normal in a child with an impending brain herniation syndrome. Clinical skills must be used to look for brain herniation syndromes.
- Over-treating children with aciclovir for herpes simplex virus encephalitis when they have a pre-existing neurological disorder (especially those with epilepsy and/or cerebral palsy) plus a non-specific viral infection: observe and investigate rather than immediately starting aciclovir.
- Over-treating children with aciclovir for herpes simplex virus encephalitis when there is another definite cause for their encephalopathy, such as a head injury or drug overdose.
- Discounting a possible infective space-occupying lesion because there is no fever or history of fever: symptoms and signs can be subtle.

When to worry

Acute problems

- Infants are at risk of an acute deterioration for many reasons (see section on acute bacterial meningitis, below): they must be carefully monitored to identify and manage complications.
- Intensive care has complications: infants with CNS infections can develop venous thrombosis with or without pulmonary embolism, aspiration pneumonia, feeding difficulties, nutritional deficiencies, ventilator- and possible tracheostomy-dependence, critical illness neuropathy or myopathy.

Chronic problems in the recovery phase:

- ongoing seizures (epilepsy),
- chronic raised intracranial pressure (often with a ventriculo-peritoneal shunt),
- movement disorders including dystonia and spasticity, new physical disabilities,
- communication and swallowing difficulties needing therapists and orthotists,
- nutritional needs and feeding difficulties (nasogastric tube feeding or percutaneous endoscopic gastrostomy feeding may be needed), and
- new learning difficulties and behavioural problems.

Introduction to neurological infectious diseases
The topic of neurological infections in infants is important because unlike many other neurological disorders, specific and potentially life-saving treatments can be given. There are several ways of thinking about this group of disorders but perhaps the most useful is to classify them into presenting clinical syndromes, then to consider specific causative organisms or other pathologies. Some organisms can cause more than one neurological syndrome. The key neurological syndromes that will be discussed here include meningitis, encephalitis and space-occupying lesions (SOLs; abscesses). There can be considerable overlap between the presentations of these syndromes. Febrile seizures are covered in Chapter 16 and congenital brain infections in Chapter 19.

Definitions
Meningitis is defined as inflammation of the brain meninges, characterized clinically by inflammatory cells in CSF. Typically the infant is febrile and fully conscious with signs of meningeal irritation but they may be encephalopathic in severe cases (see section on clinical features below).

Encephalitis means inflammation of the brain parenchyma. This is strictly a pathological diagnosis but unless a brain biopsy or post mortem is carried out, surrogate markers such as CSF microscopy or the findings of brain imaging (MRI) are used. Typically the infant is febrile and encephalopathic with an altered level of consciousness or a behavioural change. They may also have signs of meningeal irritation (see section on clinical features). They may have focal neurological symptoms or signs.

Infective space-occupying lesions include brain abscesses and extra-axial collections of pus. Lesions may be single or multiple depending on the cause. Typically the infant is febrile and will have focal neurological symptoms or signs but not in all cases (see below). There may be underlying medical problems which provide the source of infection for the SOL; for example, congenital cardiac abnormalities, ear/nose/throat infection, septicaemia (particularly if there are any catheters, or intravenous or arterial lines present).

Children who are immunocompromised may present with milder or atypical symptoms and signs for any of these infective neurological syndromes. These infants may not even be febrile. A careful history should be taken to establish whether an infant could be immunnocompromised, particularly if their illness is unexplained. This includes asking the mother about risk factors for HIV.

Acute bacterial meningitis

Incidence and etiology
The incidence of meningitis during infancy, particularly during the neonatal period, is higher than during any other period of the lifespan. The causative organisms are dependent upon age.

During the neonatal period, Group B *Streptococcus*, *Escherichia coli* and *Listeria monocytogenes*, but also other organisms, particularly Gram-negative organisms such as *Citrobacter* species, can cause devastating meningitis often complicated by the formation of abscesses. Although the organisms that most commonly cause acute bacterial meningitis (ABM) in older infants can cause ABM in neonates, these organisms are relatively rare. In infants aged 1–3 months the above organisms become less common, and by the age of 4 months *Streptococcus pnemoniae*, *Haemophilus influenza* and *Meningococcus* are the predominant organisms.

Clinical features
Classically, symptoms include a triad of a short history of fever, headache and neck stiffness. Caution is needed because a young infant may have a low or unstable body temperature and an infant cannot localize pain so is likely to be irritable in place of complaining of a headache. There may be associated photophobia but this cannot usually be detected in an infant.

Signs
- Petechial or purpuric rash in cases caused by meningococcus
- Bulging anterior fontanelle
- Meningism (e.g. Brudzinski and Kernig signs) may, in the first year of life, be absent or no more than a subtle reluctance to flex neck
- Altered level of consciousness in severe cases
- Seizures, focal or generalized, in 30%
- Focal neurological signs: cranial nerves 15%, other 10%
- Septicaemic shock, multiorgan involvement, deranged clotting, especially meningococcal infection.

Infants (and especially those who are immunocompromised) may not display typical features. A high index of suspicion is needed and an LP should be undertaken unless there is a specific contraindication (see Table 15.1). Infants with tuberculous (TB) meningitis may have a more chronic presentation. They may also present with signs of hydrocephalus or raised intracranial pressure (see section on TB meningitis).

Differential diagnosis
Other infections: viral (aseptic) meningitis (see below). Beware of diagnosing viral meningitis in a child who has received antibiotics which may lower CSF white cell count in ABM; other bacterial meningitis including listeria, cryptococcal or tuberculous (see below); other infections including Lyme disease (borelliosis), fungal meningitis, brucellosis, rickettsial infections, parasitic infections.

Non-infectious disorders: some drugs, such as trimethoprim-sulfamethoxazole, ampicillin, intravenous immunoglobulin, non-steroidal anti-inflammatory drugs; autoimmune diseases, such as collagen vascular diseases or other autoimmune diseases (rare in infancy); Aicardi–Goutières syndrome (see also Chapter 14, p. 186 and Table 19.1, p. 264); malignant meningitis; that is, meningitis due to a malignant neoplastic process.

Table 15.1 Contraindications to LP

- Glasgow Coma Scale score* <9 or deteriorating level of consciousness
- Signs of raised intracranial pressure, including:
  - Dilated pupils or absent pupillary response to light
  - Hypertension >95th centile for age or bradycardia <60/min
  - Abnormal respiratory pattern
  - Papilloedema
  - Abnormal posturing, especially decerebrate or decorticate posturing[†]
  - Absent oculocephalic (doll's eye) reflex
- Other focal neurological signs: hemi-/monoparesis, abnormal plantar responses, ocular palsies
- Glasgow Coma Scale score <13 and convulsive seizures that are recent (in preceding 30 min) or prolonged (lasting >30 min)
- Focal or tonic seizures (is it decerebrate or decorticate posturing, not a seizure?)
- Strong suspicion of meningococcal infection (typical purpuric rash in an ill child)
- State of shock
- Local superficial infection in lumbar region
- Disordered blood coagulation

See also www.nottingham.ac.uk/paediatric-guideline/Guideline%20algorithm.pdf (see Resources list).
*See Table 14.1.
[†]See Figure 15.1.

Investigations
CSF examination by LP is essential, except in the presence of a specific contraindication (Table 15.1), when ABM is suspected. See Table 15.2 for the typical changes seen in the CSF in infants with various infective neurological disorders.

Cranial imaging is often normal in a child with suspected meningitis. Clinical features rather than imaging must be used to determine whether it is safe to do a LP. CT is only needed if there are clinical contraindications to a LP (see Table 15.1) and waiting for CT to inform decisions can cause unnecessary delays in investigation and treatment. Request a CT or MRI of the brain if the child is encephalopathic or has focal neurological symptoms or signs. This is done to make an alternative diagnosis, e.g., an infective SOL, arterial ischaemic stroke or encephalitis (abnormal in approximately 30% of cases). Give contrast if possible. In meningitis, the meninges usually enhance and infective SOL will usually also enhance. However, radiologists are often reluctant to give gadolinium to infants. Imaging may also be useful in the management of a child with definite meningitis if they become encephalopathic or deteriorate in other ways or if a complication of the infection is suspected at a later stage of management.

Table 15.2 Typical cerebrospinal fluid (CSF) findings in central nervous system infections

	Viral meningo-encephalitis	ABM	TB meningitis	Fungal	Normal
Opening pressure	Normal/high	High	High	High–very high	Age <1 year – <5 cm
Colour	Clear	Cloudy	Cloudy/yellow	Clear/cloudy	Clear
Cells/mm³	Normal–high	High–very high	Mild elevation	Normal–high	<5
	0–1000	1000–50000	25–500	0–1000	
Differential	Lymphocytes	Neutrophils	Lymphocytes	Lymphocytes	Lymphocytes
CSF/plasma glucose ratio	Normal	Low	Low–very low (e.g. <0.3)	Normal–low	66%*
Protein (g/L)	Normal–high	High	High–very high	Normal–high	<0.5
	0.5–1	>1	1.0–5.0	0.5–5.0	

Normal values: a bloody tap will falsely elevate the CSF white cell count, and protein. To correct for a bloody tap, subtract 1 white cell for every 700 red blood cells/mm³ in the CSF, and 0.1 g/dL of protein for every 1000 red blood cells.

*Although a normal CSF glucose ratio is quoted as 66% only values <50% are likely to be significant.

Some important exceptions

- In viral CNS infections, an early lumbar puncture may give predominantly neutrophils, or there may be no cells in early or late lumbar punctures. In patients with acute bacterial meningitis (ABM) that have been partially pre-treated with antibiotics (or patients <1 year old) the CSF cell count may not be very high and may be mostly lymphocytes.
- Tuberculous (TB) meningitis may have predominant CSF polymorphs early in the infection.
- *Listeria monocytogenes* can give a similar CSF picture to TB meningitis, but the history is shorter.
- CSF findings in bacterial abscesses range from near normal to purulent, depending on location of the abscess, and whether there is associated meningitis or rupture.
- A cryptococcal antigen test (CRAG) and Indian ink stain should be performed on the CSF of all patients in whom cryptococcus is possible.

Investigation on CSF obtained at LP

- Measure opening pressure using a manometer or an intravenous 'giving set' (narrow-gauge flexible plastic tubing) and a tape measure to measure the vertical height above LP needle to which column of CSF in the tube rises.

- Send CSF for microscopy culture and sensitivities, glucose (with paired plasma sample), protein, lactate.

- Rapid antigen testing may be possible for several bacteria (*S. pneumoniae, N. meningitidis, H. influenzae*).

- Polymerase chain reaction (PCR) may be possible for several bacteria (*S. pneumoniae, N. meningitidis, H. influenzae*).

- Save (freeze) a sample in case further investigations are needed.

- Send for PCR for enterovirus, adenovirus and herpes simplex viruses if viral meningitis is suspected.

- Consider sending CSF for PCR for viruses shown in section on viral encephalitis as well (see below) if the child is encephalopathic.

- Send for Ziehl-Neelsen staining and TB culture (see below) if TB meningitis is suspected. Ideally, a 2–5 ml sample is needed to improve yield.

Blood investigations

- Full blood count and differential (may show low or high white cell count, left shift, atypical white cells, low or high platelets).

- Blood culture.

- C-reactive protein, renal and liver function studies.

- Rapid bacterial antigen testing (*S. pneumoniae, N. meningitidis, H. influenzae*).

- Clotting/coagulation studies if the child appears ill or has a petechial rash.

- Chest X-ray or imaging of the sinuses may be helpful depending on clinical features.

- Freeze serum for specific antibody tests. A convalescent sample will also be needed 3 weeks after the onset of the illness. A decision about which organisms to test for can be made at a later date.

Treatment

Meningitis during infancy, particularly during the neonatal period, should be treated aggressively. Since it is difficult to distinguish between viral meningoencephalitis and bacterial meningitis in neonates, give both antibacterial and antiviral (e.g. aciclovir) treatment. Antibacterial treatment needs to cover a wide range of organisms including the Gram-positive and Gram-negative organisms, and consider the possibility of antibiotic resistance, using all available local information.

Recommended antimicrobial regimens include ampicillin and an aminoglycoside such as gentamicin. However, resistance of *Escherichia coli* to ampicillin has been reported.

Cefotaxime is often added, although resistance to this antibiotic has also been reported.

Antimicrobial treatment should last for 14–21 days in neonatal meningitis, and the antimicrobials may need to be adjusted in the light of culture and sensitivity results. Repeating the LP after 24–72 h after onset of treatment may help with management. There is little evidence that corticosteroids improve the outcome in neonatal meningitis.

Supportive care is important for:

- maintaining blood pressure to ensure adequate cerebral perfusion,
- careful fluid management,
- correction of electrolyte disorders,
- respiratory support may be needed, and
- management of seizures with Phenobarbital, benzodiazepines or phenytoin may be used but it can be difficult to ensure appropriate levels.

Complications
Acute: raised intracranial hypertension and progression to a brainstem herniation syndrome (see Figure 15.1), effusions and empyema, acute symptomatic seizures, cerebritis, abscess formation, hydrocephalus, electrolyte disturbances (particularly a low sodium or a metabolic acidosis), venous sinus thrombosis leading to cerebral infarction.

Chronic: cognitive impairment/educational difficulties, behavioural problems, hemiplegia, spastic quadriplegia, dystonia, spasticity, hearing loss or visual loss, epilepsy. Seizures may be focal or multifocal and may be refractory to medical treatment (see Chapters 13 and 16). Always test hearing early in the recovery phase since early detection increases options for treatment.

Chronic bacterial meningitis
Chronic bacterial meningitis is uncommon during the neonatal period, although fungal infections are associated with neonates requiring intensive care.

TB meningitis occurs in infancy, either as a separate clinical syndrome or as part of miliary TB. Most infants present with fever, vomiting, cough and impaired consciousness. Seizures are common. Bulging fontanelle is noticeable in younger infants, paresis or opisthotonus may occur and should lead to consideration of TB. Tuberculosis and fungal infections can be transmitted during pregnancy, although congenital meningitis is uncommon. Diagnosis is often based upon a high index of suspicion, history of contacts, positive tuberculin test and evidence of TB in other organs, particularly in the lungs.

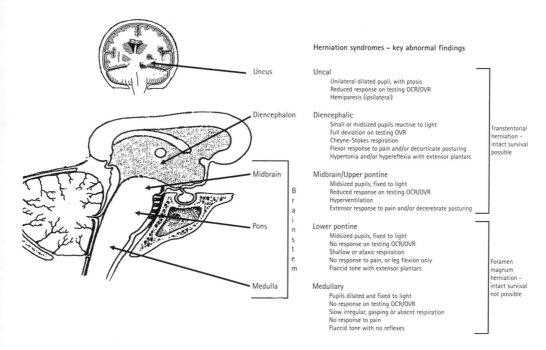

Herniation syndromes – key abnormal findings

Uncus — **Uncal**
Unilateral dilated pupil, with ptosis
Reduced response on testing OCR/OVR
Hemiparesis (ipsilateral)

Diencephalon — **Diencephalic**
Small or midsized pupils reactive to light
Full deviation on testing OVR
Cheyne-Stokes respiration
Flexor response to pain and/or decorticate posturing
Hypertonia and/or hyperreflexia with extensor plantars

Midbrain — **Midbrain/Upper pontine**
Midsized pupils, fixed to light
Reduced response on testing OCR/OVR
Hyperventilation
Extensor response to pain and/or decerebrate posturing

Transtentorial herniation - intact survival possible

Pons — **Lower pontine**
Midsized pupils, fixed to light
No response on testing OCR/OVR
Shallow or ataxic respiration
No response to pain, or leg flexion only
Flaccid tone with extensor plantars

Medulla — **Medullary**
Pupils dilated and fixed to light
No response on testing OCR/OVR
Slow irregular, gasping or absent respiration
No response to pain
Flaccid tone with no reflexes

Foramen magnum herniation - intact survival not possible

B r a i n s t e m

Figure 15.1 Mid–sagittal section of brain showing anatomy and key abnormal findings of midline herniation syndromes, and (above) coronal section showing herniation of the uncus of the temporal lobe: this compresses the third nerve (to cause a palsy of CNIII), and the contralateral cerebral peduncle (to cause an ipsilateral hemiparesis). OCR, oculocephalic (doll's eye) reflex; OVR, oculovestibular (caloric) reflex.

Laboratory investigations
- Hyponatraemia is common
- CSF pleocytosis, usually <1000 cells/mm³, mostly lymphocytes (Table 15.2)
- Increased CSF protein
- Decreased CSF glucose
- Acid-fast bacilli are often not seen and culture often not positive
- PCR can be helpful in reliable laboratories
- CT or MRI and cranial ultrasound commonly show hydrocephalus and, less often, basal enhancement and/or infarction of the basal ganglia.

Treatment
Isoniazid, rifampicin, streptomycin and pyrazamide should be started with dexamethasone, since the latter reduces neurological sequelae. The streptomycin, pyrazamide and dexamethasone are given for 2 months, and the isoniazid and Rifampicin for 18 months.

Ventriculo-peritoneal shunting is often required for hydrocephalus.

Outcome
Mortality is high and neurological sequelae are common.

Fungal meningitis
Fungal meningitis, particularly cryptococcal meningitis, commonly occurs in immune-compromised hosts and may be the first sign of an acquired immune deficiency syndrome (AIDS)-defining illness. It is seen in immune-compromised infants. The other fungi that commonly cause meningitis are *Candida albicans* and *Coccidioides immitis*. It is reported from immune-competent infants as well.

The presentation may be more insidious than TB, presenting with respiratory distress, not tolerating feeds and/or abdominal distension in low-birth-weight infants. Fundoscopic examination may reveal disseminated *Candida*. CNS signs may occur, but the meningitis is often detected during a screen for sepsis. The organisms may be seen with fungal stains of the CSF, but the organism is usually isolated from other parts of the body, and meningitis is suspected from the pleocytosis.

Treatment
Candida: amphotericin B in combination with flucytosine.

Cryptococcus: amphotericin B and flucytosine for 6–10 weeks in HIV-negative patients. For HIV-positive patients amphotericin B and flucytosine for 2 weeks and then fluconazole for 10 weeks.

Outcome
The mortality rate is very high and sequelae are common in those that survive.

Viral (aseptic) meningitis

Incidence and etiology
The epidemiology depends on geography, climate and vaccination coverage. Epidemics can occur and new viruses can emerge. Viral meningitis is common but children are not usually 'toxic' nor do they have multiorgan failure or clotting derangements. Mild elevation of the liver enzymes or pancreatic enzymes can occur with some viruses. Specific diagnosis is often not found, but the yield can be increased by sending stool or rectal swabs and throat swabs (see below).

The most common agents are

- *Enteroviruses*: (85%) including echovirus, coxsackie and poliovirus. All may cause diffuse rashes with or without more specific features:
    - Echovirus: conjunctivitis, myositis,
    - Coxsackie: Hand, foot and mouth disease, myocarditis, pericarditis, pleurisy

- ○ Poliovirus (very rare if vaccination coverage is good): isolated meningitis or meningitis before onset of typical paralytic disease.
- *Mumps*: parotitis, pancreatitis (with elevated amylase and lipase), hearing loss.
- *Herpes viruses*:
  - ○ Herpes simplex virus (HSV) type 1: usually no cold sores or skin lesions found. Usually a primary infection. For details about congenital herpes infections, see Table 19.2, p. 266,
  - ○ Varicella zoster virus (VZV): may have typical chicken pox rash with fluid-filled blisters,
  - ○ Epstein–Barr virus (EBV): pharyngitis, lymphadenopathy, splenomegaly, atypical peripheral lymphoctyes, may have abnormal liver-function tests (uncommon in infancy),
  - ○ Cytomegalovirus (CMV): may have abnormal liver-function tests and retinitis (uncommon unless immunocompromised),
- Human herpes viruses (HHV) 6&7: roseola infantum (slapped-cheek rash), febrile seizures.
- *Measles*: typical confluent rash, lymphadeonopathy, conjunctivitis, pneumonitis (rare if vaccination coverage is good)
- *Adenovirus*: conjunctivitis, respiratory infection or gastroenteritis.
- *Lymphocytic choriomeningitis virus*: subacute illness with orchitis, myocarditis, parotitis, alopecia. Need contact with rodents.
- *Arboviruses* (requires an infected mosquito or tick bite): not found in Northern Europe, consider if travel to South or Southeast Asia (Japanese encephalitis, dengue), all other continents (West Nile).

Clinical features
See section above on ABM. Altered level of consciousness is very uncommon.

Investigations
If viral meningitis is suspected, a LP is essential. A contraindication (Table 15.1) is very unlikely to exist. See Table 15.2 for the typical changes seen in the CSF in viral meningitis.

CSF analysis: see section on ABM. Similar CSF tests are needed in an infant with suspected viral meningitis.

Other investigations: see section on ABM. Similar investigations are needed in an infant with suspected viral meningitis. It is very unlikely that an infant will need cranial imaging. It is also useful to send a throat swab and a rectal swab or a stool sample for *viral* isolation (N.B. viral culture medium needed). A serum sample should be saved to compare with a convalescent sample taken 3 weeks after the onset of the illness.

Differential diagnosis: see section on ABM.

Treatment: for uncomplicated viral meningitis, no specific treatment is needed. Full recovery usually occurs within 2 weeks, although some patients may have post-viral fatigue syndrome (rare in infancy). HSV meningitis is accompanied by encephalitis and specific treatment is required (see next section). Always test hearing after recovery.

Encephalitis

Encephalitis in infancy is uncommon but the incidence in infants is higher than for older children. Even if appropriate investigations are undertaken, a definite diagnosis is only found in approximately 50% of cases. The most common causes of sporadic viral encephalitis (VE) in infants are HSV type 1, enterovirus and VZV. In some parts of the world, arboviruses or rabies virus are more common. The epidemiology depends on the on geography, climate and vaccination coverage. Epidemics can occur and new viruses can emerge.

It is very important to identify and treat an infant with VE due to HSV type 1 as the outcome is better if the child is treated early in the illness. The differential diagnosis of encephalitis is quite wide (see below).

Most common causes of viral encephalitis (VE) in infancy

The list is very similar to that given for viral meningitis above. Extra specific details are given below

HERPES VIRUSES

HSV type 1 is the most common sporadic cause of VE in the western setting. In an infant this is usually a primary infection but, despite this, the presence of the typical herpes blistering rash, cold sores or gingivo-stomatitis is unusual. Seizures and focal neurological signs are common. Presentation may be with a subtle, psychiatric presentation and low-grade fever.

HSV in neonates. The fetus is usually infected during delivery. Rarely there is postnatal infection from close contacts (usually HSV1). Some 50–75% of cases are type 2 and the remainder type 1. Asymptomatic infection is common in the mother but unusual in the infant. Preterm infants are more frequently affected. Fetal scalp electrodes are a risk factor. Damage is caused by inflammation and destruction. Many features are similar to other congenital infections including toxoplasmosis, rubella, cytomegalovirus and HSV (sometimes known as the TORCH infections). Severe cases have multiorgan involvement: predeliction for reticulendothelial system (anaemia, jaundice, haemorrhaging). Specific features include vesicular mucocutaneous lesions (often over the site of viral entry), conjunctivitis and keratitis. If infection is localized to the CNS (without visceral involvement), symptom onset is later (second or third week of life). CNS abnormalities include meningoencephalitis and/or multifocal, severe and diffuse, seizures/coma, bulging fontanelle. See also Table 19.2, p. 266.

VZV

VZV can have many neurological manifestations including postinfectious cerebellitis (common, but not in the first year of life), meningitis, an acute encephalitis (rare) and reactivation syndromes including large- and small-vessel vasculitis (see below) or neuropathies causing brainstem encephalitis including Ramsay–Hunt syndrome (facial palsy, hearing impairment/vertigo and rash affecting ear canal and palate) or involvement of other cranial nerves including ophthalmic shingles. Those with VE caused by VZV may have a concomitant VZV rash or this may appear later. The virus lies dormant in ganglia along the entire neuroaxis. Reactivation can lead to an encephalitis. In the immunocompetent host this causes a large-vessel vasculitis leading to a stroke syndrome (Chapter 14). This is common in infants and can occur up to several months after the primary infection. An immunocompromised host is more likely to get a small-vessel vasculitis leading to a progressive encephalitis. VZV is also associated with acute disseminated encephalomyelitis (ADEM), but this is very uncommon in the first year of life.

HUMAN HERPES VIRUSES 6 AND 7
HHV 6 & 7 encephalitis mainly affects young children (<2 years old) during primary infection. It usually causes a milder VE with febrile seizures and the typical roseola/slapped-cheek rash seen with HHV6. Both viruses can be reactivated in the immunocompromised.

ARBOVIRUSES
These are the most common cause of VE worldwide and are also 'emerging' diseases in previously unaffected geographical areas but the identity of the specific virus depends on geography and the presence of the specific transmitting vector. Seizures are common. Some specific virus types cause a movement disorder with parkinsonian-like features and also a flaccid paralysis 'polio-like illness' with anterior horn cell involvement. The arbovirus most likely to affect the Commonwealth of Independent States in Central and Eastern Europe and Central Asia is the tick borne encephalitis *flavivirus*. This virus is unlikely to affect infants because of lack of exposure, but in older children and adults a flaccid paralysis affecting the upper limbs and neck is seen. The clinical signs are similar to motor neuron disease. Some patients are also reported to have developed repeated and regular myoclonic seizures affecting the limbs. Patients from South or Southeast Asia may have *Dengue encephalitis*. Most patients also have the typical vascular abnormalities seen in Dengue haemorrhagic fever.

ENTEROVIRUSES
Enteroviruses commonly affect neonates and infants. Brainstem features are common. Epidemics with *enterovirus 71* strain are reported in the Asian Pacific region. These children may also have myocarditis.

MEASLES VIRUS
Causes four neurological syndromes: acute illness with the infection (the electroencephalography is abnormal in a high proportion of 'uncomplicated' measles), acute ADEM-like illness within weeks of infection, a subacute progressive encephalitis affecting the immunocompromised around 6 months after primary infection and sub-acute sclerosing pan encephalitis (SSPE) which presents years later (and therefore outside infancy) and is even rarer if immunization rates are high.

INFLUENZA TYPES A AND B (INCLUDING H1N1 'SWINE FLU' STRAIN)

Different neurological presentations are described, from mild encephalopathy with seizures to more severely affected cases with ADEM, malignant brain oedema syndrome and acute necrotizing encephalopathy (ANE; see Chapter 14, p. 187). These are rare in infants.

ROTAVIRUS

Infants with rotavirus gastroenteritis can present with clusters of seizures and this may not be associated with fever. Some cases reported with positive PCR for rotavirus ribonucleic acid (RNA) in CSF and their may be a CSF pleocytosis (usually <100 cells/ml). The outcome is good.

Non-viral causes of encephalitis

The neurological syndrome of encephalitis (as described in the definitions section above) can also be caused by acute and chronic bacterial infections such as *S. pneumoniae* and *Mycobacterium tuberculosis* but also by immune-mediated mechanisms.

All forms of *immune-mediated parainfectious CNS disorder* are very rare indeed in the first year of life. ADEM (see also Chapter 14) is the most common cause of immune-mediated encephalitis but this occurs in the first year of life only very rarely. Its diagnosis relies on brain imaging with MRI being by far the most sensitive imaging modality (Chapter 7), but it may not be possible in all settings.

Autoantibody-mediated encephalitis has been recognized in children only recently and so far reports of its occurrence in the first year of life are very rare indeed. Variants of this include *N*-methyl-d-aspartic acid receptor (NMDAR) antibody and voltage-gated potassium channel (VGKCA) complex antibody encephalitis. Some older children diagnosed with these types of encephalitis have been found to have an ovarian or other tumour. It is important to consider these disorders as the treatment is different: immunomodulatory agents including corticosteroids and plasma exchange are used. Diagnosis of immune-mediated encephalitis may not be possible in settings without the resources needed (which includes laboratories offering assays for the detection of the abnormal antibodies in serum and CSF). It is likely the specific antibody tests will soon become more widely available.

Clinical features

Classically there is a short history of fever, irritability, lethargy, encephalopathy and sometimes seizures. Focal neurological signs are often identified. Multiorgan failure or clotting abnormalities are uncommon but mild elevation of the liver enzymes or pancreatic enzymes can occur with some viruses. Specific diagnosis is often not found, but as with the investigation of children with viral meningitis, the yield can be increased by sending stool, rectal or throat swabs (see above).

There may also be a more subtle presentation with behavioural change, excessive sleepiness or lethargy for a few days. Eventually the child may have a seizure but the early symptoms can be dismissed by healthcare professionals. This is particularly the case for VE caused by HSV type 1; therefore VE should be considered in an infant with this presentation, particularly if they could be immunocompromised.

Differential diagnosis
The differential diagnosis of VE includes the same disorders shown in the section for ABM above but other disorders to consider include

- metabolic encephalopathy: particularly mitochondrial disorders, fatty acid oxidation defects and urea-cycle defects (see Chapters 13, 14 and 24). Also acquired metabolic disorders of blood biochemistry (e.g. high or low sodium, low calcium, low blood glucose);

- trauma (especially inflicted traumatic brain injury): see Chapter 14;

- spontaneous brain haemorrhage (more common in neonates than older infants) or acute arterial stroke; see Chapter 14;

- exacerbation of seizures in a child with established epilepsy or non-convulsive status epilepticus (often occurs with non-specific viral infections). Or febrile infection-related epilepsy syndrome (FIRES), a devastating non-encephalitic epileptic encephalopathy (very rare in infancy);

- endocrine disorders: consider new presentation of diabetes mellitus (rare in infants);

- toxins: accidental ingestion or poisoning; and

- CNS vasculitis is very rare indeed in infancy. Vasculitis may be associated with systemic connective tissue disorders, such as systemic lupus erythematosus or primary CNS vasculitis.

Investigations
Many of the investigations needed for VE are the same as for ABM or viral meningitis (see sections on ABM and viral meningitis above). LP is mandatory and is still useful after treatment is started as CSF HSV PCR can still be positive up to 10 days after treatment with aciclovir. Failure to get CSF analysis may result in unnecessary prolonged treatment with aciclovir.

For HSV type 2 in a neonate: examination of vesicular fluid/skin scrapings is useful; histology: multinucleated giant cells or intranuclear inclusions seen or electronmicroscopy: viral particles identified.

Viral isolation from throat, stool, urine and CSF (viral culture media swabs needed). Serology is less useful as the IgM response may be delayed.

CSF findings are similar to those of viral meningitis although the protein count may be up to 6 g/L (see Table 15.2). It may be normal if LP is performed in the first 48 h of the illness. Repeat LP if VE is still strongly suspected and first CSF analysis is normal. PCR for viral DNA/RNA is possible for many viral infections (seek local advice for which are offered) but may be negative if the LP is undertaken less than 2 days or more than 10 days after the onset of the illness. Send CSF for PCR for HSV 1 and 2 and VZV initially as VE caused by these viruses responds to treatment with aciclovir. Store CSF for further tests if these are negative. Viral isolation is sometimes possible. Measurement of IgM response to specific viruses in the CSF is also possible and may confirm the diagnosis even if viral PCR is negative. Discuss with a clinical virologist if possible.

Brain imaging
CT is usually the first-line investigation but CT can be normal in up to 30% of cases especially in the early stages of the illness. Abnormal areas will show as hypodensities with or without patchy haemorrhage. MRI is the investigation of choice as the sensitivity is good and diffusion-weighted images are particularly helpful for identifying early changes.

- HSV type 1: most commonly gives an abnormal signal (often with haemorrhage) in the temporal lobes, insular cortex, frontal lobes and thalami. Meningeal enhancement is also often present. Midline shift may be present if significant cerebral oedema is present. However, appearances may be atypical, especially in infants and children.
- HSV type 2: CT and ultrasound may identify multifocal parenchymal abnormalities.
- VZV: multiple abnormal areas of signal in the grey and white matter representing vasculitis and infarction. May be in an arterial distribution in a case associated with viral reactivation.
- Enteroviruses: may have an abnormal signal isolated to the brainstem, dentate nucleus of the cerebellum or thalami.
- Arboviruses: may have an abnormal signal in the basal ganglia and thalami.
- Rotavirus: usually normal.
- Influenza A and B: depends on the clinical syndrome caused by the virus. May be normal or have focal changes but more likely to have changes consistent with ADEM or ANE.

Electroencephalography shows diffuse slowing of the background in all cases. Epileptiform focal abnormalities may also be seen and periodic lateralizing epileptiform discharges (PLEDs) may be present later in the illness in HSV type 1 encephalitis. PLEDs are not specific and may occur in SOLs or other focal brain abnormalities.

Brain biopsy has become unnecessary for this diagnosis since the advent of PCR for viral DNA/RNA. However, it might need to be considered if the findings could change clinical management, for example if considering micro-abscesses from an embolic source, TB or a parasitic or fungal infection, vasculitis or distinction between an infective SOL or a malignant process (see section below on SOL).

Treatment
Proven HSV 1 and 2: intravenous aciclovir for 21 days. Monitor renal function. If relapse occurs, re-treat and consider prophylaxis with valaciclovir or oral aciclovir for 90 days (although there is no published randomized controlled trial to support this).

Use of steroids in VE is controversial. Some anecdotal evidence of improvement in outcome is reported. Consider using a 3–5-day pulse of methylprednisolone or dexamethasone in severe cases with raised intracranial pressure. Consider surgical decompression in cases where raised intracranial pressure is refractory to medical treatment. There are no other specific antiviral treatments currently used for VE.

For treatment of immune-mediated encephalitis (very rare in the first year of life), use 3–5 days of intravenous methylprednisolone (see also Chapter 14) before considering other treatments.

Prognosis
Prognosis depends on the cause, the severity of the clinical illness at presentation and, in VE caused by HSV type 1, the time interval before treatment was started. Mortality is reduced by 40% in HSV type 1 if aciclovir is given promptly. Neurorehabilitation is often needed in a multidisciplinary setting. Patients who have had VE caused by HSV type 1 often experience severe memory problems. In HSV type 2 in neonates the mortality is highest (30–60%) for those with disseminated infection and is lower (15%) in those with isolated CNS disease. There are high levels of sequelae in survivors of both groups.

Infective SOLs
Brain abscesses or extra-axial collections can be caused by bacteria, fungi or parasites with the most common causal organisms in infancy being staphylocci (*Staphyloccus aureus* and other staphylococcal species), *Streptococcus* (aerobic and anaerobic) and *H. influenzae*. Anaerobic organisms such as bacteroides, *Streptococcus milleri* and *Fusobacterium* are also commonly found. CNS TB should be considered. Fungi (*Aspergillus* species) and parasites have also been reported. Many abscesses will contain mixed flora (approximately 40%).

They may be caused by haematogenous or local spread; they may be single or multiple. Localization is related to an underlying predisposing factor with those spreading in the blood found in a distribution that reflects the cerebral blood supply, usually the middle cerebral artery. There may also be haematogenous venous spread from the sinuses to the frontal lobes. There may be direct invasion from infections of the sinuses or middle ear and these infections tend to cause abscesses in the temporal lobes or cerebellum.

Risk factors
● Infancy: infective SOLs are more common in infants than older children
● Congenital heart disease
● Sinus or ear infections

- Poor dental hygiene (very rare in infancy)
- Immunosuppression
- Presence of a ventriculo-peritoneal shunt
- Skull fracture
- Dermal sinuses or other channel to the CNS from head, neck or back
- Complication of bacterial meningitis
- Following aspiration of a foreign body (very rare in infancy).

Clinical features
Irritability and fever are typical with a focal neurological deficit that depends on location of lesion(s). In infancy, the fontanelle can bulge and the head circumference can increase rapidly. There may be irritability or lethargy or a reduced level of consciousness but children can appear surprisingly well and present with progressive macrocephaly. Raised intracranial pressure and brain herniation syndromes can develop. Acute neurological decompensation and signs of meningitis may supervene if the abscess ruptures into the ventricular system.

Laboratory investigations
- There may be non-specific haematological markers of infection with elevated peripheral white cell count, erythrocyte sedimentation rate and C-reactive protein.
- Blood cultures are rarely positive.
- A cardiac assessment including an ECHO should be undertaken.
- CSF examination (LP) is contraindicated due to the risk of brain herniation syndromes.
- Drainage of a suspected abscess may be required for SOLs over 2 cm in diameter. Needle biopsy sampling of SOLs under 2 cm may also be helpful to confirm the diagnosis of infection, obtain sensitivities to antibiotics and exclude other diagnoses. This clearly requires access to appropriate neurosurgical expertise and equipment, preferably including stereotactic guidance equipment.

Cranial imaging
Cranial ultrasound may be useful in a neonate. CT is useful and will detect most SOLs but lesions in the posterior fossa may be missed. Contrast should be given as extra-axial collections can be missed on an unenhanced CT scan and ring enhancement of lesions is characteristic. MRI is the modality of choice, with and without contrast if possible. Diffusion-weighted MR and MR spectroscopy can also be helpful in differentiating a single parenchymal lesion from a tumour.

Differential diagnosis
- Brain tumour
- Intraparenchymal haemorrhage
- Lymphoma or an isolated single demyelinating lesion are included in the differential diagnosis but very unlikely to occur in infancy.

Treatment

Small lesions (<2 cm in diameter) or those in whom the causative organism has been identified may be amenable to medical treatment with antimicrobials. Surgical drainage followed by prompt initiation of empirical broad-spectrum empirical antimicrobial therapy is often needed (usually for 6 weeks but longer in the immunocompromised). Surgical specimens should be sent for histology and for microbiology investigations. Typical first-choice antibiotics would include a third-generation cephalosporin and metronidazole but advice should be sought from the infectious diseases team. If an associated foreign body, such as a central line or ventriculo-peritoneal shunt, is found, it should be removed.

Outcome

Depends on severity and location of parenchymal damage. Neurorehabilitation is often necessary (see above) as 40% of children have neurological sequelae and 25% have epilepsy.

Resources

Kim KS. Acute bacterial meningitis in infants and children. *Lancet Infectious Diseases*, 2010, 10:32–42.

Sheehan JP et al. Brain abscesses in children. *Neurosurgical Focus*, 2008, 24(6):E6.

The Paediatric Accident and Emergency Research Group. *Management of the child with a decreased conscious level. An evidence-based guideline.* www.nottingham.ac.uk/paediatric-guideline/Guideline%20algorithm.pdf

Thompson C, Kneen R, Riordan A, Kelly D, Pollard AJ. Encephalitis in children. *Arch Dis Child*, 2011, June 28 [published ahead of print].

Visintin C et al. Management of bacterial meningitis and meningococcal septicaemia in children and young people: summary of NICE guidance. *British Medical Journal*, 2010, 340:c3209 (http://guidance.nice.org.uk/CG102/Guidance/pdf/English).

Chapter 16
Post-neonatal epileptic seizures

Hans Hartmann and J. Helen Cross

Key messages
- Differentiate an epileptic seizure from a non-epileptic paroxysmal event. Home videos demonstrating an event can be extremely helpful.
- Manage infants with simple febrile seizures expectantly.
- Treat an infant with status epilepticus vigorously.
- Recognize possible underlying genetic or metabolic disorders in infants presenting with epileptic seizures.

Common errors
- Diagnosing epilepsy in an infant with non-epileptic paroxysmal events.
- Treating infants with sodium-channel disorders with the wrong antiepileptic drugs.

When to worry
- When seizures occur in clusters or the infant goes into status epilepticus.
- When there are persistent focal signs.
- When the infant does not adequately regain consciousness following a seizure.
- When the infant shows developmental regression.

Definitions
Epileptic seizures are transient and fully reversible events involving a disturbance of neurological function. Epileptic seizures are caused by abnormal, excessive activity of a more or less extensive population of cerebral neurons. They need to be differentiated from non-epileptic seizures, considered in Chapter 17. This differentiation can be supported by electroencephalography (EEG) demonstrating (or not) epileptic discharges; that is, temporary paroxysmal change in EEG activity. Most epileptic seizures are brief, lasting only seconds to a few minutes. Following a seizure, the infant may be drowsy and in case of a focal motor seizure transiently show a paresis (Todd's paresis).

Status epilepticus refers to a seizure going on for more than 30 min or a condition in which the infant has a series of seizures without completely regaining consciousness in between.

Epilepsy is a common chronic neurological condition that is defined as recurrent unprovoked epileptic seizures. Febrile seizures, i.e. seizures provoked by a developing fever, are not unprovoked and do not fall within the definition of epilepsy.
The cause of epilepsy may be

- genetic: the epilepsy is the direct result of a known or presumed genetic defect(s) in which seizures are the core symptom of the disorder;
- structural/metabolic: structural lesions include acquired disorders such as stroke, trauma and infection. They may also be of genetic origin (e.g. tuberous sclerosis, many malformations of cortical development); however, as we currently understand it, there is a separate disorder interposed between the genetic defect and the epilepsy. Metabolic causes include inborn errors of metabolism;
- unknown cause: the nature of the underlying cause is as yet unknown; it may have a fundamental genetic defect at its core as yet undetermined or it may be the consequence of a separate as-yet-unrecognized disorder.

Epileptic encephalopathy refers to a condition where worsening of the child's development is thought to be related to ongoing epilepsy. This needs to be delineated from neurodevelopmental regression independent of the epilepsy because of the natural course of an underlying disorder.

Epilepsy syndromes are clinical entities that can reliably be identified by a cluster of electroclinical characteristics: seizure type(s), age at onset, family history of epilepsy, and EEG features.

Epileptic seizures

Seizure classification
Epileptic seizures can be classified as generalized or focal on grounds of the appearance of the seizure onset. Table 16.1 summarizes the classification of seizures.

Table 16.1 Classification of seizures

Generalized seizures
    Tonic-clonic (in any combination)
    Absence
        Typical
        Atypical
        Absence with special features
            ● Myoclonic absence
            ● Eyelid myoclonia
    Myoclonic
            ● Myoclonic
            ● Myoclonic atonic
            ● Myoclonic tonic
    Clonic
    Tonic
    Atonic
Focal seizures
Unknown
        ● Epileptic spasms

Generalized epileptic seizures are conceptualized as originating at some point within, and rapidly engaging, bilaterally distributed networks. Such bilateral networks can include cortical and subcortical structures, but do not necessarily include the entire cortex.

Focal epileptic seizures are conceptualized as originating within networks limited to one hemisphere. They may be discretely localized or more widely distributed. Focal seizures may originate in subcortical structures. Typical descriptors for focal seizures include the following:

- without impairment of consciousness or awareness:
  - ○ with observable motor or autonomic components (focal motor and autonomic seizures),
  - ○ involving subjective sensory or psychic phenomena only (aura);
- with impairment of consciousness or awareness (complex partial seizures); and
- evolving to a bilateral, convulsive seizure involving tonic, clonic or tonic and clonic components (secondarily generalized seizures).

Epileptic spasms are brief phenomena characterized by abrupt onset of head and arm jerks, both flexor and extensor lasting 0.2–2 s, often occurring in clusters. Spasms last longer than myoclonic jerks, but are shorter than tonic seizures.

Typical phenomena that can be observed during seizures according to the International League Against Epilepsy (ILAE) glossary of descriptive terminology for seizure semiology are shown in Table 16.2.

Table 16.2 Typical phenomena that can be observed during seizures

Term	Description
Motor	Involves musculature in any form. The motor event could consist of an increase (positive) or decrease (negative) in muscle contraction to produce a movement.
Elementary motor	A single type of contraction of a muscle or group of muscles that is usually stereotyped and not decomposable into phases.
Tonic	A sustained increase in muscle contraction lasting a few seconds to minutes
Postural	Adoption of a posture which may be bilaterally symmetrical or asymmetrical (as in a 'fencing posture').
Versive	A sustained, forced conjugate ocular, cephalic and/or truncal rotation or lateral deviation from the midline.
Dystonic	Sustained contractions of both agonist and antagonist muscles producing athetoid or twisting movements which when prolonged may produce abnormal postures.
Myoclonus	Sudden, brief (<100 ms) involuntary single or multiple contraction(s) of muscles(s) or muscle groups of variable topography (axial, proximal limb, distal).
Clonus	Myoclonus which is regularly repetitive, involves the same muscle groups, at a frequency of about 2–3/s, and is prolonged.
Tonic-clonic	A sequence consisting of a tonic followed by a clonic phase. Variants such as clonic-tonic-clonic may be seen.
Atonic	Sudden loss or diminution of muscle tone without apparent preceding myoclonic or tonic event lasting 1–2 s or more, involving head, trunk, jaw or limb musculature.
Astatic	Loss of erect posture that results from an atonic, myoclonic or tonic mechanism. Synonym: drop attack.
Automatism	A more or less coordinated, repetitive, motor activity usually occurring when cognition is impaired and for which the subject is usually amnesic afterwards. This often resembles a voluntary movement, and may consist of inappropriate continuation of ongoing pre-ictal motor activity.

Table 16.2 *Continued*

Term	Description
Hyperkinetic	Involves predominantly proximal limb or axial muscles producing irregular sequential ballistic movements, such as pedalling, pelvic thrashing, rocking movements. Increase in rate of ongoing movements or inappropriately rapid performance of a movement.
Hypokinetic	A decrease in amplitude and/or rate or arrest of ongoing motor activity.
Adapted from Blume et al. (2001).	

Clinical approach to an infant presenting with a first seizure

QUESTIONS TO BE ASKED

Was the seizure epileptic or does the infant suffer from a non-epileptic paroxysmal disorder (see Chapter 17 in this volume)?

Was the seizure possibly provoked by an acute illness, such as febrile illness or infection?

Is there evidence for an underlying chronic illness?

Is the child in stable condition following the seizure?

EXAMINATIONS ALWAYS INDICATED FOLLOWING A FIRST NON-FEBRILE SEIZURE

- Blood pressure
- Finger-prick blood test to exclude hypoglycaemia if the child is drowsy after the seizure.

EXAMINATIONS THAT MAY BE INDICATED FOLLOWING A FIRST NON-FEBRILE SEIZURE

To exclude central nervous system (CNS) infection, perform lumbar puncture, including cerebro spinal fluid (CSF) cell count and differential cell count, glucose, lactate, protein, herpes simplex virus polymerase chain reaction (PCR; always in infants with focal seizures) and bacterial culture. To exclude electrolyte disturbance, measure plasma concentrations of sodium, calcium and magnesium and if abnormal assess the likely cause in the context of the wider electrolyte and clinical picture.

IMAGING STUDIES

Such studies are usually *not* indicated following a first seizure if the child subsequently is well unless there is evidence for trauma or haemorrhaging, or the child had a first non-febrile seizure with focal signs.

EEG

EEG is usually indicated following a first non-febrile seizure, whereas EEG is usually *not* indicated following a first simple febrile seizure (see Figures 16.1 and 16.2).

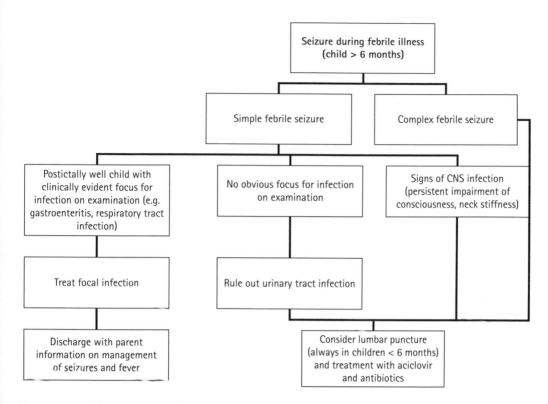

Figure 16.1 Management of the child following a first seizure during a febrile illness. CNS, central nervous system.

Febrile seizures

Febrile seizures are age-related events affecting approximately 3% of children between the age of 6 months and 5 years. It is important to characterize a febrile seizure as either simple or complex because complex febrile seizures are associated with a less good prognosis than simple febrile seizures.

Criteria for simple febrile seizures include the following:

- generalized tonic clonic seizure
- duration of less than 15 min
- no recurrence within the next 24 h
- no underlying neurological illness
- no focal features during or after seizures (approximately 30% of febrile seizures are focal).

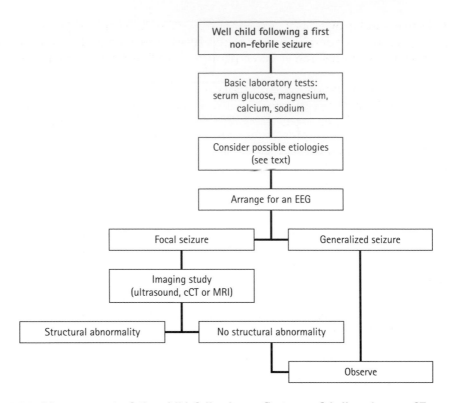

Figure 16.2 Management of the child following a first non-febrile seizure. cCT, cranial computed tomography; MRI, magnetic resonance imaging.

Criteria for complex febrile seizures include the following:

- prolonged seizures lasting 15 min or more
- repetitive febrile seizures in clusters (two or more within 24 h)
- seizures with focal features at onset or after the event
- seizures occurring in children with underlying neurological illnesses, such as cerebral palsy or developmental delay.

Most febrile seizures are brief, lasting 3–6 min. However, in 8% they are longer than 15 min and may progress to febrile status epilepticus. Children with febrile status show an increased risk of developing epilepsy. Recurrences of simple febrile seizures occur in 30–50% of cases. They are more common in those with a first-degree relative who has had febrile seizures and in those with a first febrile seizure under 1 year of age. A complex febrile seizure is a risk factor for the subsequent development of epilepsy. The overall risk for epilepsy developing after a febrile seizure is 3%. Whereas it is only 1–2% in infants who experience a simple febrile seizure, it increases to 15% in children having complex febrile seizures, according to how many and which risk factors they carry.

The intellectual and behavioural outcome following febrile seizures is good. The subsequent psychomotor development of children who were normal prior to the onset of febrile seizures is normal and children perform as well as other children at school.

ACUTE MANAGEMENT OF AN INFANT WITH A FEBRILE SEIZURE

Long-lasting febrile seizures (>10 min) are a medical emergency. If a febrile seizure has lasted longer than 5 min, emergency services should be called and pharmacological treatment should be given in the form of either rectal diazepam (5 mg for children <12 kg, 10 mg for children ≥12 kg) or buccal midazolam (2.5 mg at age 6–12 months or 5 mg at 1–5 years) or, if in the hospital, intravenous benzodiazepines. Additionally, antipyretics should be given.

PREVENTING RECURRENCE OF FEBRILE SEIZURES AND MANAGEMENT OF RECURRENCES

Antipyretic therapy in infants with a history of febrile seizures does not reduce the recurrence risk. Therefore, antipyretic therapy should be used as in children without history of febrile seizures to comfort the child and help avoid dehydration. Continuous prophylactic treatment with antiepileptic medication is not recommended for children with febrile seizures. Intermittent prophylactic treatment at the time of a febrile illness with oral diazepam (0.3 mg/kg) may, in rare cases, be indicated if the parents are exceedingly worried. In case of a further febrile seizure, parents should be advised to:

- place the infant on their side or stomach,
- give rectal diazepam (5 mg for children <12 kg, 10 mg for children ≥12 kg) if the febrile seizure has not ceased within 5 min, and
- call for professional medical assistance if this does not stop the seizure or the child does not fully regain consciousness.

OTHER SITUATION-RELATED SEIZURES

Seizures may also occur in relation to central-nervous (CNS) system metabolic disorders, trauma and infections (see Chapters 9 and 13–15). In all these situations the infant will usually show signs of an underlying acute illness before the seizure, suffer serial seizures or not recover completely following the seizure.

STATUS EPILEPTICUS

Since any seizure type can progress to status epilepticus, a wide range of clinical symptoms can be observed. Clinically it is important to distinguish convulsive from nonconvulsive status epilepticus (NCSE). Convulsive status epilepticus (CSE) is defined as either a seizure lasting for more than 30 min, or as two or more convulsions without complete recovery of conciousness in between. It is a life-threatening emergency. In population-based studies the incidence of CSE has been calculated as 14.5/100 000/year. Outcome, including mortality, further episodes of CSE, development of epilepsy and neurodevelopment, strongly depends on the etiology. It is reassuring that, in a recent population-based study, all deaths occurring in status epilepticus could be attributed to severe underlying diseases (meningitis, neurodegenerative disorders; Chin et al., 2008). Nevertheless, CSE requires vigorous diagnostic work-up and pharmacological treatment.

CSE can occur in the context of a febrile illness or without fever. In febrile CSE, it is important to exclude central nervous system (CNS) infection before CSE can be attributed to a prolonged febrile seizure. Differential diagnosis of afebrile CSE includes

- acute electrolyte imbalance, including hypoglycaemia, hypocalcemia and hypomagnesemia,
- acute head injury,
- intracranial haemorrhage,
- cerebrovascular insult,
- drug overdose,
- intoxication,
- hypoxia,
- seizures secondary to pre-existing neurological abnormality, including CNS malformation, previous brain injury and cerebral palsy,
- metabolic diseases, or
- epilepsy-related.

Diagnostic work-up in an infant with new-onset CSE should always include serum electrolytes, blood sugar, EEG, imaging (computed tomography or magnetic resonance imaging), a lumbar puncture if there are signs of infection and urine toxicology if there is a possibility of intoxication. In an infant with previously known epilepsy, diagnostic work-up should include levels of antiepileptic drugs, electrolytes and EEG. Additionally, the possibility of an acute infectious disorder causing CSE independently of the previously known epilepsy needs to be considered.

Various treatment protocols have been suggested for CSE and a treatment algorithm is given in Figure 16.3. Generally, benzodiazepines are used as first-line drugs. In the pre-hospital setting, either rectal diazepam or buccal midazolam is used. In hospital, treatment should be continued via intravenous access and, as initial treatment, a second dose of benzodiazepines is suggested. Lorazepam has been shown to be more effective in terminating the seizure than other benzodiazepines. Most treatment protocols suggest observation periods of 10 min between medications. A maximum of two doses of benzodiazepines should be given prior to the next stage. Second-line medications then include phenobarbital, phenytoin and sodium valproate. In children with a history suggestive of Dravet syndrome, phenytoin should *not* be used, because its action on sodium channels can result in a worsening of the epileptic condition. Caution should also be exercised with sodium valproate if a metabolic disorder is suspected. If the second-line medication is not successful, the infant needs to be transferred to an intensive care unit and further management may include thiopental or midazolam.

NCSE is characterized by a cognitive or behavioural change (ranging from mild confusion to coma) coupled with evidence of seizure activity on EEG that has changed

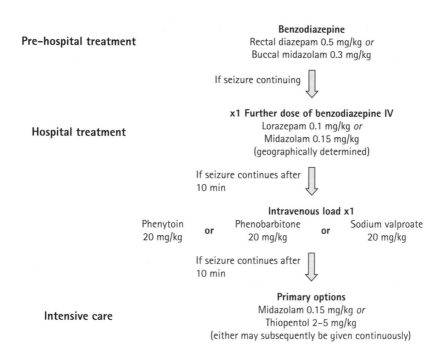

Pre-hospital treatment

Benzodiazepine
Rectal diazepam 0.5 mg/kg *or*
Buccal midazolam 0.3 mg/kg

If seizure continuing

Hospital treatment

x1 Further dose of benzodiazepine IV
Lorazepam 0.1 mg/kg *or*
Midazolam 0.15 mg/kg
(geographically determined)

If seizure continues after 10 min

Intravenous load x1

Phenytoin 20 mg/kg   **or**   Phenobarbitone 20 mg/kg   **or**   Sodium valproate 20 mg/kg

If seizure continues after 10 min

Intensive care

Primary options
Midazolam 0.15 mg/kg *or*
Thiopentol 2–5 mg/kg
(either may subsequently be given continuously)

Figure 16.3 Treatment algorithm for convulsive status epilepticus.

from baseline. It can be either generalized, i.e. absence status epilepticus, or focal. It is extremely uncommon in the first year of life, but may occur in the context of genetic or structural epilepsies, or underlying metabolic encephalopathies. Therefore, diagnostic work-up should include metabolic evaluation and treatment should focus on possible treatment of any underlying disorder in addition to antiepileptic drugs. Whether successful treatment of NCSE will result in improved developmental outcome is unclear.

Epilepsies with onset in the first year of life

The incidence of epilepsy is age-specific, being highest in young children and elderly people. During the first year of life, the incidence is around 150/100 000. Epilepsy syndromes are also age-specific. The seizure type and epilepsy may be more dependent on the child's age than on the underlying pathology.

Most causes of neonatal seizures can also cause epilepsy in infancy and therefore causes of neonatal seizures must continue to be considered in infants older than 28 days. Late presentations of pyridoxine-dependent epilepsy and pyridoxal phosphate-dependent epilepsy do occur.

Clinical approach to an infant with epilepsy

QUESTIONS TO BE ASKED

Can the seizure type be clearly described?

At what age did seizures start?

Is there a family history for epilepsy?

Was there anything remarkable during pregnancy, birth or the immediate postnatal period?

Was the infant's development normal until the manifestation of the epilepsy?

Do the seizures affect the infant's development?

PHYSICAL EXAMINATION SHOULD ESPECIALLY INCLUDE

● Measurement and determination of percentiles for body length, weight and head circumference

● Cutaneous abnormalities, especially hypo- or hyperpigmented areas; check for areas of hypopigmentation using Woods light (ultraviolet light with a wavelength of approximately 365 nm)

● External abnormalities including external genitalia

● Hepato- or splenomegaly

● Neurological examination and developmental assessment

● Eye-movement disorder.

DIAGNOSTIC PROCEDURES MUST INCLUDE

● EEG, preferably also sleep EEG

● Ophthalmologic examination of the retina (fundus)

● Magnetic resonance imaging, unless the underlying pathology is known

● Metabolic work-up, unless the underlying pathology is known

METABOLIC WORK-UP MAY, IN SELECTED CASES SHOULD INCLUDE

● Blood gas analysis

● Serum glucose and lactate

● Plasma amino acids, plasma homocysteine

● Acyl carnitine profile

● Plasma very-long-chain fatty acids

● Urinary organic acids and oligosaccharides.

If late-onset vitamin-B6-dependent epilepsy is considered

● Plasma pipecolic acid

● Urinary alpha-aminoadipic semialdehyde

● CSF protein, glucose and lactate, amino acids, neurotransmitters, folates, pterines.

Epilepsies with onset during the neonatal period or early infancy

The 2010 ILAE report (Berg et al., 2010) differentiates syndromes by age at onset. Electroclinical syndromes with onset during the neonatal period include benign familial neonatal seizures (or BFNS), early myoclonic encephalopathy (EME) and early infantile epileptic encephalopathy (EIEE; Ohtahara syndrome). Seizures in BFNS are limited to the neonatal period, and this is discussed in Chapter 13. EME and EIEE are further discussed here as the impact of the seizures in these conditions is protracted throughout infancy.

EIEE (Ohtahara syndrome)

Children typically present during the first weeks of life with tonic epileptic spasms and other seizures including partial and myoclonic seizures. EEG shows a suppression-burst pattern during wakefulness and sleep. Infants usually become inactive and floppy, and they do not show developmental progress. During the course of the disease, infants usually show severe neurological abnormalities such as a cerebral palsy. EIEE is often associated with cortical malformation or structural brain damage. Rarely, underlying metabolic etiologies may be identified. More recently genetic causes have been described. The epilepsy usually does not respond to antiepileptic treatment and in about 75% it evolves into West syndrome between 2 and 6 months of age.

EME

As with EIEE, seizures may start during the first weeks of life. However, the predominant seizure type is erratic myoclonia, which may be both epileptic and non-epileptic. The EEG also shows a suppression-burst pattern. In contrast to EIEE, underlying metabolic disorders are often identified, especially nonketotic hyperglycinaemia and other amino acid disorders. The clinical course of the disorder is severe, with infants developing neurological abnormalities and developmental arrest. Antiepileptic treatment usually is not effective.

Epilepsies with onset in infancy

The following epileptic syndromes typically start during infancy.

West syndrome

West syndrome is an age-related epileptic encephalopathy affecting children between the ages of 3 and 24 months characterized by a specific seizure type referred to as epileptic spasms. Children usually present with the abrupt onset of head and arm jerks, both flexor and extensor, lasting 0.2–2 s. A clustering of spasms is often seen and may especially occur after sleep/wake transition. The infant may become upset and cry during the events which appear to impair consciousness only briefly. Most infants subsequently show developmental impairments. The diagnosis of West syndrome is confirmed by EEG showing hypsarrhythmia (high-voltage, chaotic and asynchronous pattern with multifocal epileptiform discharges) but this may be present only in an EEG recording made when the child is asleep. West syndrome is seen with many underlying etiologies and associated conditions, including those listed in Table 16.3.

Table 16.3 Underlying etiologies and associated conditions seen in West syndrome

Genetic
    Chromosomal abnormalities (trisomy 21)
    X-linked disorders (e.g. ARX, CDKL5)
Structural
    Hypoxic ischaemic encephalopathy
    Congenital infections
    Trauma
    Disturbed brain development with malformations related to
        abnormal proliferation of neurons of glia
        abnormal neuronal migration
        abnormal cortical organization
    Neurocutaneous disorders
    Intracranial haemorrhage
    Infection
Metabolic
    Pyridoxine dependency
    Nonketotic hyperglycinaemia
    Peroxisomal disorders
    Amino acid disorders, especially untreated phenylketonuria
    Organic acid disorders, especially glutaric acidaemia type 1
    Biotinidase deficiency
    Mitochondrial disorders

ARX, aristaless-related homeobox; CDKL5, cyclin-dependent kinase-like 5.

Investigations need to be directed to exclude any specifically treatable disorder as soon as possible. These include especially some metabolic diseases or intoxications. Prognosis of West syndrome mainly depends on the etiology, but there is also evidence that rapid recognition and control of seizures will improve outcome.

If no specifically treatable disorder can be identified then treatment of West syndrome can be attempted with hormonal therapy (adrenocorticotropic hormone or oral prednisolone) or vigabatrin. Hormonal therapy has a higher success rate but vigabatrin seems to be especially effective in patients with tuberous sclerosis.

Benign infantile familial and non-familial seizures
Benign familial infantile seizures clinically are characterized by clusters of seizures with an age at onset of 3–20 months (peak 5–6 months). Seizures are usually brief and predominantly focal with motor arrest, impairment of consciousness, staring and automatisms. Between the seizures the infants behave normally. The EEG will show

abnormalities only during a seizure; the inter-ictal EEG is normal. Patients respond extremely well to low dosages of carbamazepine, valproate or phenobarbitone, which can be withdrawn after 1 year.

Dravet syndrome (synonym: severe myoclonic epilepsy in infancy)
This is an epilepsy syndrome of lifelong duration with onset in early infancy. Clinically it is characterized by three stages:

1. Infants develop normally until early-onset febrile seizures occur mostly between 3 and 12 months, often febrile status epilepticus. Fever after vaccinations may trigger seizures but this does not alter the natural history of the condition (McIntosh et al., 2010).
2. Subsequently, with a peak age at onset of 12 months, they develop febrile and non-febrile clonic seizures, myoclonic seizures, atypical absences with some impairment of consciousness often accompanied by myoclonic jerks and head drops, and complex focal seizures. Status epilepticus is common. Children show impairment of cognitive function and ataxia.
3. Later children show intellectual disability, and often tonic-clonic seizures persist.

In about 80% of infants with Dravet syndrome, mutations of a gene encoding a sodium-channel protein (*SCN1A*) can be found. This is very important because many antiepileptic drugs act by inhibiting the function of sodium channels. These drugs (phenytoin, carbamazepine, oxcarbazepine and lamotrigine) must not be used in patients with seizures suggestive of Dravet syndrome because they may aggravate seizures, promote status epilepticus and worsen developmental outcome.

Myoclonic epilepsy in infancy
This is an age-specific epilepsy presenting in infancy. It is characterized by brief myoclonic jerks affecting head, eyeballs, upper extremities and the diaphragms. Jerks can be single or clustered and may be elicited by tactile or acoustic stimuli. Consciousness is usually not disturbed. The inter-ictal EEG is usually normal, and the ictal EEG may show generalized spikes or polyspikes. Whereas the myoclonic seizures usually remit during early childhood, 10–20% of children may show generalized tonic-clonic seizures later. Antiepileptic treatment with valproate or levetiracetam is usually effective.

Migrating partial seizures of infancy
This is a rare disorder usually starting within the first months of life. Children present with unprovoked seizures showing both motor and autonomic symptoms occurring in clusters. Seizures are characterized by 'migration' of the focality +/– the EEG during the seizure. Secondarily generalized seizures are common. It is important to recognize this disorder because of the extremely poor prognosis. Regardless of treatment, children go on to show a wide spectrum of seizure types and developmental regression. It is not yet clear whether this condition arises from one or from several different causes.

Treatment options for epilepsy in the first year of life

Medical treatment

Infants with epilepsy will usually require medical treatment. Treatment with antiepileptic drugs should be considered after a second epileptic seizure. If a structural (e.g. hydrocephalus) or metabolic (e.g. phenylketonuria) cause for the epilepsy can be identified, this needs to be treated appropriately. If the cause for epilepsy is genetic or unknown, or if causative treatment of a structural or metabolic epilepsy is not possible or unlikely to be successful, antiepileptic treatment should be initiated. Valproate should be avoided when an underlying metabolic cause remains likely. Therapeutic principles are summarized in Table 16.4.

Table 16.4 Therapeutic principles of the treatment of epilepsy

Epilepsy or epileptic syndrome	First-line treatment	Second-line treatment	Comments
Structural	CBZ, OXC	LTG, VPA, corticosteroids	
Metabolic			Treatment generally according to the underlying cause
West syndrome	Prednisolone/ACTH or VGB (first choice in patients with tuberous sclerosis)	VGB or corticosteroids	
Benign infantile familial and non-familial seizures	CBZ, OXC	PB	Treatment may be stopped at age 1 year
Dravet syndrome	VPA	Clobazam, Stiripentol	Avoid CBZ, OXC, LTG, PHT
Myoclonic epilepsy in infancy	VPA, Levetiracetam		Treatment may be stopped after 1 year
Migrating partial seizures of infancy	VPA, Levetiracetam		Treatment usually ineffective

ACTH, adrenocorticotropic hormone; CBZ, carbamazepine; LTG, lamotrigine; OXC, oxcarbazepine; PB, phenobarbitone; PHT, phenytoin; VGB, vigabatrin; VPA, valproate.

Surgical treatment
Surgery is an option for infants who suffer from epilepsy as the result of a unilateral structural abnormality. All infants with a unilateral structural abnormality should be referred for surgical assessment where available regardless of response to treatment in view of the high risk of relapse and consequence of seizures on neurodevelopmental progress. However, at the very least it should be considered when two drugs have been tried without achieving freedom of seizures, especially if there is evidence of West syndrome or another epileptic encephalopathy.

Alternative therapies
A ketogenic diet may be an option for infants who do not respond to first- or second-line medical treatment and in whom surgical treatment is not an option. Because of the possible side effects and risks, especially in children with underlying metabolic disorders, its use should be restricted to specialized units.

Reference

Berg AT et al. Revised terminology and concepts for organization of seizures and epilepsies: report of the ILAE Commission on Classification and Terminology, 2005–2009. *Epilepsia*, 2010, 51(4):676–685.

Blume WT et al. Glossary of descriptive terminology for ictal semiology: report of the ILAE task force on classification and terminology. *Epilepsia*, 2001, 42(9):1212–1218.

Chin RFM, Neville BGR, Peckham C et al. Treatment of community-onset, childhood convulsive status epilepticus: a prospective, population-based study. *Lancet Neurology*, 2008; 7:696–703 [erratum *Lancet Neurology*, 7:771, 2008; Note: dosage error in text].

McIntosh AM, McMahon J, Dibbens LM et al. Effects of vaccination on onset and outcome of Dravet syndrome: retrospective study. *Lancet Neurology*, 2010; 9:592–598.

Resources

Eltze C, Cross JH. Treatment of the neonate or infant with catastrophic epilepsy. In *Therapeutic strategies in epilepsy*, French J, Delanty N (eds). Oxford, Clinical Publishing, 2009, pp. 63–83.

Kossoff EH et al., and Charlie Foundation, and the Practice Committee of the Child Neurology Society. Optimal clinical management of children receiving the ketogenic diet: recommendations of the international ketogenic diet study group. *Epilepsia*, 2009, 50:304–317.

Lux AL et al. The United Kingdom Infantile Spasms Study comparing vigabatrin with prednisolone or tetracosactide at 14 days: a multicentre, randomised controlled trial. *Lancet*, 2004, 364(9447):1773–1778.

Lux AL et al., and United Kingdom Infantile Spasms Study. The United Kingdom Infantile Spasms Study (UKISS) comparing hormone treatment with vigabatrin on developmental and epilepsy outcomes to age 14 months: a multicentre randomised trial. *Lancet Neurology*, 2005, 4(11):712–717.

Panayiotopoulos CP. *The epilepsies: Seizures, syndromes and management*. Chipping Norton, Bladon Medical Publishing, 2005.

Roger J et al. (eds) *Epileptic syndromes in infancy, childhood and adolescence*, 4th edn. New Barnet, John Libbey, 2005.

Yoong M, Chin RFM, Scott RC. Management of convulsive status epilepticus in children. *Arch Dis Child Educ Pract Ed*, 2009, 94:1–9.

Chapter 17

Non-epileptic paroxysmal disorders in infancy

John B.P. Stephenson and Alla Nechay

Key messages

- Most paroxysmal events are non-epileptic.
- Most – but not all – are benign.
- Precise description and a video of events are of most value for correct diagnosis.
- Most do not require medications of any kind.
- Psychological support and comforting of the family is the main treatment.

Common errors

- To use electroencephalography between episodes to decide whether it is epilepsy.
- To give antiepileptic medications ('anticonvulsants') without being certain that the infant has epilepsy.
- To give other 'brain medicines' of no proven value.

When to worry

- Suspicion that the intracranial pressure might be high.
- Episodes of stiffness with startle (hyperekplexia).
- All episodes occur when only the mother is present.
- *Note*: all these are rare.

Breath-holding spells (prolonged expiratory apnoea)

Definition
An episode in response to pain or annoyance that begins with grunting expiration followed rapidly by deep cyanosis with loss of consciousness and rigid extension. After an inspiratory groan the infant or toddler is briefly dazed and usually cries on regaining consciousness. In English this is usually called a cyanotic breath-holding spell (or CBHS).

Clinical approach
If there are jerks or non-epileptic spasms they are irregular. The diagnosis is made from the clinical history. It may be difficult to distinguish this type of reflex syncope from reflex anoxic seizures/reflex asystolic syncope but this distinction is not important. What is important is *not* to diagnose epilepsy: epileptic seizures are never directly provoked by discomfort or frustration.

Note: when we talk about anoxic seizures we mean events that look like epileptic seizures but are due to lack of oxygen or oxygenated blood going to the brain. By contrast, epileptic seizures occur when there is sudden excessive hyper-synchronous neuronal activity. So, in an anoxic seizure due to syncope cerebral activity is markedly reduced, whereas in an epileptic seizure cerebral activity is markedly increased.

Management
Reassurance that episodes will terminate spontaneously is most important. Parents are often very frightened by what they see and need support. No medications or other treatments are of any value. Remission usually occurs before school age.

Reflex anoxic seizures (or reflex asystolic syncope)

Definition
An episode of stiffening and loss of consciousness in response to pain or surprise, especially an unexpected bump on the head, assumed to be due to reflex arrest of cardiac action, that is to say reflex asystole.

Clinical approach
Episodes of reflex anoxic seizure resemble episodes of cyanotic breath-holding except that there is no more than mild cyanosis, and the latency between the stimulus (pain or surprise) is shorter, maybe only 10 s. The child is often described as going grey or looking as if they had died.

Management
If there is any concern that there might be a long QT syndrome it is wise to obtain a 12-lead ECG to confirm that the QT interval corrected for heart rate (QTc) is normal. Reassurance about the excellent prognosis is the keystone to management.

Anoxic-epileptic seizures without epilepsy

Definition
Anoxic-epileptic seizure (AES) is a rare sequence of two paroxysmal events when a true epileptic seizure follows a triggering non-epileptic syncope. In most cases the trigger for the true epileptic seizures is neurally mediated syncope with either reflex asystole (reflex anoxic seizures) or prolonged expiratory apnoea (cyanotic breath-holding spells).

Clinical approach
The duration of the triggering syncope (the anoxic seizure) is usually less than 30 seconds. The resultant epileptic seizure usually lasts more than 2 minutes (sometimes up to 40 min). In the majority of cases the triggered epileptic seizures are reported as clonic. Sometimes the epileptic component resembles a myoclonic absence. Syncope-triggered epileptic seizures are easily distinguished from the much more common anoxic seizures:

- AES are long, many minutes rather than less than 1 min in duration, and
- the jerks in AES are rhythmic rather than irregular.

The syncopes and epileptic component typically remit in preschool years and are not usually associated with learning disability.

Most children with AES do not have epilepsy, that is, their epileptic seizures are only provoked by syncopes. Any individual with AES has, mostly, simple syncopes leading only to anoxic seizures, and only a minority of syncopes trigger epileptic seizures.

Management
Because AES are uncommon in most affected children, rescue medication, such as a benzodiazepine, is commonly sufficient to abort the epileptic component.

Tonic attacks with acutely raised intracranial pressure
Synonyms include extensor posturing (e.g. in meningitis, encephalitis, hydrocephalus).

Definition
Although clonic epileptic seizures (with rhythmic jerking) may occur in infections of the central nervous system or acute hydrocephalus, it is important to recognize tonic attacks in which there is stiffening in extension because these usually indicate dangerously high intracranial pressure.

Clinical approach
It can be argued that lumbar puncture is contra-indicated in this situation but that is debatable. What seems important is not to give antiepileptic drugs, in particular not to give rectal or intravenous diazepam.

Management
It is wise to avoid antiepileptic drugs such as diazepam, treat the infection, consider mannitol and perhaps other ways of safely lowering intracranial pressure.

Imposed upper airways obstruction

Definition
Episodes covertly induced by the mother by occluding the infant's airway (synonym: smothering). Only rarely is the father the perpetrator.

Clinical approach
The mother presents as a very caring competent concerned parent. Episodes always begin in her presence and the onset is never observed by others, but the mother shows the limp pale cyanosed infant to neighbours or friends or nurses or doctors. She often becomes skilled at cardiopulmonary resuscitation. The diagnosis depends on an absolutely exact history. It may be very difficult as no one else sees the suffocation by hand, pillow, cling-film, or by pressing the infant's face against the mother's bosom. If the infant is in hospital and nurses are charting episodes it is essential to determine whether what is written on the 'seizure chart' is a direct observation of the nurse or a transcription of what the mother has told the nurse. This disorder may be regarded as a dangerous form of fabricated or induced illness by carers.

Management
If the mother is separated from the infant or *constantly* observed, the episodes will cease. Multi-disciplinary assessment may well recommend involvement of psychiatry, social and specialist police services (see Chapter 14 on inflicted traumatic brain injury).

Alternating hemiplegia of childhood

Definition
Alternating hemiplegia of childhood (AHC) is a disease of early childhood, typically presenting with attacks of hemiplegia of one or another side or bilaterally symmetrical. Hemiplegias usually start at 6–18 months of age, usually accompanied by autonomic phenomena, but stiffening (tonic episodes) and bouts of nystagmus (which may be unilateral) commonly begin in the neonatal period or soon after.

Clinical approach
Paroxysms of hemiplegia and/or tetraplegia happen once or twice per week, and may be accompanied by tonic or dystonic episodes, disorders of eye movements (episodic strabismus, monocular nystagmus), choreoathetosis, crying and autonomic presentations. Episodes always disappear with sleep and are absent after awaking. Non-epileptic symptoms in children with AHC include developmental impairment, muscular hypotonia, choreoathetosis and ataxia. Hot and warm baths, strong emotions and physical fatigue may provoke attacks of AHC. Usually the disease progresses, at

least during initial period. Etiology of AHC is not defined so far, but vascular, metabolic and congenital mechanisms (channelopathies) may play a role in mechanism of development of the disease. Special investigations are not informative, but if moyamoya is thought possible then brain magnetic resonance imaging (with or without magnetic resonance angiography) will be necessary.

Differential diagnosis

- Partial epilepsy with Todd paresis
- Hemiplegic migraine
- Paroxysmal dyskinesia
- Mitochondrial encephalomyopathy, lactic acidosis and stroke-like episodes (MELAS)
- Vascular abnormalities (including moyamoya).

Management

Blockers of calcium channels (flunarizine) may be effective in prophylaxis of attacks of AHC. Benzodiazepines may be effective in aborting of attacks of AHC and reduce the frequency of events. Limitation of provoking factors is recommended.

Hyperekplexia

Definition

Hyperekplexia is a rare disorder in which there is excessive startle. In the neonatal period the infant is both stiff and easily startled, with excessive brainstem reflexes including a positive nose-tap test.

Clinical approach

Hyperekplexia is easy to overdiagnose as all normal infants may show startle. If there is a positive family history of dominantly inherited startle with sudden falls then the diagnosis is not too difficult. With no family history one has to be very careful and precise. Affected newborns not only startle excessively to sounds but have prominent head-retraction reflex on tapping the tip of the nose, immediately followed by a flexor spasm. This response to nose tap does not habituate, so that repeated nose taps elicit repeated head retraction and flexor spasms. A dangerous complication is severe apnoeic syncope (accompanied by severe quivering stiffness) that may be fatal if untreated.

Management

If possible, DNA should be obtained for analysis of the hyperekplexia genes. Medical staff, nurses and parents should be taught the Vigevano manoeuvre: if the infant becomes stiff and apnoeic, he or she is flexed by bringing the head towards the feet. Oral clonazepam is usually helpful, but the condition often spontaneously improves later in the first year.

Benign neonatal sleep myoclonus

Definition
Flurries of myoclonia that only occur during sleep with onset in the neonatal period, usually between day 1 and day 16.

Clinical approach
Benign neonatal sleep myoclonus (BNSM) is a common condition occurring in perhaps 2% of the general population and in nearly 70% of infants of opioid-dependent mothers. The only harm that may come to the infant is if a diagnosis of epilepsy is wrongly made: if antiepileptic drugs are given the myoclonus worsens and intensive care may be needed. It is thus most important that all doctors who deal with newborns are very familiar with BNSM, and preferably have seen videos of the condition.

The myoclonus appears as flurries of myoclonia affecting the limbs (though rarely the face also). The flurries last no more than 0.5 s and to the casual observer look like a single jerk. Bouts of jerking may continue for up to 30 min or more, but cease if the infant wakes up or is made to wake up. They may be triggered by rocking the infant.

Management
No investigations are required. In particular an electroencephalogram is not indicated nor any type of brain scan or blood test. No antiepileptic drugs ('anticonvulsants') must ever be given. The parents should be reassured that the jerkings are harmless and will probably cease by age 3 months (rarely up to 10 months or so).

Fejerman syndrome: shuddering, benign non-epileptic infantile spasms, benign myoclonus of early infancy

Definition
Isolated or repeated movements involving the upper limbs that may be shudders, spasms or jerks or even loss of tone, of *non*-epileptic nature.

Clinical approach
The history will be of a normally developing infant having sudden movements of the upper limbs and upper body that may occur singly or occur in clusters. These movements may be shudders (resembling a shiver) or spasms (resembling epileptic infantile spasms) or jerks (that look like myoclonus). Sometimes there is loss of tone (as in negative myoclonus or an astatic epileptic seizure). The infant is not disturbed by these events (which only occur in the awake state) and if there is a series or cluster, the cluster terminates if the infant is distracted. No developmental regression occurs and after a while – perhaps some months – episodes cease.

Management
No investigations are usually required, but home video – for instance using a mobile phone – may be very helpful to clarify the diagnosis. An additional value of a home

video is that it may be shown to a more experienced paediatric neurologist to confirm your impression.

Infantile masturbation/gratification

Definition
Rhythmic repetitive lower limb movements, in particular thigh adduction, accompanied by a 'distant' or absorbed facial appearance.

Clinical approach
Infantile masturbation is highlighted because it has been often mistaken for epilepsy due to usual presentation with paroxysmal movements of recurrent character. Infantile masturbation can also mimic other conditions such as abdominal pain, paroxysmal dystonia and dyskinesia. Masturbatory activity in infant and young children is difficult to recognize because it has a spectrum of different behaviour patterns which often do not involve manual stimulation of the genitalia. Misdiagnosis consequently might lead to unnecessary investigations and treatment. The condition is more often seen in girls than in boys. Usually it starts at age under 1 year of life. Episodes are often observed when the child is sitting in a car seat, when he/she is bored or tired and in relation to sleeping. During the events of masturbation, children exhibit different types of behaviour: dystonia-like posturing of different parts of the body, grunting, flushing and sweating; rocking could also be observed in these children. Episodes may last from several seconds up to several hours, sometimes many times per day. Children never lose consciousness during the events and can be distracted from the activity by parents, although sometimes unwillingly. Careful history-taking is very important key to the diagnosis.

Management
Home-video recording is of most help in understanding the nature of the episodes and extremely important for prevention of unnecessary investigation and treatment of these children. Parents prefer the term gratification (or even benign idiopathic infantile dyskinesia) to infantile masturbation as there is less social stigma attached to these terms. It is debatable whether these episodes, which involve predominantly the lower limbs rather than the upper limbs, are different in nature from Fejerman syndrome.

Paroxysmal torticollis

Definition
Paroxysmal torticollis of infancy is a benign disorder characterized by recurrent and transient episodes of cervical dystonia of unknown etiology.

Clinical approach
Attacks of head tilt to one or other side are often accompanied by vomiting, pallor, ataxia and irritability, settling spontaneously within hours or days. The disorder, which disappears within the first few years of life, is often misinterpreted and the child undergoes numerous pointless tests.

Management
Investigations are usually not informative although rarely *CACNA1A* mutations have been detected. Usually head tilt becomes less prominent after infancy, being replaced by vertigo and eventually by migraine headaches.

Summary and conclusions
In this chapter we have given brief descriptions of most of the common non-epileptic conditions that may occur in infants. We have concentrated on conditions (not necessarily disorders) that may be confused with epilepsy. Most are seen in otherwise healthy infants of normal development, although some if not all may be seen in those with slow or deviant development.

The important point that we emphasize is that such non-epileptic conditions should not be misdiagnosed as epilepsy (the definition of which includes recurrent epileptic seizures). In particular, it is essential not to prescribe 'anticonvulsants' (that is, antiepileptic medications) nor sedatives nor other brain-altering drugs. Exceptions to this rule are the rare disorders AHC, in which flunarizine may help, and hyperekplexia, in which clonazepam is the treatment of choice.

It should be borne in mind that in almost all of the conditions we describe in this chapter the only harm that may come to the infant comes from the doctor – paediatric neurologist or otherwise – who does not recognize the non-epileptic nature of the events and prescribes medications that may impair the infant's brain function. This chapter aims to prevent such unfortunate iatrogenic consequences.

Home video, nowadays often on the ubiquitous mobile phone, greatly assists in the diagnosis of many of these conditions. Once an event has been captured on video, this may also be viewed by other paediatric neurologists with more experience. Other investigations such as electroencephalography and brain imaging should be used with great care and caution, as false positives are frequent. Diagnosis should be *clinically* based on your skills as a doctor.

Resources
Horrocks IA, Nechay A, Stephenson JBP, Zuberi SM. Anoxic-epileptic seizures: observational study of epileptic seizures induced by syncopes. *Archives of Disease in Childhood*, 2005, 90:1283–1287.

King MD, Stephenson JBP. *A handbook of neurological investigations in children.* London, Mac Keith Press, 2009.

Mineyko A, Whiting S, Graham GE. Hyperekplexia: treatment of a severe phenotype and review of the literature. *Canadian Journal of Neurological Sciences*, 2011, 38:411–416.

Stephenson JBP. *Fits and faints.* London, Mac Keith Press, 1990.

Uldall P et al. The misdiagnosis of epilepsy in children admitted to a tertiary epilepsy centre with paroxysmal events. *Archives of Disease in Childhood*, 2006, 91:219–221.

Chapter 18
Macrocephaly, including hydrocephalus

Colin Kennedy

Key messages
- Distinguish a large head from an excessive rate of head growth.
- Manage normally developing macrocephalic infants expectantly.

Common errors
- Diagnosing hydrocephalus without imaging.
- Diagnosing hydrocephalus without enlargement of lateral ventricles.
- Intervening in a normally developing macrocephalic infant.
- Diagnosing craniosynostosis when the head shape is normal (unlikely).

When to worry
- Excessive rate of head growth.
- Marked separation of the cranial sutures.
- Lethargy, persistent unexplained vomiting, sunsetting.
- Focal neurological signs in association with macrocephaly.

Definition
Macrocephaly (synonym: macrocrania) can be defined as an occipitofrontal head circumference (OFC) more than three standard deviations above the mean level (i.e. >99.6th centile). Excessive rate of head growth (crossing centiles) is more likely to be associated with underlying pathology than a large head increasing in size appropriately (i.e. parallel to the centiles). Macrocephaly can be due to an increase in the volume of any cranial component.

Clinical approach to assessment of head size and shape

Head size
Measurement of OFC requires only a measuring tape, preferably a disposable paper tape, and a centile chart appropriate to the sex of the infant of head circumference against age. These are essential items for any neurologist and can be most reliably found if both are carried with the examiner in all clinical settings. WHO centile charts for head circumference, height and weight can be found at the end of this book (see Appendix 1).

Centile charts for head circumference do vary so that whichever growth standard is chosen, is likely to lead to children being spuriously labelled as having abnormal head growth because the centiles in the reference population differ slightly from the centiles in the local population (Baxter, 2011; Wright et al., 2011). The WHO 2007 head circumference growth standards (see Appendix 1) are suitable.

As with length and weight, both measurement and centile must be documented. Documentation in the medical record of OFC, with date, forms part of the basic medical assessment of all infants, whether in the hospital or the community. This history can be very valuable not only at the time but also later as evidence for the likely age at which abnormal growth first became evident. Measurement on more than one occasion enables determination of growth rate. This often points the physician helpfully towards the diagnosis (e.g. birth asphyxia, congenital infection, hydrocephalus, brain tumour, possible inflicted injury, Rett and other syndromes).

Head size is more closely related to parental head size than to the child's own weight or height. Genetic factors are the major determinant of head size in a well-nourished healthy infant. Parental head size and centiles give a clear indication of where the child's head size lies in relation to its genetic target. If only one parent is available to be measured, supply the family with a paper tape so they can inform the health team of a home measurement.

Careful measurement of OFC avoids many unnecessary investigations in children with familial tendency to small or large heads including those with benign external hydrocephalus (see below). Rarely, a 'normal' head size may indicate excessive or insufficient head growth depending on the genetic target.

Signs that may be associated with macrocephaly or abnormal head shape

- Separation of the cranial sutures is a useful sign in obstructive hydrocephalus in young infants.
- Fullness and firmness of the anterior fontanelle can be useful additional signs but are not quantifiable and occasionally misleading.
- A normally shaped head is unlikely to be seen in primary craniosynostosis.
- Ridging of the sutures is a sign of synostosis and must be distinguished from overlapping of the sutures. In the latter case, the ridge has only one edge and relative movement between the bones can be felt by pressing on the lower of the bones that meet along the ridge. This is much easier to interpret than plain radiographs on which overlapping bones may appear more dense and thus mimic the appearance of ossification.

Investigation of macrocephaly

The first step is to consider whether, on the clinical assessment described above, there is

- no reason for concern,
- need for continued monitoring of head growth in the community, or
- need for special investigation.

Almost all intracranial causes can only be identified on cranial imaging. Ultrasound is good for defining the size of the cerebral ventricles but less good at describing the extracerebral and subdural spaces or abnormalities of the cerebral parenchyma. Therefore computed tomography (CT) or magnetic resonance imaging is needed to confirm ultrasound findings except in cases of hydrocephalus *where the cause is already known*, for example intraventicular haemorrhage (IVH).

A list of causes macrocephaly in infancy is given in Table 18.1. Head centile charts are shown in Appendix 1 in this volume.

Megalencephaly

Definition

This is excessive brain size, not precisely defined, and most cases without neurological impairment are familial with a male preponderance. Head growth is determined by brain growth in a healthy child so megalencephaly leads to macrocephaly (synonym: macrocrania). Although brain size more than three standard deviations above the mean is associated with an increased relative risk of some intellectual impairment, this would be found in only a small percentage of individuals with megalencephalic neurological impairment. There is need, therefore, for thorough consideration of other causes of developmental impairment as in a child with normal brain size, as well as consideration of genetic causes of megalencephaly with developmental impairment, such as the phosphatase and tensin homologue (*PTEN*) cancer predisposition gene.

Table 18.1 Causes of macrocephaly in infancy

Cause	Clinical or imaging feature	Possible other feature	Comment/ management
Cephal-haematoma	Boggy mass	May be calcified, not boggy, if chronic	NB risk of infection if tapped
Extravasation of IV infusion into subcutaneous tissue	Recent scalp vein infusion	Pitting oedema	Stop infusion
Subdural haematoma	Consider inflicted injury	May be mimicked by traumatic CSF fistula	CT, skeletal survey, eye exam if unexplained Surgery only if very large or severe symptoms
Growing fracture	Cystic non-tender mass, bony defect	Trauma with dural laceration	Surgical
Benign external hydrocephalus	Head size above mean at birth	Parental macrocephaly	See text Outpatient observation; consider glutaric aciduria
Obstructive hydrocephalus	IVH	Preterm infant; usually communicating	See text
	Aqueduct/fourth ventricle obstruction	Myelomeningocoele, Dandy–Walker syndrome or other cerebral malformation, adducted thumbs	Surgical; consider genetics
	Infection; tumour; occasionally haemorrhage	Toxoplasma (perinatal); after bacterial meningitis	Also chronic ventriculitis in preterm infants

Table 18.1 *Continued*

Cause	Clinical or imaging feature	Possible other feature	Comment/ management
Megalencephaly	Parental macrocephaly	Developmentally normal	Syndromes (e.g. related to *PTEN* gene) with dysmorphism and/ or impairments
Rarer causes	Tumour mass effect	Vomiting, lethargy or focal neurological signs	Often supratentorial
	Hydranencephaly		May appear surprisingly neurologically normal but not for long
	Walker–Warburg syndrome	Dysmorphic, eye and developmental impairments	ERG, molecular genetics
	Canavan disease	Irritability and white matter abnormality	Urine organic acids, see Chapter 9
	Alexander disease	Other neurodevelopmental or white matter abnormality	Molecular genetic testing for GFAP gene (limited availability)
	Neurocutaneous	Hypomelanosis of Ito*, NF1, SWS	
	Vein of Galen malformation	Hydrocephalus, bruit	Interventional neuroradiology
	Thickened bones	Osteopetrosis and other rare syndromes	

Table 18.1 *Continued*

Cause	Clinical or imaging feature	Possible other feature	Comment/ management
	Achondroplasia, basilar impression	Short limbs or abnormal skull base	Communicating or non-communicating hydrocephalus

*Hypomelanosis of Ito is a neurocutaneous condition in which characteristic whorls of skin depigmentation provide a clue to associated cerebral malformation.
CSF, cerebrospinal fluid; ERG, electroretinogram; IV, intravenous; IVH, intraventicular haemorrhage; NF1, neurofibromatosis; PTEN, phosphatase and tensin homologue; SWS, Sturge–Weber syndrome.

Hydrocephalus

Definition and terminology

Hydrocephalus is here used to mean ventricular expansion due to elevated cerebrospinal fluid (CSF) pressure, which implies 'obstruction' to the flow of CSF. Much confusion surrounds this term because of the broader meaning of hydrocephalus to mean simply excess CSF fluid in the head, of which one cause is atrophy of the cerebral parenchyma, for example after severe asphyxia. In such cases in infancy, the key clinical feature is absence of excessive head growth. This is sometimes referred to as *hydrocephalus ex vacuo*, which is not included within the narrower definition of hydrocephalus used in this book.

The longstanding division of hydrocephalus into 'communicating' and 'non-communicating' refers to communication between the CSF spaces within the brain and those on the outside of the brain and spinal cord. This is useful in that cases of non-communicating hydrocephalus are likely to have a pressure gradient between the head and spine and so it is therefore relatively less safe to treat these patients with therapeutic lumbar puncture than those with communicating hydrocephalus. Compared with later infancy, these risks are smaller in the early months because of the tendency for intracranial volume to increase with intracranial pressure and thus reduce any pressure gradient. In general such risks are greatest with rapid changes in pressure, such as rare instances of cerebral arterial haemorrhage in the posterior fossa, acute cerebellitis or fulminant bacterial meningitis.

Note that 'obstructive' is *not* identical in meaning to non-communicating since obstructive hydrocephalus can be either non-communicating, with obstruction at the foramen of Munro or the aqueduct (with a small fourth ventricle) or at the outflow from the fourth ventricle (with a large fourth ventricle), or communicating, with obstruction at the level of the arachnoid villi.

Obstructive hydrocephalus may lead to an increase in intracranial pressure. Reference ranges for CSF pressure in infancy, as a proxy for intracranial pressure, are very scant. Mean CSF pressure of newborns was said to be around 3 cm of CSF (see Whitelaw and Aquilina, 2011) and a pressure above 5 cm is probably abnormal at this age.

Signs additional to excessive head growth associated with hydrocephalus
In a young infant these are

- lethargy or reduced conscious level,
- persistent and otherwise unexplained vomiting or apnea, and
- loss of upgaze then episodes of forced downgaze (sunsetting).

A variety of non-specific clinical features may also be seen, including irritability, poor feeding, early developmental impairment, poor head control, apnoea and bradycardia.

At a late stage

- spasticity of limbs, and
- extensor posturing (tonic attacks; see also Chapter 17, p. 242).

Porencephaly
This refers to resorption of brain parenchyma after haemorrhage or other parenchymal insult leaving a CSF-filled space. This is not hydrocephalus although the two conditions may occur together.

Ventricular dilatation
This is not of itself an indication of raised intracranial pressure and even progressive increase in size can be due to atrophy (e.g. after birth asphyxia).

Ventricular index
The *ventricular index* is the distance in millimetres between the medial and lateral margins of the lateral ventricle at the level of the foramen of Monro (Figure 18.1). Reference ranges (Figure 18.2) can be used to compare serial measurements of the ventricular index with the 95th centile for age and thus compare with the expected increase in diameter of the lateral ventricles with age. Monitoring of ventricular size is useful in post-haemorrhagic ventricular dilatation (PHVD; see below) and has been used as an inclusion criterion in trials of therapeutic intervention but should be combined with monitoring of head size and assessment of the coronal sutures and fontanelle to distinguish increase in ventricular index due to atrophy or porencephaly from that due to hydrocephalus.

Epidemiology of hydrocephalus
The incidence of hydrocephalus in the first year has been carefully tracked in Sweden over several decades (see Table 18.2). In 1999–2002, the incidence was 0.66 per 1000 live births. Male infants outnumbered females almost 2 to 1. Infants born at more than

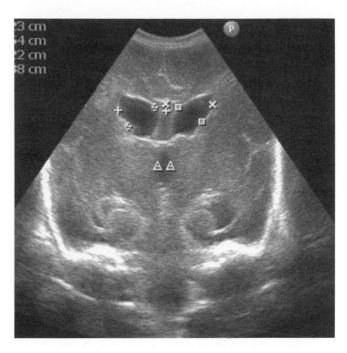

Figure 18.1 Cranial ultrasound scan showing moderate dilatation of the lateral ventricles. Coronal view with calipers showing anterior horn width (denoted by square calipers), third ventricular width (triangular calipers) and ventricular index (X and + calipers) measurements. From Whitelaw and Aqualina (2011) with permission.

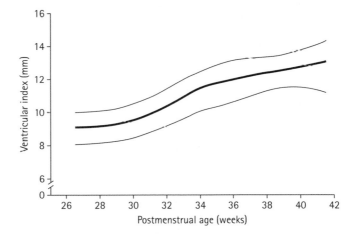

Figure 18.2 Cross-sectional chart of ventricular index against gestational age. Smoothed centiles are 3rd, 50th and 97th centiles (from Levene, 1981, with permission).

36 weeks' gestation accounted for 56% of all cases of hydrocephalus and there was a large increase in incidence (23 compared with 0.26 per 1000) in extremely preterm infants, born at less than 28 completed weeks of gestation, when compared with term infants (Persson et al, 2007). The number of cases in extremely preterm infants was higher than in previous birth cohorts, coinciding with a decrease in their mortality. The incidence of myelomeningocoele (MMC) is also higher in most countries without antenatal screening for MMC so that the relative contribution of the different causes will show geographical variation.

Table 18.2 Incidence of hydrocephalus in the first year in Swedish infants

Hydrocephalus in first year in 1999–2002 birth cohort in western Sweden	
Hydrocephalus with myelomeningocoele	0.18 per 1000
Hydrocephalus	0.48 per 1000
Malformations	49%
Intracranial haemorrhage	41%
Other	10%
After Persson et al. (2007).	

PHVD

In preterm infants most cases of hydrocephalus are secondary to haemorrhaging from immature germinal matrix vessels in the subependymal layer lateral to the lateral ventricles. Such IVH is classified as grade 1 if confined to that location, grade 2 if also seen within the ventricle and grade 3 if associated with PHVD. In addition to causing PHVD, haemorrhage can rupture into brain parenchyma with increased risk of long-term neurological sequelae.

PHVD occurs in approximately 35% of patients with IVH and, of these 35%, approximately 15% require shunt insertion for control of raised intracranial pressure. Severe IVH with its complications and periventricular leukomalacia remain the major determinants of brain injury in preterm infants, and the neurodevelopmental outcome of infants with severe PHVD is extremely poor.

Surgical treatment of PHVD in the form of ventriculoperitoneal shunt insertion is effective in treating symptoms or signs of raised intracranial pressure but has a high incidence of shunt blockage or infection in small, ill infants and carries lifelong risks associated with late infection or shunt failure. Endoscopic third ventriculostomy has been used but is unlikely to be an effective form of treatment in the majority of cases because of the communicating nature of the hydrocephalus. Moderate to severe PHVD is often managed at first by intermittent removal of CSF, but randomized trials have suggested that serial removal of CSF (by ventricular taps with or without placement of a ventricular reservoir or by lumbar puncture) does not reduce the progression to eventual shunt placement. A randomized trial of the use of acetazolamide and frusemide for PHVD showed that this treatment was ineffective and dangerous, with increased incidence of associated motor disability at follow-up (see Whitelaw and Aquilina, 2011).

Hydrocephalus due to cerebral malformation
The anatomy of cerebral malformations can usually be ascertained on CT although magnetic resonance imaging is preferable. The most common are those associated with MMC and aqueduct stenosis. Cystic dilation of the fourth ventricle with hypoplasia or agenesis of the vermis constitute the Dandy–Walker malformation: both features should be indentified on imaging before making this diagnosis in which the long-term neurodevelopmental outcome is good in a proportion of promptly treated cases. Hydrocephalus associated with open MMC commonly becomes clinically apparent soon after surgical closure of the MMC and requires prompt treatment to preserve the surgical closure.

Surgical treatment is the only active treatment option. Endoscopic third ventriculostomy is more physiological and has a lower complication rate than ventriculoperitoneal shunting, in which infection rates are highest in the youngest infants. However, the endoscopic method is only an option for non-communicating hydrocephalus and has a relatively lower success rate in infants than in older children.

A helpful brief summary of the neurosurgical aspects of current management of hydrocephalus makes the important point that delayed recognition of shunt malfunction remains an important and preventable cause of death in current practice (Kandasarmy et al., 2011).

Idiopathic (or 'benign') external hydrocephalus
This disorder is dominantly inherited and parental macrocephaly is a cardinal feature. Key clinical features are

- at least one parent with macrocephaly,
- OFC at birth above the mean for gestational age,
- excessive head growth deviating above and away from centiles, and
- no other neurological abnormalities in a well infant.

Typically the anterior fontenelle is large and may also be full. Some cases present with bulging of the fontanelle in a relatively well infant, typically brought on by a minor viral respiratory infection. Affected infants often come to medical attention because of excessive head growth. In some cases, the trajectory of head growth is dramatically above and away from the 99th centile (Figure 18.3).

Imaging
Medical concern about head growth is often increased by cranial imaging which shows enlarged, and sometimes anteriorly very large, extracerebral CSF spaces of CSF intensity/density. On CT these can be difficult to distinguish from subdural collections although complete symmetry, widened, rather than flattened, cerebral sulci and a broad interhemispheric fissure are typical features. Plump, rather than markedly expanded, lateral ventricles are also typical of benign external hydrocephalus (Figure 18.4).

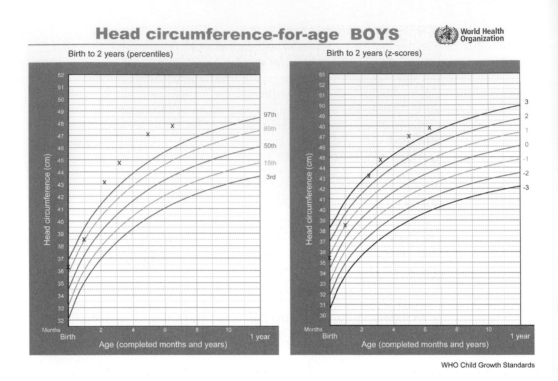

Figure 18.3 Trajectory of head growth from birth in a well male infant whose father and paternal grandfather had OFCs of 60.0 and 62.0 cm. At the time of the most recent measurement he was sitting alone, passing objects from hand to hand and babbling communicatively. The two charts are based on identical data plotted against (a) centiles and (b) z scores. This shows how perception of the need to take action might be influenced by the specifics of chart construction. (See colour plate 2)

Other investigations

No other investigations are required in most cases although consideration should be given to checking urine organic acids to exclude dominantly inherited glutaric aciduria, which can lead to both cerebral atrophy and subdural haemorrhage but without acute presentation. Some history of neurological difficulties in the affected parent or child is likely in such cases. There is no indication to undertake lumbar puncture but if CSF pressure is measured it may be above the reference range for infants. This is, however, 'normal' for infants with the other features described and does not require any intervention.

Management

In the absence of developmental problems other than delayed sitting, cranial imaging can often be avoided and investigation can be confined to monitoring of the child's clinical progress in the community. Developmental progress is normal except that independent sitting can be delayed. Motor milestones revert to normal once the child

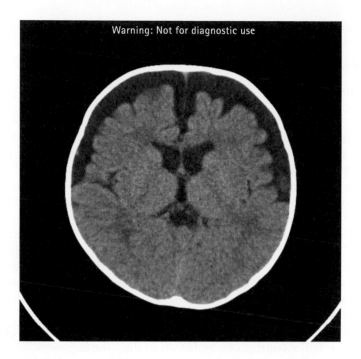

Warning: Not for diagnostic use

Figure 18.4 CT scan at age 7 months of the same infant whose head growth is shown in Figure 18.3. This shows plump cerebral ventricles and enlarged frontotemporal extratemporal CSF spaces. Identical attenuation in these spaces with that in the cerebral ventricles, enlargement of the interhemispheric fissure and the fact that the cerebral sulci appear enlarged rather than compressed are important features. The appearances are typical of benign enlargement of the extracerebral spaces (also known as benign external hydrocephalus). No intervention is required.

is able to stand independently. Medium- and long-term neurological outcome is completely normal with macrocephaly.

Pathophysiology
Pathophysiology is not fully known but the underlying condition includes megalencephaly associated with a CSF pressure that is higher than that seen in the general population but not associated with any of the clinical problems that might be seen with raised CSF pressure in other conditions. Imaging appearances normalize after infancy, possibly related to lower-pressure CSF and cerebral venous drainage in the erect posture. This condition is *not* related to idiopathic intracranial hypertension in which the child is symptomatic, head growth is normal and the ventricles are, by definition, not enlarged (Alvarez et al., 1986).

Idiopathic intracranial hypertension (IIH) is not a condition of infancy and absence of enlargement of the cerebral ventricles is part of the case definition. No cases of IIH were reported in the first year of life in a recent 3-year survey of the condition conducted among all paediatricians and paediatric neurologists in the UK.

Craniosynostosis

Definition
This refers to premature fusion of the sutures between the cranial bones while the brain is still growing and may be associated with ridging of the affected suture (see the section on signs at the beginning of this chapter). This can occur in a number of syndromic conditions with associated dysmorphism. Primary synostosis of all sutures could lead to microcephaly with normal head shape but is rare and more often leads to turricephaly. Scaphocephaly (literally, keel head), due to sagittal synostosis, is the most common and is the only single-suture synostosis likely to require treatment within the first few months of life. Dolichocephaly, brachycephaly, trigonocephaly and plagiocephaly follow from sagittal, coronal, metopic and unilateral (coronal or lambdoid) synostosis respectively. Secondary microcephaly with sutural fusion may be symmetrical when the rate of head growth is greatly reduced secondary to cerebral atrophy with or without reduction in CSF volume e.g. birth asphyxia or shunt placement for PHVD (see above) with associated encephalomalacia. This is not, strictly speaking, craniosynostosis unless the brain growth is being constrained by fusion of the sutures.

Treatment
Surgical treatment of craniosynostosis is clearly indicated only in certain dysmorphic syndromes or when accompanied by raised intracranial pressure. In these cases subspecialist craniofacial expertise is needed. Some cosmetic benefit for the more severe examples of fusion of a single suture are best considered in the light of the views of the child and parents and balanced against the risks of surgery.

Abnormal head shape without synostosis
Abnormal head shape in the absence of synostosis may be postural; for example, dolichocephaly in extremely preterm infants, brachycephaly in some cases of profound motor impairments and plagiocephaly with chest deformity resulting from asymmetrical postural preferences in infancy. These posturally induced deformities of head shape can be corrected by increasing time in non-preferred postures. Sleeping in the supine position is, however, effective in reducing the risk of sudden infant death and should be continued in all infants. Symmetrically abnormal head shape is also seen in a number of genetic syndromes.

Common myths about assessment of the cranium and ventricles
Myths about cranial imaging. One myth is that a diagnosis of hydrocephalus is possible without cranial imaging. It is not possible to diagnose hydrocephalus without establishing that there is enlargement of the cerebral ventricles and reason to think that the enlargement is pressure-driven.

Myths about size of the third ventricle. Another myth is that diagnosis of neurological conditions can be based on the dimensions of the third ventricle. There are no reference ranges for the dimensions of the third ventricle that can usefully distinguish normal from abnormal in the absence of enlargement of the lateral ventricles. In an individual with expanded lateral ventricles the third ventricle also dilates and serial measurements of its diameter in such an individual can sometimes be easier to compare with each other than lateral ventricular measurements because the dimensions of the third ventricle are less influenced by positioning of the head in the scanner.

Myths about the anterior fontanelle. Another myth is that diagnosis of neurological conditions can be based on anterior fontanelle dimensions. Considerable variation exists in the size and age at closure of the anterior fontanelle and, in the absence of dysmorphism, these variations do not show useful associations with neurological conditions and do not require investigation. Small, early-closing fontanelles may raise the question of craniosynostosis, especially if there is ridging of the sutures (see elsewhere in this chapter and Chapter 19). Large, late-closing fontanelles are a feature of some dysmorphic syndromes (e.g. with macrocephaly in *PTEN* mutation).

Myths about a cavum septum pellucidum. Another myth is that diagnosis of neurological conditions can be suspected in the presence of a cavum spetum pellucidum. The presence of a cyst between the leaflets of the septum pellucidum is a normal variant and does not require intervention.

References

Alvarez LA, Maytal J, Shinnar S. Idiopathic external hydrocephalus: natural history and relationship to benign familial hydrocephalus. *Pediatrics*, 1986, 77: 901–907.

Baxter P. Head size: WHOse growth charts? *Developmental Medicine and Child Neurology*, 2011, 53: 3–4.

Kandasarmy J, Jenkinson MD, Mallucci CL. Contemporary management and recent advances in paediatric hydrocephalus. *British Medical Journal*, 2011, 343: 146–151.

Levene MI. Measurement of the growth of the lateral ventricles in preterm infants with real-time ultrasound. *Archives of Disease in Childhood*, 1981, 56:900–904.

Persson EK, Anderson S, Wiklund LM, Uvebrant P. Hydrocephalus in children born in 1999-2002: epidemiology, outcome and ophthalmological findings. *Child's Nervous System*, 2007, 23:1111–1118.

Whitelaw A, Aquilina K. Management of posthaemorrhagic ventricular dilatation. *Archives of Disease in Childhood: Fetal and Neonatal Edition*, doi:10.1136/adc.2010.190173.

Wright CM. Inskip H, Godfrey K et al. Monitoring head size and growth using the new UK-WHO growth standard. *Archives of Disease in Childhood*, 2011, 96:386–388.

Resources

Aicardi J (ed.). *Diseases of the nervous system in childhood*, 3rd ed. London, Mac Keith Press, 2009.

Levene MI, Chervenak FA (eds). *Fetal and neonatal neurology and neurosurgery*, 4th ed. London, Churchill Livingstone, 2009.

Chapter 19
Microcephaly, including congenital infections

Richard Chin and Vlatka Mejaski-Bosnjak

Key messages
- Distinguish a small head from a slow rate of head growth.
- Manage normally developing infants with microcephaly expectantly.

Common errors
- Intervening in a normally developing infant with microcephaly.

When to worry
- Seizures in association with microcephaly.
- Difficulties with coordination and or balance.
- Slow to or failure to attain developmental milestones.
- Successive plots of occipitofrontal head circumference cross the centiles downwards.
- Dysmorphic features.
- Focal neurological signs in association with microcephaly.

Definition

Microcephaly can be defined as occipitofrontal head circumference (OFC) less than at least two standard deviations below the mean level (below the 2nd centile) for the individual's age and sex. Using this definition, 2% of the general population will have microcephaly. The term *microencephaly* denotes an undersized/-weighted brain. Microcephaly can be present at birth (primary) or develop postnatally (secondary). Primary microcephaly is usually a static developmental anomaly, whereas secondary microcephaly indicates a progressive neurodegenerative condition.

Reduced rate of head growth (crossing centiles) is more likely to be associated with underlying pathology than a small head increasing in size appropriately (i.e. parallel to the centiles). It can be due to either genetic (congenital) or environmental (acquired) causes and can be an isolated finding or part of a syndrome. It is a common myth that microcephaly is always related to low intelligence.

Causes of microcephaly

- Congenital/genetic: isolated, chromosomal, syndromal or neurometabolic (see Table 19.1 for examples).
- Acquired/environmental (see Table 19.2 for examples):
  - *perinatal infections*: toxoplasmosis, rubella, cytomegalovirus, herpes simplex virus ('TORCH'), varicella, coxsackie B virus, syphilis, human immunodeficiency virus (HIV), post-meningitis;
  - *intrauterine exposure* to alcohol, tobacco, marijuana, cocaine, heroin, radiation or prescription drugs including anticancer/antiepileptic drugs;
  - *perinatal metabolic/endocrine imbalances*: hypoglycaemia, hypothyroidism, hypopituitarism, hypoadrenocorticism, maternal phenylketonuria, hypernatremic dehydration;
  - *prenatal maternal illness or pregnancy factors*: systemic illness, anaemia, malnutrition, small for gestational age/extreme preterm birth/neonatal intensive care unit survivors/hypoxic ischaemic encephalopathy, periventricular leukomalacia/intracranial haemorrhage.

Clinical approach to assessment of head size and shape

Head size

The principles of measuring and documenting serial OFCs is addressed in Chapter 18 in this volume. In summary, sequential OFCs should be measured accurately (readily done with a measuring tape) and documented. Comparison should be made with the rest of the population using suitable age and sex growth charts (see Appendix 1). Parental OFCs should also be measured. Differences in head size between ethnic groups should also be taken into account.

Table 19.1 Congenital/genetic causes of microcephaly in infancy

Cause	Clinical or imaging features	Comment/management
Isolated		
Benign familial microcephaly	AD; small OFCs in family members with normal development, function normally, proportionately small body size, normal development; normal MRI	Reassurance, community monitoring of development
AR primary microcephaly	AR; non-progressive intellectual disability, normal neurology; slight reduction in white matter	Molecular genetics
Chromosomal disorders		
Cri du chat (5p deletion)	Characteristic meowing kitten cry in infants; feeding problems, low birth weight, severe developmental delay, cardiac defects	Dysmorphology database (e.g. OMIM), geneticist, karyotyping, molecular genetics
Cornelia de Lange	Long eyelashes, bushy eyebrows and synophrys (joined eyebrows); short stature. GIT and behaviour problems.	
Trisomy 21 (Down)	Congenital heart disease, malignancies, thyroid disorders, seizures, GIT problems	
Trisomy 18 (Edward)	Prominent occiput, talipes equinovarus or rocker bottom feet, congenital heart disease	
Trisomy 13 (Patau)	Eye, musculoskeletal, urogenital defects.	
Syndromic disorders		
Rett	Female infant development and head size normal until 6–18 months, then regression, loss of purposeful hand movements and decreased head growth; hand stereotypies and breathing irregularities	Dysmorphology database (e.g. OMIM), Geneticist, Molecular genetics; can be mistaken for autism

Table 19.1 *Continued*

Cause	Clinical or imaging features	Comment/ management
Aicardi–Goutières	AR; seizures, chillblains, intellectual disability; calcified basal ganglia	CSF lymphocytosis, raised alpha interferon in plasma and CSF, molecular genetics
Cerebro-oculo-facio-skeletal syndrome	AR; arthrogryposis, cataracts	Ophthalmology assessment
Seckel syndrome	AR; IUGR, postnatal dwarfism, bird-like face, beak-like nose	Dysmorphology database (e.g. OMIM), geneticist, molecular genetics
Cockayne	AR; deafness, photosensitivity, retinitis pigmentosa	DNA-repair defect, ophthalmology assessment, molecular genetics
Rubinstein–Taybi syndrome	AD; short stature, severe learning difficulties, broad first digits, malignancies	Dysmorphology database (e.g. OMIM), geneticist, molecular genetics
Neurometabolic syndromes		
Smith–Lemli–Opitz	AR; syndactyly of the second and third toes, cleft palate, learning difficulties, behaviour problems	Low cholesterol, high 7DHC levels
3-Phosphoglycerate dehydrogenase deficiency	Intractable seizures and severe developmental delay	CSF amino acids, plasma amino acids, urine organic and amino acids

AD, autosomal dominant; AR, autosomal recessive; CSF, cerebrospinal fluid; 7DHC, dehydrocholesterol; GIT, gastrointestinal tract; IUGR, intrauterine growth retardation; OMIM Online Mendelian Inheritance in Man (www.ncbi.nlm.gov/omim).

Table 19.2 Acquired/environmental causes of microcephaly in infancy

Cause	Clinical or imaging features	Comment/management
Perinatal infections		
CMV	Most common intrauterine infection affecting 1% of liveborn neonates by vertical mother–fetus transmission. 7–10% evident at birth: IUGR, sepsis like syndrome, marked microcephaly, chorioretinitis. Permanent sequelae in 40–58% of infants with symptomatic infection: SNHL (+++) intellectual disability, seizures, psychomotor delay, ASD Neuroimaging. CT: periventricular calcification, MRI: alteration of white matter, cortical dysgenesis (polymicrogyria), cerebellar hypoplasia in early-onset infection.	Laboratory diagnostic: IgM, IgG, PCR-CMV DNA (amniotic fluid, serum/ Guthrie card). Therapy: antiviral drug: ganciclovir IV for 6 weeks might improve hearing outcomes. Passive immunization of pregnant infected women Active immunization under investigation
HSV	Occurs in 1/3000 deliveries due to peripartum transmission, caused by HSV-2. Triad of cutaneous, neurological (microcephaly, spasticity, seizures), eye (chorioretinitis, microphthalmia) findings present at birth; brain CT/MRI reveal multiple areas of haemorrhagic necrosis	Laboratory diagnostic: HSV DNA in CSF by PCR. Antiviral drug, aciclovir therapy. Risk of transmission during third trimester can be reduced by caesarean section delivery
Toxoplasmosis	Prevalence in neonates of 0.08%, often asymptomatic. Severe neonatal disease: 'sepsis-like syndrome', chorioretinitis. Long term morbidity: severely impaired vision, spasticity, intellectual disability, microcephaly, hydrocephalus, seizures, SNHL. Neuroimaging reveals disseminated calcifications in caudate nuclei, choroid plexus, subependyma (CT), MRI detects active inflamatory lesions.	Antenatal IgM, PCR on amniocentesis fluid at 16–18 weeks. Sulfadiazine, pyrimethamine therapy. Antepartum screening available: education programmes focus on handling raw meat with protective gloves, avoiding outdoor cats

Rubella	Nowadays very uncommon as result of vaccine-induced elimination of wild rubella viral transmission. Confirmed infection in first trimester of pregnancy results in damage of 50–90% of the fetuses: 'sepsis-like syndrome', meningoencephalitis. Permanent manifestation: intrauterine/postnatal IUGR, congenital heart disease, SNHL, visual impairment (cataracts, microphthalmia, retinopathy), microcephaly	Universal infant immunization with live attenuated MMR virus vaccine; and targeted vaccination of adolescent girls
HIV	Weight, length, OFC growth are all affected in HIV-infected children. (HIV "wasting syndrome"). Decrements in OFC are early and sustained.	HIV-screening should be used in risk population of pregnant women (IV drug abusers); RNA-PCR
Toxins		
Alcohol	Fetal alcohol spectrum disorders, teratogenic effect on developing fetus, in 1–3/1000 newborns; both moderate and high level of alcohol intake in early pregnancy result in altered fetal growth and morphogenesis. Characteristic facial phenotype, microcephaly, growth deficiency, delayed development and intellectual disability (most common non-genetic cause of intellectual disability), ASD. Neuroimaging: overall reduction in brain volume and central nervous system disorganization, structural abnormalities of corpus callosum, caudate, hippocampus, brain malformation. MRI shows regional increases in cortical thickness, and disorganization of white matter.	No specific therapy Elimination of alcohol intake preconception. See also Chapter 21

Table 19.2 *Continued*

Cause	Clinical or imaging features	Comment/management
Cocaine	A commonly misused drug. Pregnancy may be complicated by spontaneous abortion, preterm birth, placental abruption, fetal asphyxia, IUGR, stillbirth (increased catecholamines, vasoconstriction, derangements of homeostasis of neurotransmitters). Often polydrug use and biomedical risk factors (poor maternal nutrition, stress). Neonatal morbidity: tremulousness/lethargy, excessive startle responses, neonatal seizures. Microcephaly is the most common brain abnormality. Long-term morbidity: SIDS, epilepsy, CP, neurobehavioural deficits, developmental delay, learning difficulties, visual problems (optic nerve hypoplasia/atrophy coloboma). Neuroimaging: intracranial haemorrhage, hypoxic ischaemic lesions, cerebral infarction, disturbance of midline prosencephalic development and neuronal migration	Screening: determination of cocaine metabolite in meconium/gastric aspirate/urine. No specific pharmacological intervention is warranted in neonatal period Prevention of cocaine exposure *in utero* (socioeconomics and education)
Tobacco	Increased prevalence of smoking among youngest and oldest pregnant women particularly of lower educational achievement Higher rate of pregnancy complication: placental insufficiency, fetal growth restriction	Education of women of child-bearing age remains the most important method of prevention
Heroin and methadone	The incidence of low birthweight among newborns of heroin-addicted women is approximately 50%, mostly due to IUGR. 40% are microcephalic. Unfavourable outcome is often related to associated factors: poor prenatal care, maternal undernutrition, intrauterine infections (HIV). 10–35% of children of methadone users are of low birth weight, of whom 40% are small for dates. Low average mean developmental scores. Both heroin and methadone addiction sharply increase risk for SIDS and seizures but seizures are more common in methadone exposure.	Toxicology screen Characteristic withdrawal syndrome observed among about 60% of passively addicted newborns present within first 24 h in 65%: coarse tremulousness (quite dramatic), irritability, hypertonus, excessive sucking, diarrhoea, sweating Treatment: supportive therapy, narcotic agent, phenobarbital

Perinatal hypoxic ischaemic/haemorrhagic brain injury

HIE	1–2/1000 live term births experience HIE and 0.3/1000 have significant neurological residua (CP, intellectual disability, epilepsy, sensory impairments, behavioural problems). Temporal characteristics, severity of hypoxia ischaemia and gestation determine the type of neuropathology that result: selective neuronal necrosis (cortical, basal ganglia/thalamus, brainstem), parasagittal cerebral, focal and multifocal cerebral injury. Neuroimaging: cranial ultrasound (basal ganglia, multifocal ischaemic injury) in neonatal age and early infancy. MRI is modality of choice (diffusion-weighted in first days), for assessment and follow-up of structural reorganization.	Laboratory diagnosis: CSF-/blood-/brain-specific isomer of creatine kinase, lactate acid, uric acid, magnesium, interleukin-6 EEG: voltage suppression/slowing, 'burst-suppression' Therapy: monitor glucose level, control of seizures, neuroprotection (see text)
PVL	PVL is the major form of brain injury and leading cause of chronic neurological disability in survivors of preterm birth. In 25% of preterm survivors, major consequences are CP and visual impairments. By school age, 25–50% manifest a broad spectrum of cognitive and learning difficulties. Predilection for periventricular white matter (focal cystic necrotic lesions, diffuse disturbances of myelination). Predisposing factors include: hypoxia, ischaemia and maternal–fetal infection.	Cranial neonatal brain ultrasound/MRI. Therapy: supportive care, prevention of neonatal complication, treatment of infection. Neuroprotection (see text)

ASD, autistism-spectrum disorder; CMV, cytomegalovirus; CP, cerebral palsy; CT, computed tomography; EEG, electroencephalography; HIE, hypoxic ischaemic encephalopathy; HIV, human immunodeficieny virus; HSV, herpes simplex virus; IUGR, intrauterine growth retardation; IV, intravenous; MMR, measles, mumps, rubella; MRI, magnetic resonance imaging; PCR, polymerase chain reaction; PVL, periventricular leukomalacia; SIDS, sudden infant death syndrome; SNHL, sensorineural hearing loss.

Signs
The sutures close earlier than normal in microcephaly, but closure does not result in abnormal ridges. Microcephaly resulting from craniosynostosis can be apparent from the abnormal head shape, usually oxycephaly (turricephaly) and the readily palpable ridging of the sutures. These ridges are symmetrical, unlike the assymetrical one-sided ridge felt between skull bones that are overlapping but not fused. Scalp rugae may accompany some microcephaly of prenatal onset that causes collapse of the skull.

Investigation of microcephaly
A systematic consideration of each of the etiological categories listed is required. The clinician should search for risk factors in the mother's habits, lifestyle, nutrition and overall health. Details of the pregnancy and birth and the infant's developmental progress should be sought and documented, along with serial OFCs, to allow for a longitudinal assessment of the child and whether there is

● any reason for concern,
● need for continued monitoring of head growth in the community, or
● need for special investigation.

If a pathological type of microcephaly is suspected, magnetic resonance imaging of the brain should be sought. Magnetic resonance imaging is superior to computed tomography for displaying most abnormalities of grey and white matter, abnormalities of neuronal migration, sulcation and gyration, and to reveal the pattern of myelin deposition or demyelination. The pattern of abnormalities may help in determining the underlying cause for microcephaly, for example periventicular leukomalacia from perinatal hypoxic brain injury. Computed tomography may be more useful, however, in revealing calcifications in the brain with distinct patterns seen in intrauterine cytomegalovirus, toxoplasmosis, rubella, and varicella infections (see Table 19.2).

Chromosomal abnormalities are commonly associated with neurological consequences including microcephaly. Thus chromosomal analysis is highly recommended. If there is a strong clinical suspicion despite negative karyotyping, molecular genetic analysis may be required. Further special investigations for specific diagnoses are listed in Tables 19.1 and 19.2. Head centile charts are shown in Appendix 1.

Neuroprotection
Neuroprotection may help reduce the incidence of acquired microcephaly from perinatal hypoxic ischaemic brain injury. This is discussed in detail in Chapter 12 but in summary the main strategies are to induce hypothermia (head or total body cooling), and to optimize brain perfusion/oxygenation through maintaining normal levels of oxygenation (do not hyperoxygenate), blood pressure, haemoglobin, fluid balance, glucose and calcium.

Experimental studies have lead to the use of several agents for neuroprotection including calcium-channel blockers, magnesium sulphate, vitamin C, vitamin E, allopurinol, erythropoietin and melatonin. However, there remains controversy over their efficacy and/or safety, and there is insufficient evidence to support a general policy for their usage.

Resources

Back SA. Perinatal white matter injury: The changing spectrum of pathology and emerging insights into pathogenetic mechanism. *Mental Retardation and Developmental Disabilities Research Reviews*, 2006, 12:129–140.

Baxter PS, Rigby AS, Rotsaert M, Wright I. Acquired microcephaly: Causes, patterns, motor and IQ effects, and associated growth changes. *Pediatrics*, 2009, 124:590–595.

Chantry CJ, Byrd RS, Englund JA. Growth survival and viral load in symptomatic childhood human immunodeficiency virus. *Pediatric Infectious Disease Journal*, 2003, 22:1038–1038.

Evrard P, Gressens P, Volpe JJ. New concept to understand the neurological consequences of subcortical lesions in the premature brain. *Biology of the Neonate*, 1992, 61:1–3.

Fan X, van Bel F. Pharmacological neuroprotection after perinatal asphyxia. *Journal of Maternal-Fetal and Neonatal Medicine*, 2010, 23(S3):17–19.

Keegan J et al. Addiction in pregnancy. *Journal of Addictive Diseases*, 2010, 29:175–191.

Ledger WJ. Perinatal infections and fetal/neonatal brain injury. *Current Opinion in Obstetrics and Gynecology*, 2008, 20:120–124.

Legido A et al. Perinatal hypoxic ischemic encephalopathy: Current and future treatments. *International Pediatrics*, 2000, 15(3):143–151.

Mendelson E et al. Laboratory assessment and diagnosis of congenital viral infections: Rubella, cytomegalovirus, varicella-zoster, herpes simpley, parvovirus 19 and human immunodeficiency virus (HIV). *Reproductive Toxicology*, 2006, 21:315–382.

Scott HJ, Kimberlin DW, Whitley RJ. Antiviral therapy for herpes virus central nervous system infections: Neonatal herpes simplex virus infection and congenital cytomegalovirus infection. *Antiviral Research*, 2009, 83:207–213.

Tarrant A et al. Microcephaly: A radiological review. *Pediatric Radiology*, 2009, 39:772–780.

Volpe JJ. *Neurology of the newborn*, 5th ed. Philadelphia, Elsevier, 2008.

Chapter 20
The floppy infant
Ulrika Ådén and Thomas Sejersen

Key messages

- Determine whether there is cognitive delay in combination with the motor delay, and whether the hypotonia is combined with dysmorphic features.
- If the clinical evaluation points to hypotonia without weakness, but with impaired responsiveness/cognition, a central cause should be investigated
- If the clinical evaluation shows hypotonia combined with weakness, a neuromuscular disease should be investigated.

Common errors

- Assessing muscular tone and strength as normal or abnormal when the reverse is true. Assessment needs to be made in many infants to get a sense of what is normal and what is not.
- Assessing 'head lag' in forward traction without assessing in ventral suspension: the combination of both enables floppiness to be distinguished from excess extensor tone.
- Failing to consider systemic illness such as sepsis or heart failure as a cause of floppiness.

When to worry

- When a child shows signs of signs of weakness in respiratory muscles.

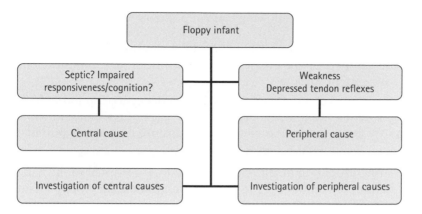

Figure 20.1 Schematic illustration of investigating whether the floppiness is due to central or peripheral cause.

Introduction
An infant who presents with generalized hypotonia, either during the neonatal period or later during the first year of life, is often referred to as a floppy infant. Hypotonia is the most common motor abnormality during the neonatal period. Several causes may be taken into consideration. First, systemic diseases like sepsis and heart failure must be ruled out. In infants with dysmorphic features, a number of different syndromes, of which Down syndrome is the most common, must be kept in mind. In other infants, central and peripheral neurological diseases must be considered (Figure 20.1). Hypotonia may be combined with some degree of muscle weakness, and one of the important issues when evaluating a floppy infant is to assess whether there is only hypotonia (most cases), or if there is also weakness. In later assessments it is also helpful to determine whether the child has motor delay alone or in combination with cognitive delay. This approach will give a rationale to the diagnostic evaluation of these children.

Definition
The measures of floppiness or muscle tonus and strength are subjective in their nature and the examiner will need to gain experience in order to assess what is normal and what is not. Hypotonia is usually detected when an infant has head lag when pulled to sitting position and when older infants have difficulties in keeping the head upright in ventral position. The infant's posture must also be evaluated in 'ventral suspension' (i.e. while supporting the infant's weight by resting his or her anterior chest wall on the examiner's hand). In this posture, the legs, arms and head will droop into a paper-clip shape if floppy but will be held up against gravity if the 'head lag' is due to an excess of extensor tone in the neck muscles.

A floppy infant may have the following clinical pointers:

- 'head lag' when pulled to sit (Figure 20.2a): the examiner grasps the infant's hands and gently pulls the infant to sitting position. This indicates both hypotonia and to some extent weakness;
- 'shoulder suspension test' (Figure 20.2b): a tendency to 'slip through' the examiner's hands when held under the arms. Lack of resistance in shoulders indicates weakness. Lack of axial control of posture indicates hypotonia;
- 'frog-legged' posture (Figure 20.2c), which indicates weakness;
- 'ventral suspension' (Figure 20.2d): when the infant is lifted prone and supported by the examiner's hand under the chest and abdomen, the floppy infant cannot maintain limb posture against gravity and assumes the position of a rag doll;

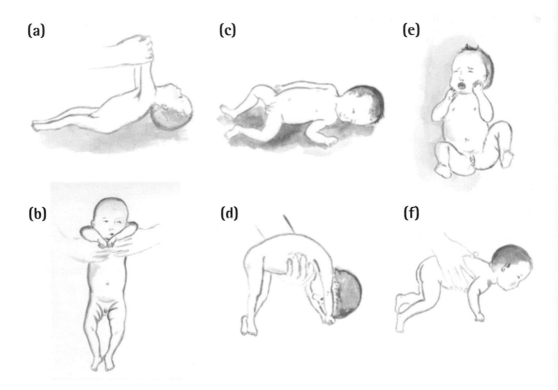

(a) **(c)** **(e)**

(b) **(d)** **(f)**

Figure 20.2 Illustration of floppy infant (a–d), and a normal child of similar age (e, f). Head lag is noted during traction in lying position (a), lack of axial control and lack of resistance in shoulders in 'shoulder suspension test' (b), 'frog-legged' posture (c) and inability to lift head and limbs against gravity in the 'ventral suspension' test (d). Note spontaneous limb movements and lack of frog-legged posture (e) and ability to move limbs and head against gravity (f) in the normal child. Illustration by Rebecka Lagercrantz.

- 'scarf sign': in supine position, either hand is placed across the neck to reach past the opposite shoulder. In a floppy infant, the elbow easily crosses the midline; and
- diminished resistance to passive movement of the limbs and increased range of movement of the peripheral joints.

Clinical approach

If the origin of hypotonia is central, the infant usually has

- altered responsiveness/cognition,
- decreased Moro and grasp reflexes,
- ability to lift the extremities from the underlying table; that is, no muscle weakness, and
- increased *or* decreased deep tendon reflexes (biceps, triceps, brachioradialis, knee and ankle jerk).

If the origin of hypotonia is peripheral, the infant typically has

- normal level of responsiveness/cognition,
- inability to lift the extremities from the underlying table; that is, weakness, and
- absent deep tendon reflexes (biceps, triceps, brachioradialis, knee and ankle jerk).

Origin of hypotonia

Significant hypotonia usually has an underlying cause (condition or disease), although in some cases no reason is identified and the hypotonia resolves spontaneously (benign congenital hypotonia). An infant suffering from congenital heart disease and congestive heart failure will use its energy to maintain circulation and respiration and will appear hypotonic. Thus it is necessary to bear this diagnosis in mind and complete a cardiovascular assessment.

Sepsis must be considered (but these infants will also show other signs of systemic infection) and infection parameters should be assessed in the basic work-up. For the remaining causes of hypotonia, a useful way of diagnostic thinking is to distinguish between central nervous system origin (more common) and peripheral neurological or muscular disease (less common).

Some origins within the central nervous system

- hypoxic ischaemic encephalopathy;
- syndromic (Down syndrome, Prader–Willi syndrome, neuronal migration disorders, gene mutation/duplication/deletion syndromes and chromosomal aberrations); dysmorphic features may be a clue;
- vascular: intracranial haemorrhagic or ischaemic stroke;

- metabolic: encephalopathy due to hypoglycaemia, hyperbilirubinaemia, electrolyte disturbances, neurometabolic disorder;
- drug side effects, iatrogenic, toxins;
- endocrine: such as hypothyroidism; or
- trauma: such as spinal cord trauma from difficult assisted delivery at birth.

Some important origins of/associations with hypotonia in the peripheral nervous system and muscles

- spinal muscular atrophy (SMA) type I (very severe hypotonia and weakness but alert),
- neurogenic arthrogryposis multiplex congenita (fixed joint position at birth combined with weakness and hypotonia; varied etiologies),
- neonatal myasthenia gravis,
- congenital myotonic dystrophy,
- congenital muscular dystrophies,
- congenital myopathies (e.g. central core disease, nemaline myopathy, myotubular myopathy), or
- metabolic myopathies (e.g. mitochondrial myopathies).

Other causes include

- sepsis, botulism,
- congestive heart failure,
- connective tissue disorders (e.g. Marfan syndrome, Ehler–Danlos), and
- benign congenital hypotonia.

Medical history
Family history should include the following:

- affected parents or siblings,
- consanguinity,
- stillbirths,
- maternal disease.

Pregnancy and delivery history should include the following:

- drug exposure,
- fetal movements,
- polyhydramniosis,
- perinatal asphyxia (Apgar scores),

- respiratory effort,
- ability to feed.

Physical examination
- Level of responsiveness/cognition, seizures
- Level of spontaneous activity
- Character of cry (often weak with pronounced peripheral weakness in SMA; hoarse cry in hypothyroidism)
- Dysmorphic features
- Arthrogryphosis, resistance to passive movements over joints
- Hepatosplenomegaly (in storage diseases like Pompe disease)
- Cardiovascular examination
- Cranial nerve function
- Clinical pointers to floppiness (see Definition section above)
- Posture, muscle tone, fasciculations
- Power (antigravity movements)
- Deep tendon reflexes
- Primary neonatal reflexes
- Asymmetry

Clinical presentation in neuromuscular diseases may include

- respiratory problems including paradoxical chest movement in respiration,
- sucking/swallowing problems,
- facial weakness (congenital myotonic dystrophy, myotubular myopathy, congenital muscular dystrophy),
- ptosis (myotubular myopathy, myasthenia),
- fasciculation of tongue (SMA), and
- arthrogryposis (congenital myotonic dystrophy, denervation syndromes).

Work-up
The initial work-up of the floppy infant depends upon the medical history and findings in the clinical evaluation. Investigations for floppiness suspected to be of central origin include the following:

- glucose, electrolytes, blood gas, complete blood count, bilirubin, septic screen including lumbar puncture,
- electroencephalography (EEG)/ambulatory EEG,
- ultrasound/computed tomography/magnetic resonance imaging,
- metabolic screening,

- infection: toxoplasmosis, rubella, cytomegalovirus, herpes simplex virus (TORCH),
- karyotype if dysmorphic features, and
- fluorescence *in situ* hybridization (FISH) or DNA methylation studies (e.g. Prader–Willi syndrome).

Investigations for suspected peripheral causes should include the following:

- examination of parents, (e.g. for myotonia),
- serum enzyme levels (creatine kinase),
- electromyography, nerve-conduction velocity,
- muscle biopsy,
- specific genetic tests, such as DNA triplet (CTG) repeats for congenital myotonic dystrophy, *SMN1* gene deletion for SMA, and
- administration of short-acting acetylcholinesterase inhibitor (e.g. edrophonium chloride) and/or trial of oral therapy if myasthenia is suspected.

Management and treatment

It is essential to evaluate a cause of hypotonia to outline investigations, management and treatment. Ethical aspects and prognosis are especially important to consider. In children with chronic hypotonia the following basic strategies may be considered:

- ventilatory support,
- treatment for respiratory infections,
- nutritional support,
- prevent and correct contractures,
- support/aids for sitting/walking, and
- therapy for speech/or alternative communication.

Prognosis

The prognosis of infants with neonatal hypotonia is entirely dependent upon the etiology and varies immensely.

Resources

Bodensteiner JB. The evaluation of the hypotonic infant. *Seminars in Pedatric Neurology*, 2008, 15:10–20.

Dubowitz V. *The floppy infant*, 2nd ed. Cambridge, Cambridge University Press, 1980.

Prasad A, Prasad C. The floppy infant: Contribution of genetic and metabolic disorders. *Brain & Development*, 2003, 25(7):457–476.

Volpe JJ. *Neurology of the newborn*, 5th ed. Philadelphia, Elsevier, 2008.

Chapter 21

Early developmental impairment and neurological abnormalities at birth

Richard W. Newton, Ilona Autti-Rämö and
Audrone Prasauskiene

Key messages

- The first consultation with parents to discuss significant neurodevelopmental impairment in their infant child is a major life event for them: see them together, if possible, and choose your words with care.

- Negative attitudes and exclusion by society are major contributors to disability and inability to participate in everyday life and social activities.

- All children need love, opportunity, setting of limits regarding what constitutes acceptable behaviour, and encouragement.

- There is no safety limit for drinking during pregnancy. Binge drinking should be avoided if becoming pregnant is possible.

- Alcohol consumption during pregnancy can lead to a large variety of symptoms ranging from a severely malformed infant with typical facial features to a child with normal phenotype but a specific learning disorder.

- Open spinal defects in myelomeningocoele should be closed within 24 h of birth.

- Progressive hydrocephalus has to be treated by ventriculo-peritoneal shunting, not by prescribing acetazolamide (Diacarb) or any other diuretics.

Common errors

- Failing to recognize that most children with early developmental impairment do have a long-term future with positive aspects.
- Failing to consider alcohol exposure as an etiological factor and thus failure to recognise fetal alcohol spectrum disorder.
- Not performing spinal X-ray or magnetic resonance imaging (MRI) to define the level of the lesion in spina bifida (very important for management and prognosis).
- Not initiating clean intermittent catheterization in spina bifida.

When to worry

- In general, when there is a deterioration in development.
- In fetal alcohol syndrome, when alcohol consumption within the family is not moderated, there is risk of maltreatment and neglect of the child.
- In myelomeningocoele, when irritability or sleepiness, bulging or pulsing fontanelle, vomiting or poor feeding is observed.

Box 21.1 Terminology derived from the International Classification of Functioning, Disability and Health: Child and Youth Version (ICF–CY; WHO 2007)

In the context of health:

- Bodily functions are the physiological functions of body systems (including psychological functions).
- Body structures are anatomical parts of the body such as organs, limbs and their components.
- Impairments are problems in body function or structure such as significant deviation or loss.
- Activity is the execution of a task or action by an individual.
- Participation is involvement in a life situation.
- Activity limitations are difficulties an individual may have in executing activities.
- Participation restrictions are problems and individual may experience in involvement in life situations.
- Environmental factors make up the physical, social and attitudinal environment in which people live and conduct their lives.

As indicated in Box 21.1, the ICF has two *parts*, each with two *components*.

Part 1. Functioning and Disability

(a) body functions and structures

(b) activities and participation

Part 2. Contextual Factors

(c) environmental factors

(d) personal factors.

Each component can be expressed in both positive and negative terms.

Definitions

The terms disorder, impairment, disability and disadvantage (handicap) have precise meanings that should be used in a consistent way by professionals. Between 1980, when WHO first published an 'International Classification of Impairments, Disabilities, and Handicaps' and the present time, the emphasis has shifted away from a purely medical view and towards a social model of disability. The ICF-CY (WHO 2007; Box 21.1) provides a common language for those involved in facilitating functioning for persons with body impairments and activity limitations. It also provides concepts and terms for describing the functional consequences in everyday life of having body impairments and activity limitations. It describes levels of functionality, identifies strengths and weaknesses and encodes them. The tool is culturally adaptable and helps clinicians target intervention based on individual performance in each developmental domain, *viz*: motor abilities, communication, cognition, social skills, emotional regulation/behaviour, and self-care skills/adaptive functioning.

This social model allows an interdisciplinary perspective on disability that reflects the views of many professionals and, more importantly, the views of disabled people themselves. It proposes that barriers, negative attitudes and exclusion by society (purposefully or inadvertently) are the things which define who is disabled within a particular society. It recognizes that many people with a physical or intellectual impairment may be disadvantaged in specific situations unless society takes steps to minimize these disadvantages. This model does not deny the existence of individual limitations or impairments but instead emphasizes that these should not be the cause of individuals being excluded. The disadvantage of a particular impairment is situationally specific and many people are disabled not by the impairment but rather by the lack of help the society in which they live (including their doctors) feels able to offer.

Thus, the extent to which a disorder, impairment or disability imposes a disadvantage on an individual depends not only on its severity but also on

- attitudes and ambitions of the child and family,
- the financial resources of the family,

- secondary problems created by professionals including doctors,
- the prejudices of the society in which the person lives,
- adaptations of the physical environment, and
- legislation in support of the disabled.

Non-fatal disabling conditions are one of the main causes for children receiving intervention and inter-disciplinary habilitation services. To maintain quality, such services need to use the ICF-CY 2007 language and framework that is shared by all professionals involved. Goals for intervention and rehabilitation have become less focused on body impairments and typical development (activity) and more focused on child functioning within context (i.e. participation). This requires involvement of family members and other persons in a child's natural environment in deciding upon and implementing interventions.

In this chapter we use the term early developmental impairment (Francoeur et al., 2010) to replace global developmental delay. The latter term is misleading to parents (as it implies their child will 'catch-up') and it is often inaccurate as many children have difficulties confined to only a few areas of development and are not 'globally' affected. The WHO (ICF-CY) addresses this issue with its International Classification of Function for Children and Youth.

The challenge for the clinician is

- to understand the underlying biology (i.e. cause),
- to explain this to parents,
- to use it to generate a probability statement to predict future outcome,
- to establish, regardless of cause, the developmental strengths and weaknesses of the individual child, and
- to create, with the help of allied professionals, such as remedial therapists and teachers, family-focused love, opportunity and encouragement to allow children to reach their potential.

Epidemiology

Definition and incidence of developmental impairment
Developmental impairment is defined as a developmental/intelligence quotient (DQ/IQ) of less than 70, a visual acuity of less than 6/60, a hearing loss of greater or equal to 90 decibels or severe non-ambulant cerebral palsy. International classifications identify ranges of function based on standard scores of DQ/IQ.

Currently two diagnostic criteria for fetal alcohol spectrum disorders (FASD) are in use: the Institute of Medicine criteria (Hoyme et al., 2005) and the 4-digit diagnostic code (Diagnostic Guide for Fetal Alcohol Spectrum Disorders, 2004). A comparison of these criteria when diagnosing FAS has been made by Astley (2006) and the main differences between these two diagnostic systems are (1) required number of characteristic facial features, (2) the definition of central nervous dysfunction and (3) the definition of the amount/level of prenatal alcohol exposure.

Assessment is based not only on DQ/IQ scores but also takes into consideration a young person's adaptive functioning so that attainment is not measured rigidly. For example, it must be acknowledged that a person with developmental cognitive impairment may function well socially or in certain work settings. Most DQ/IQ standard scoring systems identify the bottom 2% of the population (more than 2 standard deviations from the mean) as being in the impaired group. In practical terms we should regard children as having early developmental impairment when they show significant limitations in two or more domains of development before the age of 5 years in cases where those difficulties are not better explained by another developmental disorder (e.g. autistic-spectrum disorder, a cerebral palsy).

Causes of developmental impairment
- Genetic disorders
- Acquired brain injury – pre-, peri- or postnatal
  - Infection
  - Vascular disease (e.g. arterial ischaemic stroke)
  - Hypoxia ischaemia
  - Maternal drug abuse (e.g. alcohol)
- Social deprivation (e.g. poor diet or health care, or physical abuse).

Presentations in infancy
Obvious congenital abnormalities:

- neural tube defects.

Antenatal:

- poor growth
- oligo- or polyhydramnios
- reduced fetal movement
- breech or other malpresentation.

Neonatal:

- poor Apgar scores, but quick response to resuscitation.

Unusual appearance at birth:

- dysmorphism
- synostosis (see Chapter 18)

- micro- and macrocephaly (see Chapters 18 and 19)
- limb defects.

Unusual neonatal behaviour:

- sleepiness
- failure to wake for feeds
- poor suck: often difficulty with breast but not bottle feeds
- poor cry
- irritability, presence of withdrawal symptoms.

Obvious neurological abnormalities:

- hypotonia – EDI is an important cause of the floppy infant syndrome (see Chapter 20)
- hypertonia
- unusual patterns of tone (e.g. increased extensor tone, arching)
- unusual patterns of movement (e.g. jerky, dystonic)
- seizures.

Later detection:

- all of the above
- poor visual function
- poor hearing function
- delay in achieving developmental milestones
- irritability, inconsolable when upset
- disturbed behaviour and/or social behaviour
- obvious dysmorphism.

Additional points in the history:

- family history?
- consanguinity?

Clinical approach

History
Seek more information on all of the above points.

Examination
Use the clinical method (see Chapter 5).

Investigations
In blood: full blood count, chromosomal karyotype, amino acids, thyroid function tests, possibly lactate. In urine, mucopolysaccarides, organic acids. Additional investigations should be tailored to the specific clinical features. Some investigations will not be available in all centres.

Principles of management

What to tell the parents: giving the news of developmental impairment
Parents want news about diagnosis

- together,
- as soon as possible,
- sympathetically and in private, and
- with accuracy and honesty.

They also want

- help with how to pass on the news to family and friends, and
- to have the infant /child present.

Language to use and language to avoid is outlined below.

- Remember parents will take note of every word.
- Do not be too negative about future prediction if deterioration is not evident.
- Do not provide information or advice that you are not confident about. It is better to say that you or perhaps nobody knows an answer to a particular question than give false 'expert' opinions.
- Compare: 'I am very sorry but I have some very bad news for you. Your child has Down syndrome' with 'I have some news you were not expecting. Your child has a condition known as Down syndrome. This may be something you have heard of but know little about. I shall do the best I can to explain something about it to you and then explain how we can help.'
- Do not be too positive.
- Present a balanced view on therapies.
- Parents may believe that remedial therapy may 'heal'. Rather, explain that therapy maximizes developmental potential and limits secondary complications.
- Warn them of the unproven and at times harmful effect of alternative therapies (see below).

Remember the following:

- Parents are going through a major life event in receiving advice about their infant. Consequently they will recall little of this first consultation and may misunderstand some of what they do remember.

- Always try to see both parents together at important interviews.
- See if an advocate is available to attend with them (health visitor, social worker, ward nurse or a friend they know well).
- See them again soon to answer any questions they may have.

Help them understand their own feelings.

- Many parents show features of bereavement after the birth of a child with a developmental impairment. Tell them that the intensity of this grief will decrease with time.
- The family will learn to find a way to find happiness and joy, and to laugh again.
- Mothers and fathers may work through their grief at a different pace. Help them understand each others' feelings.

What to tell the parents: how to deal with uncertainty
- Uncertainty is stressful: parents want to know what the future holds for the child as soon as possible. However, this may not be possible. Tell them they will need to be brave and patient.
- A diagnostic label is no more than a probability statement; for example, the range of ability in Down syndrome is broad, from profound to borderline developmental impairment.
- It is not unusual to have to wait until the infant is 10 or more months old before a preliminary estimate of future developmental performance can be made, although this depends on the type and degree of impairment.

Treatment and therapy

What to tell the parents: give them a plan
- What they can do and who can help.
- Disabled children need what all children need: love, opportunity, setting of limits regarding what constitutes acceptable behaviour, and encouragement
- Encourage parents to have confidence as their child's main carers, teachers and therapists.
- Remedial therapists/community workers will explain how to maximize learning opportunity by teaching positioning, postures, interactive play and the provision of seating or toys.
- Therapists will assess and explain how parents can help and advise on specific interventions.

Specific diagnoses
In the remainder of this chapter we will consider in turn epilepsy, neural tube defects, fetal alcohol spectrum disorders, Down syndrome and finally other specific genetic syndromes. In the newborn period poor feeding, failure to wake for feeding, a weak cry

and ultimately failure to thrive are common. Delayed milestones then become more evident over the subsequent months. For each condition recognizable features, presentation and a guide to future health surveillance will be reviewed. Remember that all these syndromes may present with a history of reduced fetal movement, malpresentation or polyhydramnios.

THE CHILD WITH EPILEPSY
Manage as for all the epilepsies as follows:

- confirm it is an epilepsy (history, electroencephalography)
- identify/classify the epilepsy if possible
- explain the biology to the family
- teach first aid
- use an anti-epileptic drug, in most cases, if epilepsy is confirmed.

THE CHILD WITH A METABOLIC DISORDER
- Investigate and treat the treatable; for example, pyridoxine dependency, the biotin- or folinic acid-responsive disorders (see Chapter 13).

THE CHILD WITH A SURGICALLY TREATABLE DISORDER
- Developmental disability should not be regarded as a contraindication to appropriate treatment (e.g. in neural tube defects: see below);
- hydrocephalus and spina bifida;
- recognized comorbidities; for example, cardiac defects in Down syndrome; tracheo-oesophageal fistulae; anal atresia.

Common myths are outlined in Box 21.2.

Neural tube defects

Incidence
There is marked geographical variation: fetal incidence of neural tube defect is 17 per 10 000 pregnancies; live birth incidence is 5.7–6.7 per 10 000 live births. The difference in these figures is due to termination of pregnancy and deaths *in utero*, particularly in cases with severe defects.

Cause
Multifactorial

- *Genetic*. Risk of recurrence for non-syndromic sibling of proband: from 3 to 5%; 0.7% with pre-conceptional folate supplementation.
    - Folate-dependent metabolic pathway gene polymorphisms (e.g. *PCMT1*, *MTHFR*, methionine synthase and methionine synthase reductase).
    - Folate-independent pathways (lipomyelomeningocoeles are folate-resistant).

Box 21.2 Common myths

Early assessment or imaging accurately predicts future development

For many children a diagnostic label is associated with a wide range of potential. The passing of time allows a more accurate assessment of potential to emerge. The best indication of how a child will make progress in future is how they are making progress at present, rather than what imaging shows. Ultimately, many young people with a developmental impairment may achieve some degree of independence as adults if given the right opportunity and encouragement.

Intensive intervention alters outcome

Instead emphasize love, opportunity and encouragement (which all children need to reach their potential). Concentrate on treating the treatable (see above), help parents to identify realistic goals and what activities to include in their play with the child to encourage the next developmental step.

Brain stimulants/mega-vitamins/sicca-cell injections/stem cells alter outcome

There is no evidence base for any of these but there are cases of reported harm being done to children treated with them.

- ○ Syndromes such as 22q11 microdeletion, X-linked and autosomal dominant Mendelian disorders (e.g. Currarino triad: sacral, anal and urological anomalies).
- *Folic acid deficit*: dietary.
- *Maternal factors*: obesity, diabetes with hyperinsulinaemia, first-trimester fever, antiepileptic drugs: valproate, phenytoin, carbamazepine, polytherapy; retinoins.

Presentation:

- *Antenatal:* combined test (ultrasound with maternal alpha-foeto-protein) gives 99% sensitivity (see below under Down syndrome).
- Fetal ultrasonography (18–20 weeks of pregnancy):
- Head:
  - ○ concavity of the frontal bones (the 'lemon sign'); present in 50% from 16 to 24 weeks' gestation;
  - ○ ventriculomegaly (moderate to severe), present in 70% from late second trimester and up to 90% by term;
  - ○ Chiari II malformation: from 16 weeks' gestation the 'banana sign' reflecting abnormal anterior cerebellum with obliteration of cisterna magna; very few false positives.
- Spine:
  - ○ C- or U-shaped vertebrae in sagittal views.

There is raised maternal alpha-fetoprotein (AFP) at 16–20 weeks of pregnancy in 70–75% of cases of open spina bifida. If AFP is raised, acetylcholinesterase will be raised in amniotic fluid. Serial fetal ultrasound monitors growth and development.

Management at birth: what to tell the parents

Unlike many conditions considered below, the presence and potential impact of this condition will be immediately obvious to the doctor. The immediate situation needs handling with skill. Parents need a calming and reassuring statement, such as "Your infant has been born with some under-development of part of the back-bone. We need to examine the area thoroughly, perhaps do some tests and then we will be able to work out how best to help." Following the clinical assessment and explanation of the management plan can then follow. It is important for all staff concerned to be calm, positive and reassuring.

In due course they can be counselled on the immediate, medium- and long-term care plan. They need information on the primary and secondary complications of the condition (see below) and the recurrence risk for future children and prenatal diagnostics.

Assessment of the newborn with spina bifida

Involve a neurosurgeon, a renal or urological specialist and spinal orthopaedic surgeon.

Clinical assessment

The lesion may be obvious or subtle. In the routine examination of the back look for the following:

- an open lesion and its configuration
- large midline lipoma, preventing positioning or care in the supine position
- asymmetrical natal cleft
- dermal sinus above the natal cleft (distinguish from benign sacral dimple in the coccygeal region)
- midline naevus; for example hair patch (a subtle dermal sinus may also be present)
- kyphosis or scoliosis
- talipes equinovarus (may be asymmetrical).

Any of these may be present, signifying an open or occult neural tube defect. Then, identify the level of the spinal lesion, the major determinant of morbidity.

- Radiological level: use X-ray or magnetic resonance imaging (MRI) of spine; MR has no known risks related to exposure to the magnetic fields and is preferable to computed tomography in infants who are at higher risk than older children of long-term risks associated with exposure to radiation.
- Neurological level: often higher than the anatomical level, and determines future disability. Assess muscle bulk, spontaneous anti-gravity movements, spinal reflexes, abnormal spread of reflexes, and sacral sensation (see Table 21.1).

Table 21.1 Clinical signs related to level of lesion

Site of lesion	Clinical view	Functional prognosis
Thoracic lesion	Innervation of the upper limb and neck musculature and variable function of trunk musculature are present with no volitional lower limb movements. Patients with thoracic malformations tend to have more involvement of the CNS and associated cognitive deficits. Sensation is disordered below hips.	Wheelchair is used for independent movement from early childhood.
Upper lumbar lesion (L1–L2–L3)	Variable hip flexor and hip adductor strength is characteristic, some sensation below hip joint and absence of hip extensors, hip abductors, and all knee and ankle movements are noted.	Long orthosis (knee-ankle-foot orthosis) and crutches for ambulation. For longer distances uses wheelchairs.
Lower lumbar lesion (L4–L5)	Hip flexor, adductor, medial hamstring and quadriceps strength is present; strength of the lateral hamstrings, hip abductors and ankle dorsiflexors is variable; and strength of the ankle plantar flexors is absent. This means that voluntary knee flexion movements and foot dorsiflexion and eversion (turning outwards) movements are possible.	For independent walking usually needs ankle-foot orthosis and, in some cases, crutches or sticks. In later childhood. may be mobile by wheelchair.
Sacral lesion	The power in foot flexors and/or hip extensors (gluteus maximus) may be moderately reduced.	Usually walks independently. Sometimes might need foot orthosis.

Also note the following:

- associated central nervous system (CNS) malformations;
- measure head circumference serially;
- bone or joint deformities; for example, congenital hip dislocation (20%), kyphosis, and talipes equinovarus. Refer to specialist orthopaedic team;

- dermal sinus tract. Leads to risk of CNS infection. Often associated with underlying spinal malformation. Needs referral to neurosurgeon;
- non-neurological anomalies (e.g. check anus, heart);
- bowel dysfunction. Assess anal tone. Neurogenic constipation often present (also effects of concurrent anorectal anomalies);
- bladder dysfunction: often incomplete bladder emptying against outflow resistance, leading to secondary reflux nephropathy. Check for a good urinary stream – measure urine output by weighing nappies – urgent urology/nephrology opinion if poor.

Recommended pre-surgical care for open lesions is to

- cover wound with sterile gauze, wash daily with normal saline, changing dressing when soiled;
- give ampicillin 200 mg/kg/day in two divided doses, gentamycin 5 mg/kg/day in two doses with or without cloxacillin 100 mg/kg/day in two doses until wound clean and dry;
- treat for meningitis if fever and/or seizures and/or depressed conscious level.

The lesion should be closed as soon as possible and always in 24 h.
For post-surgical care the surgical site is inspected every day for any signs of infection and cerebrospinal fluid leak.

Longer-term sequelae
Part of longer-term sequelae goes beyond the first year of life and so is outside the scope of this handbook. Nevertheless, the given information should be very helpful for planning long-term goals and a treatment/habilitation scheme.

The child needs to be monitored closely for the development of secondary complications. This is the role of the general paediatrician, involving community-based medical services (general practitioners or neurodevelopmental paediatricians) or specialist services (neurosurgery, orthopaedics, nephrology or urology) as necessary.

- *Hydrocephalus* occurs in 80% of myelomeningocoele cases, often precipitated by surgical closure of the back lesion. It requires ventriculo-peritoneal (VP) shunting, often with some urgency because of rapid progression. It is uncommon in other variants. Monitor head circumference weekly for first month then monthly; assess pressure symptoms, irritability or sleepiness, bulging or pulsing fontanelle, vomiting, poor feeding; serial cranial ultrasound should be performed at 2 and 6 weeks and 4 months.
- *Chiari type II malformation:* occurs in 80–100% of cases, and the main cause of hydrocephalus. Symptoms relate to brainstem compression and lower cranial nerves dysfunction: dysphagia, repetitive vomiting, impaired suction, impaired gag reflex, dizziness, characteristic weak or squeaky cry or stridor caused by vocal cord palsy, apneoic episodes, nystagmus, bradycardic episodes, repeated aspirations

leading to pneumonia. Torticollis, opisthotonus, facial weakness and motor disorders may occur (5–10%). They may become apparent only after lesion closure and may be associated with increasing ventriculomegaly.

- *Cord-tethering syndrome:* back pain, mixed upper and lower motor neuron signs, enlarging area of sensory disturbance, incontinence. Symptoms may start appearing at any age, especially during periods of rapid growth.

- *Syringomyelia:* caused by subarachnoid obstruction to cerebrospinal fluid flow (11–77%). Signs and symptoms are similar to those of Chiari type II malformation, tethered cord or VP shunt malfunction. Syringomyclia and tethered cord are treated surgically.

- *Bladder and bowel dysfunction* (affects 97%): the neurogenic bladder leads to overflow and urge incontinence, bladder dysynergia, and vesicoureteral reflux with a risk of urinary tract infections, upper tract dilatation and chronic renal insufficiency. Manage with continence advice, regular catheterizations, medication (pro- or anticholinergics) and surgical procedures (intravesical botulinum toxin injections; vesicostomy; bladder augmentation and bladder neck procedures). Regular renal/urology team follow-up should include:

  ○ renal function tests, blood pressure measurement and urine culture 3 monthly;

  ○ pre- and post-micturition ultrasound scan of the urogenital tract 3–6 monthly, as a measure of residual urine;

  ○ antibiotic prophylaxis is indicated;

  ○ bladder catheterization is discussed;

  ○ examination for cryptorchism with referral for surgical treatment if necessary;

  ○ assessment and treatment of bowel movement disorders;

  ○ management of bowel dysfunction; constipation with overflow soiling; faecal impaction may worsen urinary dysfunction. Managed with continence advice, diet, laxatives and enemas. Refer to paediatric surgeons. Conduit procedures for anterograde colonic washouts may be required.

- *Orthopaedic problems:* kyphoscoliosis (20–40%) with secondary cardiorespiratory complications, hip dislocation, knee contractures, pathological fractures from bone demineralization, internal and external tibial torsion, foot deformities (clubfoot, equinovalgus, cavus, calcaneovarus, calcaneovalgus) are common. Orthopaedic assessment for each of the above at 3, 6 and 12 months. Treatments include bracing, rigid orthoses, spasticity management, physiotherapy and surgery.

- *Latex allergy:* the risk which increases with age is minimized by avoiding latex articles, educating parents and using silicone or vinyl as a substitute. Up to 70% have latex allergy. Allergy symptoms: tearing of the eyes and runny nose, sneezing,wheeziness, skin rashes, urticaria, itching or swelling at the site of contact; in severe cases there are respiratory disorders, and rarely anaphylactic shock.

- *Trophic skin lesions:* poorly healing, pressure ulcers on pelvic ischia and feet in the area of sensory deficit. The risk is minimized by frequent inspection (by parents or the child) of at-risk areas; noting redness of 45 min duration or more; keeping skin clean and dry; wearing footwear inside and outside; care with choice of clothing and footwear; care with braces and orthoses; maintaining weight symmetry while lying or sitting in a wheelchair with frequent position changes, Nursing care to affected areas.

- *Growth disorders*: short stature seen in 50–60%, usually related to skeletal deformity and hypothalamic-pituitary dysfunction, which can predetermine premature puberty and lack of growth hormone. Shortage of growth hormone is diagnosed in 10–20% patients with myelomeningocoele. Either inadequate nutrition or obesity may occur.

- *Tumours*: teratoma and benign dermoid cysts may present late with paraparesis.

- *Dental hygiene*: arrange dental care with advice to parents on diet, teeth-cleaning.

- *Seizure control*: seizures occur in 10–30% and are related to associated brain malformations, or may be a sign of shunt malfunction or infection.

Note that deterioration of neurological status, rapid progression of a scoliosis, disparity between the myelomeningocoele level and neurological level, emergence of asymmetry of neurological signs and a suspicion of Chiari type II malformation, should each lead to an urgent MRI of the spinal cord/head with neurosurgical referral as appropriate.

Outlook
- *Ambulation*: lesion level predicts ambulatory ability. Cognitive, perceptual and coordination impairments, spasticity and bone deformities may also limit activity. Ankle dorsiflexion (L5) strength predicts community ambulation: outdoors walking and independent transfers. Use ankle orthoses and foot care only. Knee extension (L3–L4) strength predicts household ambulation: standing for transfers, walking short distances with hip-knee-ankle-foot orthoses, rigid gait orthoses and wheelchair for longer distances. Poor trunk stability and hip flexion (T6–L2) predicts impaired ambulation: therapeutic weight bearing with orthoses. Wheelchair indoors for mobility. Ambulation may deteriorate in later childhood.

- *Cognition*: The majority of children with myelomeningocoele do not have overt developmental impairment. Mean IQ is lower than average, about 90. Performance IQ is typically below verbal IQ. Recurrent VP shunt infections predict lower IQ. Monitor head circumference monthly; assess pressure symptoms, irritability or sleepiness, bulging or pulsing fontanelle, vomiting, poor feeding; serial cranial ultrasound at 2, 6 and 13 weeks and 5 months. Urgent referral is needed for VP shunt if hydrocephalus is confirmed.

- *Vision and hearing*: test as a routine, as for all children with a developmental impairment.

- *Psychosocial issues*: puberty and sex education, self-image problems, educational and occupational exclusion.

- *Mortality and morbidity*: increased risk of death in infancy with high spinal lesions, open lesions and multiple malformations. Causes of increased mortality: decompensated hydrocephalus, VP shunt infection; renal failure; peri-operative (particularly scoliosis surgery). The majority of children can expect to survive well into adulthood: 30% of adults continue to require daily additional help. Quality of life affected by sequelae and functional limitations rather than level of lesion per se.

Creating opportunity and encouragement for the child
This is best achieved by helping parents adjust to their child's condition. Remedial therapists will help minimize the disadvantages attendant on the child's impairment (it is important to emphasize that they do not 'put the problem right') by the provision of aids and advice to parents and teachers on how to create opportunities for improved function. Excellent communication between home, hospital and school is required. All professionals involved should direct parents to information specific to their child's condition (associations, websites, etc.). A suggested approach to habilitation is given in Table 21.3.

Fetal alcohol spectrum disorders (FASD)
Marked geographical variation occurs in prevalence of FASD within and between countries. Estimated worldwide prevalence is 9 in 1000 live births but even higher prevalence rates have been observed (Italy 35/1000, Croatia 40/1000).

Alcohol is a teratogen. In early pregnancy binge drinking (five or more units on one occasion) can lead to severe organ malformation or be lethal; and in later pregnancy is especially detrimental to growth and CNS development. No universal safety limit (time, kind or amount) has been identified. The longer the mother drinks the poorer the outcome: every day without alcohol benefits the child. There is biological variability (genetic, nutrition, socioeconomic) and each woman and fetus is different but there is no way to foresee the limit for a harmful dose in individual cases. The evidence of harm is clearer the more the mother drinks per occasion and/or per week; binge drinking is especially detrimental. One unit is 330 ml of beer, 120 ml of wine or 40 ml of spirits (beware: strengths vary), and the only safe advice is *do not drink when pregnant or planning pregnancy.*

A specific pattern of prenatal growth deficiency, developmental impairment, and craniofacial abnormality caused by prenatal alcohol exposure originally confined to the fetal alcohol syndrome (FAS), now viewed as a spectrum of disorders (FASD) including FAS, partial FAS, alcohol-related neurodevelopmental disorder and alcohol-related birth defects (see Table 21.4).

Presentation
In the newborn period with symmetrical growth retardation (but head small relative to length, especially as infancy progresses), dysmorphism including small palpebral fissures, smooth philtrum and a thin upper lip (see http://depts.washington.edu/fasdpn/htmls/lip-philtrum-guides.htm). There may be microcephaly already at birth, postnatal head growth often slowed. Feeding and weight-gain are often poor.

Table 21.3 A suggested approach to habilitation in spina bifida and contributions from individual team members

Team member	Issues concerned	Tests	Therapy
Physiotherapist	Muscle strength and range of joint movement of lower limbs, correct body posture, selection of compensatory aids and orthoses	Assessment of muscle strength with the help of manual muscle testing. Assessment of range of motion in the joints of lower limbs with the help of goniometry. Assessment of senses with the help of ASIA sensory topographic scheme. Follow-up of skin status (trophic ulceration).	Passive movements of lower limbs, muscle stretching exercises, position, training of head control, waist-pelvis control, and sitting balance; strengthening of muscles of lower limbs, etc. Instructions to parents and other family members on the care of an infant with myelomeningocoele. Application of positions in routine activity. Selection and adaptation of compensatory aids (sitting chair, standing frame) and adaptation of orthoses.
Occupational therapist	Fine motor and self-care skills	Clinical follow-up (fine motor skills as infant moves or plays). Focus should be given to child's posture, coordination, transferring movements (e.g. from bed to chair). To inform a remedial programme it may be useful to examine muscle tone, primitive reflexes (i.e. balance reaction, asymmetry) and muscle strength. Functional tasks (formed in order to measure or assess the mobility in joints, muscle function and strength, tone and coordination of movements)	Hand function and hand–eye coordination is encouraged through play. Special seating is adapted for feeding and playing; special feeding instruments are selected, if necessary.

Table 21.3 *Continued*

Team member	Issues concerned	Tests	Therapy
Speech and language therapist	Assess non-verbal and then verbal communication		Games and nursery rhymes which encourage the child to attribute meaning to signs (language) and the rhythms of speech; helped by Portage, a UK-based home-visiting early education service for pre-school children but equivalents are found in many European countries
Social worker	To identify social need according to ability		To share experiences of parents who have overcome any attendant difficulties; and provide information on the benefit system

ASIA, American Spinal Injury Association.

Table 21.4 A comparison of Institute of Medicine (IOM) and four-digit diagnostic criteria for fetal alcohol syndrome

	IOM	Four-digit diagnostic code
Growth retardation	Pre- or postnatal height or weight ≤10 centile, corrected for racial normative values if possible	Pre- or postnatal height or weight ≤10th centile, corrected for racial normative values and midparental height if possible
Characteristic pattern of minor facial anomalies	Two out of three: 1. palpebral fissure length ≤10th centile, 2. philtrum rank 4 or 5, 3. upper lip rank 4 or 5	All three: palpebral fissure length ≤10 centile, philtrum rank 4 or 5, upper lip rank 4 or 5
CNS	Evidence of deficient brain growth or abnormal morphogenesis, including at least one of the following: 1. structural brain abnormalities 2. head circumference ≤10th centile	Evidence of at least one of the following: structural brain abnormalities or microcephaly ≤−2SD Neurological abnormality: seizure disorder of prenatal origin or hard neurological signs significant brain dysfunction: three or more domains of brain functions ≤−2SD of mean
Alcohol consumption during pregnancy	Confirmed pattern of excessive intake characterized by substantial regular intake or heavy episodic drinking *or* without confirmed maternal alcohol exposure	Confirmed prenatal alcohol exposure, a specific pattern is not required

After Astley (2006).

Some children exposed to binge drinking in early pregnancy have organ malformations, especially renal or cardiac abnormalities; late onset is common with developmental impairment, specific learning disorder or behavioural difficulties first observed at preschool/school age.

Diagnosis may be difficult, especially if alcohol consumption is concealed. Ask about consumption before and during pregnancy and how it changed when pregnancy was confirmed. These questions are routine but reliable answers require confidentiality and trust.

Newborn problems: irritability, tremulousness and marked startle reflex amount to a neonatal withdrawal syndrome which may require sedation, constipation and feeding problems.

Health surveillance issues: developmental and at times behavioural difficulties emerge through childhood. They may not be evident in infancy. A high percentage of children with FASD do not carry characteristic dysmorphism. If FASD is suspected, screen heart and kidney for associated abnormalities and vision and hearing for impairment.

Down syndrome
Incidence is about 1 in every 700 live births. The cause is trisomy 21.

Diagnosis
Prenatally by amniocentesis or chorionic villus biopsy following maternal AFP screen linked to maternal age. Recommendations from the Serum Urine and Ultrasound Screening Study (SURUSS) and NICE guidelines currently recommend the following:

- Combined test: nuchal translucency scanning plus serum measurement of free beta-human chorionic gonadotrophin (hCG) and pregnancy-associated plasma protein A (PAPP-A) should be offered to women at between of 11 weeks and 13 weeks + 6 days of gestation.
- The quadruple test: this measures free beta-hCG, AFP, inhibin-A and uE3 and is the best to offer for women presenting in the second trimester (see Table 6.2, p. 64).

A method for the prenatal diagnosis of chromosomal abnormalities is being developed using the allelic ratios of polymorphisms present within the methylated promoter of a DNA sequence on chromosomes 13, 18 and 21. This should allow maternal blood tests to replace the invasive chorionic villus biopsy and amniocentesis methods we currently use.

Postnatally through distinctive dysmorphism: microcephaly, brachycephaly, mongoloid slant to the eyes, single palmar crease, wide space between great and second toe, small ears, macroglossia.

Hypotonia, an important cause of the floppy infant.

Issues for early infancy
Poor feeding, congenital heart disease common, ideally screen with echocardiogram (usually atrioventricular canal defects), may need urgent treatment. Transient myeloproliferative disease; duodenal atresia.

Long-term health surveillance issues
Long-term cardiovascular surveillance; atlanto-axial instability (usually after infancy). Intellectual disability. Hearing and vision problems are common, arrange screening. Screening for hypothyroidism.

Other common associations
Celiac disease; hypothyroidism often associated with thyroiditis; enhanced risk of acute myeloid leukaemia (more than 50-fold increased risk compared to the general population); immunodeficiency, impaired cellular immunity predisposes to bacterial or fungal infections; dry skin may require Oilatum emollient in the bath and moisturising creams (later psoriasis and eczema is more common).

Clinical features and presentation: hypotonia is striking. Feeding difficulties are marked and often require tube feeding. Dysmorphism includes an almond-shaped palpebral fissure, an elongated face, prominent nose and smooth philtrum. Undescended testicles and small feet.

Long-term health surveillance: the behavioural phenotype leads to excessive weight gain with compulsive eating after the age of 2. Excessive weight gain may be associated with sleep disorders (often obstructive sleep apnoea) and the emergence of scoliosis. Delayed puberty and short stature are associated.

Specific genetic syndromes
If the clinical phenotype refers to a specific genetic syndrome, the clinical geneticist should be consulted about further investigations. Defer labelling a condition as a specific syndrome until specific evidence from further investigations, if potentially available, supports the diagnosis.

Prader–Willi syndrome
Incidence is 1 in 12000–15000 live births. The cause is chromosome 15p deletion (paternal) or uniparental disomy (maternal).

Presentation: marked hypotonia with feeding problems and poor weight gain in infancy (often requiring tube-feeding). Often happy, placid babies with short stature, small hands and feet and fair skin.

Dysmorphism: distinctive facial features: narrow face, almond shape eyes, small mouth with thin upper lip and down-turned corners.

Long-term health surveillance: severe obesity (often between 1 and 6 years) due to obsessive over-eating with associated diabetes, hypertension, chronic venous insufficiency, cellulitis, and hypoventilation. *Hypogonadism, undescended testicles*, small penis, delayed puberty. Also, *strabismus*, scoliosis, osteoporosis (with childhood fractures in some cases), disturbed sleep and sleep apneoa, enuresis, dental problems, including soft tooth enamel, thick saliva, poor oral hygiene, bruxism (teeth grinding).

Behaviour problems may include temper tantrums, violent outbursts, obsessive/compulsive or oppositional defiant behaviour.

Phenylketonuria
There is marked geographical variation. Incidence is 1 in 15 000 live births. The cause is an inborn error of metabolism: phenylalanine hydroxylase deficiency (autosomal recessive).

Phenylketonuria is normally detected through neonatal screening at 6–14 days after birth. If undetected it may present with seizures, albinism and a 'musty odour' to the infant's sweat and urine. Strict diet can prevent progression of the disease. Untreated children are normal at birth but then present with an evolving developmental impairment and acquired microcephaly. Seizures are common.

Rett syndrome
Incidence is 1 in 10 000–22 000 live births. The cause is mutations in the *MECP2* or more rarely the *CDLK5* or *FOXG1* genes and is seen almost exclusively in females.

Development is typically normal until the age of 6 months or so, then development slows, purposeful hand use is lost and there is a deceleration of head growth. Hand stereotypes appear such as wringing and/or repeatedly putting hands into the mouth and holding the shoulders abducted with the hands at the level of the mouth. Developmental plateau and then regression then follows with the long-term emergence of a dystonia, avoidance of eye contact, lack of social skills, a loss of communication skills and in the teenage years scoliosis. Seizures are common.

Neurocutaneous syndromes
The incidence of neurofibromatosis type 1 (NF1) is 1 in 3000–4000 live births; that of tuberous sclerosis is 10–16 per 100 000 live births.

Causes are listed below:

- NF1: mutation of chromosome 17q11.2 encoding neurofibromin.
- NF2: mutation of chromosome 22q12 encoding NF2 (Merlin).
- Tuberous sclerosis: autosomal dominant pattern with variable penetrance. Two-thirds result from new sporadic genetic mutations. Mapped to two genetic loci, *TSC1* and *TSC2*. *TSC1* encodes for the protein hamartin, and is located on chromosome 9q34; *TSC2* encodes for the protein tuberin, and is located on chromosome 16p13.3.

The café-au-lait patches associated with neurofibromatosis or depigmented patches associated with tuberous sclerosis may be evident in the newborn period requiring further clinical assessment followed by special investigation as necessary.

Apart from non-specific features such as evolving developmental impairment throughout infancy, it would a be unusual for the neurocutaneous syndromes to present with medical problems in infancy. The one exception is in the context of the epileptic spasms and hypsarrhythmia that make up West syndrome, of which tuberous sclerosis is a common cause.

The velo-cardio-facial syndrome
Incidence is 1 in 4000 live births. The cause is a deletion in chromosome 22q11.2.

Presentation and signs: may present in the newborn period with cyanosis related to an associated congenital heart disease, craniofacial dysmorphism with a round face, prominent parietal bones and a bulbous nasal tip. The face appears long and hypotonic with narrow palpebral fissures, puffy upper eyelids, a squared nasal root and a narrow alar base with thin alae nasi. There may be cleft palate, hypospadias and long tapering fingers.

Other features: nasal regurgitation, hypocalcaemia, poor feeding.

Long-term health surveillance: check for cardiac abnormalities and disorders of calcium metabolism. Monitor growth and development (short stature seen in about 30%).

Angelman syndrome
The incidence is 1 in 12 000–20 000 live births. The cause is 15q11–13 deletion (maternal) or uniparental disomy (paternal).

Angelman syndrome is often not diagnosed in the newborn period.

Presentation: as infancy progresses, developmental impairment becomes more obvious. The behavioural phenotype is one of a happy demeanour. Spontaneous laughter is a characteristic but inconstant feature. Children often have jerky arm movements due to cortical myoclonus hand flapping movements, are restless with a short attention span and may have episodes of over-breathing or hyperventilation.

There is evolving microcephaly, seizures may develop in infancy (usually by 3 years of age) associated with large-amplitude posterior slow waves and spikes on the electroencephalogram.

Characteristic facial appearance includes a broad jaw. A wide based stiff-legged ataxic and apraxic gait evolves.

Long-term health surveillance: classification management of seizures.

Klinefelter syndrome
The incidence is 1 in 500–1000 males. The cause is karyotype 47, XXY.

Presentation in the newborn period or early infancy rare. Developmental impairment emerging in the second half of infancy with an emphasis on low tone and delayed motor development. Later in childhood language impairment emerges in 25–85% of published studies.

Long-term health surveillance: hypogonadism with the effects emerging at puberty.

Turner syndrome
The incidence is 1 in 2500 females. The cause is karyotype 45, X.

Presentation and signs: may be indentified antenatally with a heart or renal abnormality, cystic hygroma or ascites.

Dysmorphism: symmetrical growth retardation, lymphoedema of hands and feet, shield like chest with wide-spaced nipples, low hairline, low set ears, small finger nails.

Health surveillance: visual impairment from scleral or corneal abnormalities or glaucoma; screen for heart abnormalities.

Developmental impairment emerges throughout infancy.

Triple X syndrome
The incidence is 1 in 1000 live births in females. The cause is karyotype 47, XXX.

Unusual to present in the newborn period or infancy. Indeed, may not present throughout life! Associated with hypotonia and delayed development in some. The clue to the diagnosis is often disorders of menstruation after puberty.

Williams syndrome
The incidence is 1 in 20 000 live births. The cause is a deletion on chromosome 7 which may include several genes to give a varying phenotype: *CLIP2*, *ELN* (connective tissue abnormalities and cardiovascular disease, specifically supravalvular aortic stenosis), *GTF2I*, *GTF2IRD1* (facial features) and *LIMK1*.

Newborn period and presentation: dysmorphism: an elfin facial appearance with a low nasal bridge. There may be failure to thrive and low muscle tone. Presentation often occurs after infancy with developmental impairment, good verbal skills but poor understanding.

Health surveillance issues: cardiac abnormalities including supravalvular aortic stenosis and transient hypercalcaemia.

Fragile-X syndrome
The incidence is 1 in 4000 males; 1 in 8000 females. The cause is mutations in the *FMR1* gene encoding fragile X intellectual disability 1 protein, which probably has a role in synapse development. CGG triplet repeats are expanded in the *FMR1* gene and ability relates to the size of the expansion.

Presentation: even though this is an X-linked disorder both males and females can be affected. Recognizable dysmorphism becomes more evident with impairment; but features are very variable. Look for prominent ears, macrocephaly with a prominent forehead, flexible finger joints, high palate, pes planus. Pubertal enlargement of testicles and a long face. Impairment ranges from mild learning disabilities to severe intellectual disability. There are developmental delays, especially speech and language (most often in males). Later in childhood there may be identified attention deficit hyperactivity disorder (ADHD) or poor attention span, or autism and autistic behaviours, such as hand flapping, hand biting and chewing on clothes.

Long-term health surveillance: much related to behaviour. Social and emotional problems, such as aggression in males or shyness in females with frequent tantrums; may get anxious, but often have a good sense of humour.

In common with many children with developmental impairments they may be very sensitive to stimuli such as sound.

References

Astley SJ. Comparison of the 4-Digit Diagnostic Code and the Hoyme Diagnostic Guidelines for Fetal Alcohol Spectrum Disorders. *Pediatrics*, 2006, 118:1532–1545.

Diagnostic guide for fetal alcohol spectrum disorders. The 4 digit code. University of Washington. 3rd edition 2004. http://depts.washington.edu/fasdpn/htmls/4-digit-code.htm

Francoeur E, Ghosh S, Reynolds K, Robins R. An international journey in search of diagnostic clarity: early developomental impairment. *Journal of Developmental & Behavioral Pediatrics*, 2010, 4:338–340.

Hoyme HE, May PA, Kalberg WO, Kodituwakku P, Gossage JP, Trujillo PM, Buckely DC, Miller JH, Aragon AS, Khaole N, Viljoen D, Jones KL, Robinson LK. A practical clinical approach to diagnosis of fetal alcohol spectrum disorders; clarification of the 1996 institute of medicine criteria. *Pediatrics* 2005, 115:39–47.

WHO. *International Classification of Functioning, Disability and Health: Child and Youth Version*. Geneva, WHO, 2007.

WHO. *International Classification of Impairments, Disabilities and Disadvantages (Handicaps)*. Geneva, WHO, 1980.

Resources

Bjorck-Akesson E et al. The ICF-CY as a tool in child habilitation/early childhood intervention – feasibility and usefulness as a common language and frame of reference for practice. *Disability and Rehabilitation*, 2010, 32(S1):S125–S138.

Chapter 22
Cerebral palsy

Florian Heinen and Peter Baxter

Key messages
- Cerebral palsy (CP) can be diagnosed in the first year(s) of life.
- It has no cure but does have appropriate multidisciplinary management, especially functional therapy (e.g. physiotherapy) and communicating the diagnosis to the parents to allow realistic expectations about development. Physiotherapy is necessary but lacks specificity.
- Diagnosis of CP has three aspects: clinical type and pattern (Surveillance of Cerebral Palsy in Europe), severity (Gross Motor Function Classification System) and etiology (history, pathoanatomical distribution and timing of lesion; imaging).
- Essentials for development: binding, family involvement and educating parents.

Common errors
- False positive: misdiagnosing transitory neurological phenomena or a single missed milestone at a single timepoint as 'early or likely CP'.
- False negative: diagnosis is not confirmed within the first year of life.
- Misleading communication; pressure, not support: 'you must do this to avoid that'.
- Therapeutic misconceptions, or 'the-more-you-give-the-more-you-get medication' (vitamins, minerals, 'cognitive enhancers', etc.).

When to worry
Risk factors
- History of preterm delivery and/or birth complications.
- Birth <32 weeks of gestational age or birthweight <1500 g.
- Neonatal seizures, encephalopathy, hyperbilirubinaemia or hypoglycaemia.
- Suspected or proven pathological sonography (e.g. periventricular leukomalacia, infarction, thalamic lesions).

Possible signs

- Reduced spontaneous motor behaviour, including sucking and feeding.
- Abnormal muscle tone; for example, initial hypotonia, later hypertonia with persistent excess of extensor tone in trunk and neck, scissoring, or fisting (thumb in palm, poor head control).
- Delayed motor milestones beyond stated limit (but see also Common errors, above): head control 4 months; rolling over 5 months; sitting unsupported 9 months; standing with assistance 14 months; walking alone 18 months.
- Characteristic 'catch' on fast passive movement at the ankle, suggesting spasticity.
- Pathologically brisk deep-tendon reflexes together with other upper motor neuron signs.
- Persistent motor reactions: Moro, asymmetric tonic neck reflexes, etc.

Definition

Owing to the complexity of the biological systems involved (cortico-subcortico-spino-muscular) no single definition is available that covers all aspects of cerebral palsy (CP). The following three suggestions have good practical use.

CP

CP describes a group of permanent disorders of the development of movement and posture, limiting activity, that are attributed to non-progressive disturbances that occurred in the developing fetal or infant brain. The motor disorders of CP are often accompanied by disturbances of sensation, visual perception, cognition, communication or behaviour, epilepsy and/or secondary musculoskeletal problems.

This definition highlights on the one hand the priority of the motor system disorder and on the other the important comorbidities. Within the first year of life the motor system is the easiest developmental ability to observe and examine (AACPDM, 2007).

Spasticity (hypertonia)

The US Pediatric Motor Disorder Task Force proposed the following definition of spasticity (compared to dystonia or rigidity). Hypertonia is used as 'headline'. 'Spasticity' is defined as hypertonia in which one or both of the following signs are present: (a) resistance to externally imposed movement increases with increasing speed of stretch and varies with the direction of joint movement and/or (b) above a threshold speed or joint angle, resistance to externally imposed movement rises rapidly.

'Dystonia' is defined as a movement disorder in which involuntary sustained or intermittent muscle contractions cause twisting and repetitive movements, abnormal postures, or both (Sanger et al., 2003). Dystonia is not velocity-dependent.

Upper motor neuron syndrome

Damage to the motor areas and/or pathways of the central nervous system may give rise to a specific type of movement disorders arising rostral to (i.e. above the level of) the lower motor neuron and subsumed under the term of upper motor neuron syndrome (UMNS). In the context of this syndrome, an easily triggered muscle stretch reflex and a velocity-dependent increase of muscle tone upon passive stretching (pathological tonic stretch reflex) of affected motor segments are considered the most important clinical criteria for the presence of spasticity.

Classic descriptions of UMNS differentiate between clinically negative and clinically positive symptoms: negative symptoms include paresis, impaired coordination and impaired control of movement together with easy fatigability of the limb(s). Positive symptoms include spasticity, abnormal posture (spastic dystonia) and – over time – changes in the mechanical properties of muscles with a tendency to develop contractures, which are initially dynamic and later fixed.

Clinical approach

While taking the history (especially the 'When to worry' points above), observe the infant's spontaneous motor behaviour, eye contact and visual behaviour ('go by the eyes'), interaction with their parents and adaptive motor behaviour, for example undressing.

With the child on a stable warm surface, offer objects that are suitable for the first year of life and observe visual interest, reaching, grasping, etc. Then perform a flexible and adaptable neurological examination including (a) cranial nerves, (b) muscle stretch (i.e. deep-tendon) reflexes, (c) motor reactions and (d) milestones. Use the formalized help of the Basic Neurological Examination as orientation to differentiate normal from abnormal neurological development (see Tables 22.1–22.5, below).

Make special note of the head size, response to visual and auditory stimuli, head control, pronator and thumb adductor tone, hip joint mobility (especially abduction), slow (range of motion) and fast (modified Tardieu test) ankle dorsiflexion (known in some countries as 'flexion'), presence or absence and symmetry of the Moro response, asymmetric tonic neck reflexes and defensive responses.

Use the data from these assessments to decide the following. Can CP be diagnosed? Yes, no or needs further monitoring?

Note: hypertonia or spasticity are rarely present in the neonatal period or in the so-called honeymoon period of the first 3 months of life. In unilateral CP, even when there is a demonstrated cause such as a porencephalic cyst, an infant may not show any features at all until after 3 months, when it is noted that the affected arm is not being moved or used as much as the other side, and there is a tendency to hold it pronated and fisted (with the thumb adducted across the palm). Neglect of a limb can be an early feature. In bilateral CP truncal hypotonia and poor head control are the main signs in the first few months of life, and may be difficult to differentiate from other causes of neonatal hypotonia (see also Chapter 20). Some can also show asymmetric axial tone with head lag when being pulled to sit but reasonable head control when held prone. Bottom shuffling can be a later presenting feature. Many with severe early-onset problems can be unsettled infants who cry a lot.

If yes, is the type according to Surveillance of Cerebral Palsy in Europe (SCPE) (Cans et al., 2007)

- bilateral or unilateral,
- spastic, dyskinetic (i.e., dystonic or choreo-athethoid), or ataxic?

Note: within the SCPE terminology 'hypotonic' CP is no longer considered a diagnostic option (see Chapter 20).

Note also it is well known that mixed types exist. Use the predominant one in diagnosis. If you or your team are not familiar with the SCPE system, details are available on an educational DVD: see Resources.

Decide the severity using the following Gross Motor Function Classification System (GMFCS) levels (before the age of 2 years)
See Table 22.1. Within the second half of the first year you will be able to use the GMFCS to get an idea of severity. Re-evaluate every time you see the child.

Table 22.1 Gross Motor Function Classification System (GMFCS)

GMFCS level	Features
Level I	Infants move in and out of sitting and floor sit with both hands free to manipulate objects. Infants crawl on hands and knees, pull to stand and take steps holding on to furniture. Infants walk between 18 months and 2 years of age without the need for any assistive mobility device.
Level II	Infants maintain floor sitting but may need to use their hands for support to maintain balance. Infants creep on their stomach or crawl on hands and knees. Infants may pull to stand and take steps holding on to furniture.
Level III	Infants maintain floor sitting when the low back is supported. Infants roll and creep forward on their stomachs.
Level IV	Infants have head control but trunk support is required for floor sitting. Infants can roll to supine and may roll to prone.
Level V	Physical impairments limit voluntary control of movement. Infants are unable to maintain antigravity head and trunk postures in prone and sitting. Infants require adult assistance to roll.

Communicate your estimated GMFCS level to the parents, therapists and carers and – if you like – use the GMFCS treatment curves to communicate an idea about the perspective of the developmental curve of the child beyond the first year of life (see Resources and Figure 22.1) (Heinen et al., 2010).

Etiology

Known etiology plays a crucial role for any planning and the communication of concepts. Etiology is (if available) based on neuroimaging (ultrasound, computed tomography and especially magnetic resonance imaging (MRI) scans), from which the nature and thus probable timing of the lesion can be decided (see Table 22.2).

In general about 1–2/1000 live-born children are diagnosed with CP by the age of 3–5 years. Of these, approximately half are born at term and the other half pre-term. In those born before 32 weeks gestation or with birthweights below 1500 g, the prevalence rises to 80–100/1000 live births. Post-neonatal causes account for approximately 5% of children with CP.

Clinicoradiological correlates (Krageloh-Mann and Horber, 2007) are listed in Table 22.3.

Figure 22.1 Types of treatment for children with bilateral spastic CP by age and severity of impairment. The first Figure plots motor performance on y axis against age in years on x-axis. The five curves shown correspond to the five levels (I–V) of the Gross Motor Function Classification System (GMFCS, Russell et al., 2003; Palisano et al., 2008). A careful history and repeated clinical assessments provide the basis for estimating the likely trajectory and brain imaging within the first two years will provide additional information. The graph provides parents, caretakers and the multidisciplinary team with a vehicle for discussion of management options for the individual child and a means of visualizing the projected future course of the child's motor development. The basal green curve represents therapist input to which orthoses/aids (bright green), oral medication (yellow), botulinum toxin (orange), intrathecal baclofen (red) and orthopaedic surgery (blue) can be added as necessary. The thickness of the lines A to D indicates an approximation to the percentage (0–25%, 25–50%, 50–75%, 75–100% respectively) of patients having the need for each type of therapy with a broken line indicating an intermittent requirement.
The second Figure gives the indications, principles and summary of limitations of the different treatment options indicated by the different coloured lines in the first Figure, illustrated by examples. Indications for selective dorsal rhizotomy are not shown. For each treatment, the potential for benefit has to be weighed against the limitations. These Figures can be downloaded from Heinen et al, 2010, supplementary data, the European Journal of Paediatric Neurology.
(Supplementary data) (Heinen et al., 2010). BSCP, bilateral spastic cerebral palsy. (See colour plate 3)

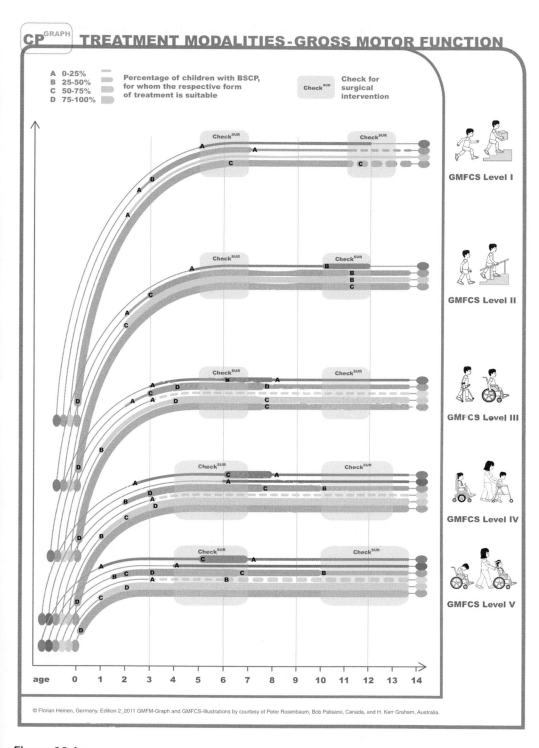

Figure 22.1a

INDICATION, PRINCIPLE & LIMITATION

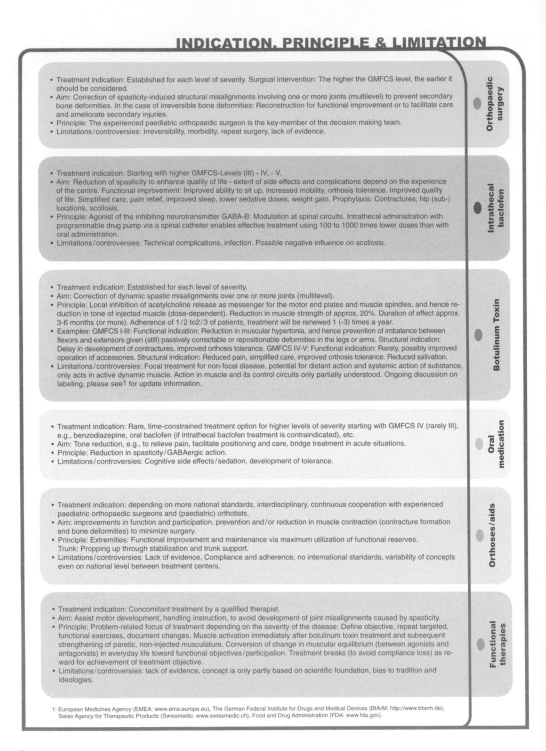

Orthopaedic surgery
- Treatment indication: Established for each level of severity. Surgical intervention: The higher the GMFCS level, the earlier it should be considered.
- Aim: Correction of spasticity-induced structural misalignments involving one or more joints (multilevel) to prevent secondary bone deformities. In the case of irreversible bone deformities: Reconstruction for functional improvement or to facilitate care and ameliorate secondary injuries.
- Principle: The experienced paediatric orthopaedic surgeon is the key-member of the decision making team.
- Limitations/controversies: Irreversibility, morbidity, repeat surgery, lack of evidence.

Intrathecal baclofen
- Treatment indication: Starting with higher GMFCS-Levels (III) - IV, - V.
- Aim: Reduction of spasticity to enhance quality of life - extent of side effects and complications depend on the experience of the centre. Functional improvement: Improved ability to sit up, increased mobility, orthosis tolerance. Improved quality of life: Simplified care, pain relief, improved sleep, lower sedative doses, weight gain. Prophylaxis: Contractures, hip (sub-) luxations, scoliosis.
- Principle: Agonist of the inhibiting neurotransmitter GABA-B: Modulation at spinal circuits. Intrathecal administration with programmable drug pump via a spinal catheter enables effective treatment using 100 to 1000 times lower doses than with oral administration.
- Limitations/controversies: Technical complications, infection. Possible negative influence on scoliosis.

Botulinum Toxin
- Treatment indication: Established for each level of severity.
- Aim: Correction of dynamic spastic misalignments over one or more joints (multilevel).
- Principle: Local inhibition of acetylcholine release as messenger for the motor end plates and muscle spindles, and hence reduction in tone of injected muscle (dose-dependent). Reduction in muscle strength of approx. 20%. Duration of effect approx. 3-6 months (or more). Adherence of 1/2 to 2/3 of patients, treatment will be renewed 1 (-3) times a year.
- Examples: GMFCS I-III: Functional indication: Reduction in muscular hypertonia, and hence prevention of imbalance between flexors and extensors given (still) passively correctable or repositionable deformities in the legs or arms. Structural indication: Delay in development of contractures, improved orthosis tolerance. GMFCS IV-V: Functional indication: Rarely, possibly improved operation of accessories. Structural indication: Reduced pain, simplified care, improved orthosis tolerance. Reduced salivation.
- Limitations/controversies: Focal treatment for non-focal disease, potential for distant action and systemic action of substance, only acts in active dynamic muscle. Action in muscle and its control circuits only partially understood. Ongoing discussion on labeling, please see[1] for update information.

Oral medication
- Treatment indication: Rare, time-constrained treatment option for higher levels of severity starting with GMFCS IV (rarely III), e.g., benzodiazepine, oral baclofen (if intrathecal baclofen treatment is contraindicated), etc.
- Aim: Tone reduction, e.g., to relieve pain, facilitate positioning and care, bridge treatment in acute situations.
- Principle: Reduction in spasticity/GABAergic action.
- Limitations/controversies: Cognitive side effects/sedation, development of tolerance.

Orthoses/aids
- Treatment indication: depending on more national standards, interdisciplinary, continuous cooperation with experienced paediatric orthopaedic surgeons and (paediatric) orthotists.
- Aim: improvements in function and participation, prevention and/or reduction in muscle contraction (contracture formation and bone deformities) to minimize surgery.
- Principle: Extremities: Functional improvement and maintenance via maximum utilization of functional reserves. Trunk: Propping up through stabilization and trunk support.
- Limitations/controversies: Lack of evidence, Compliance and adherence, no international standards, variability of concepts even on national level between treatment centers.

Functional therapies
- Treatment indication: Concomitant treatment by a qualified therapist.
- Aim: Assist motor development, handling instruction, to avoid development of joint misalignments caused by spasticity.
- Principle: Problem-related focus of treatment depending on the severity of the disease: Define objective, repeat targeted, functional exercises, document changes. Muscle activation immediately after botulinum toxin treatment and subsequent strengthening of paretic, non-injected musculature. Conversion of change in muscular equilibrium (between agonists and antagonists) in everyday life toward functional objectives/participation. Treatment breaks (to avoid compliance loss) as reward for achievement of treatment objective.
- Limitations/controversies: lack of evidence, concept is only partly based on scientific foundation, bias to tradition and ideologies.

1: European Medicines Agency (EMEA: www.ema.europe.eu), The German Federal Institute for Drugs and Medical Devices (BfArM: http://www.bfarm.de), Swiss Agency for Therapeutic Products (Swissmedic: www.swissmedic.ch), Food and Drug Administration (FDA: www.fda.gov).

Figure 22.1b

Table 22.2 Timing of pathogenetic lesions

Probable time of insult	Approximate gestational age	Radiological or pathological findings
First and second trimester	Before 24 weeks	Malformations
Early third trimester and neonatal	25–34 weeks	Predominantly white matter disorders such as periventricular leukomalacia, intraventricular haemorrhage
Late third trimester	35 weeks to 28 days post term	Cortical-subcortical and deep grey-matter lesions, basal ganglia lesions
Post-neonatal	28 days post term to 2 years	Traumatic, ischaemic, vascular or infectious lesions

Table 22.3 Correlation of clinical and neuroradiological findings

Type of CP	MRI positive	
Bilateral spastic	90%	60% periventricular leukomalacia (90% if preterm) 15% cortical or subcortical/basal ganglia/thalamus lesions (4% if preterm) 10% malformations (1.5% if preterm) 3% unclassified
Unilateral spastic	90%	35% periventricular leukomalacia (85% if preterm) 30% infarction 20% malformations 5% unclassified
Dyskinetic	60–70%	50% basal ganglia/thalamus lesions 15% periventricular leukomalacia Rare: basal ganglia lesions ('kernicterus')
Ataxic	40–50%	Cerebellar hypoplasia (not correlated with clinical severity)

From Krageloh-Mann and Horber (2007).

Approximately 16% of children with CP have normal findings on MRI. In most, no other explanation can be found, but conditions such as dopa-responsive dytonia or hereditary spastic paraparesis should be considered especially if there is a positive family history. If the diagnosis by history and clinical course is CP, additional metabolic testing is not indicated unless there are clinical features suggestive of a neurometabolic disease (e.g. progression, involvement of organs other than the central nervous system, episodes of worsening/crises).

Management and follow-up

Management relies on close collaboration between parents and professionals. This is best achieved by a multidisciplinary team who meet together with parents to report progress and plan interventions. It is important to understand the beliefs and resources of the parents and their motivation for 'do's and don'ts' (Heinen et al., 2010). Provision for the child's non-neurological health needs is beyond the scope of this book but their feeding and nutrition is a key element of their well-being and must be given specific consideration (see Sullivan, 2009).

Motor function

Motor functions and signs can change markedly in the first few years of life. Some children with CP cannot be diagnosed until the age of 3 years or older, while in others the type or severity can change. In one study of at-risk infants, 50% of those suspected to have CP at 12 months of age did not have it when reviewed at the age of 7 years, although there was an increased prevalence of comorbidities such as learning disability, behaviour difficulties and epilepsy.

Management of the motor problems primarily relies on physiotherapy. There are several different 'schools' of physiotherapy which advocate different methods (e.g. Bobath, Conductive Education, Montessori, Vojta). None of these have been proved to be superior to the others.

In the first 2 years of life other interventions such as muscle relaxants (baclofen, diazepam, etc.), botulinum toxin, orthoses and orthopaedic surgery are usually *not* indicated. However, severe extensor spasms can improve with oral baclofen and positioning (slight flexion of the neck). Other forms of spasticity reduction such as intrathecal (i.e. into lumbar cerebrospinal fluid using an implanted infusion pump) baclofen or dorsal root rhizotomy are impractical in this age group.

Complementary medications and interventions are widely used but there are no data to prove or disprove any benefits, and they can be costly.

On follow-up, predict the motor development over the next 3–6 months – this is best done together with the physiotherapist – and communicate realistic developmental and therapeutic goals. A written Goal Attainment Scale (GAS; Table 22.4) can help in monitoring progress. It will need assessing and updating at each visit. You can define specific goals for different domains of International Classification of Functioning,

Table 22.4 Goal Attainment Scale

Goal Attainment Scale	Level of attainment
−2	Much less than expected
−1	Somewhat less than expected
0	Expected level of outcome
+1	Somewhat more than expected
+2	Much more than expected

Disability and Health (ICF) levels (body structure and function, activity and participation, environmental and personal factors). Videos at home and in the standardized clinical setting are also useful when documenting progress (e.g. from mobile phones).

The GMFCS levels should also be reviewed at each visit. These measures can be used to build motor development curves (Palisano et al., 2008).

Consider hip assessment at each visit. This is best by ultrasound in the first year and thereafter by radiographic imaging. The method of choice to detect inadequate positioning of the head of femur is measuring the Reimers Migration Index (MI), a standardized radiographic imaging of the pelvis in patients *older than 1 year of age*. MI <10% right/left is normal in healthy children. Different definitions for subluxation and luxation of the hip joint exist, but in general a hip at risk in children with CP is defined as a MI ≥30% (with additional information gained using GMFCS levels or Ashworth scores). If this is the case, involve an orthopaedic surgeon for hip management. Different hip surveillance programmes can prevent hips from (sub-) luxation over time when started early enough (Hagglund et al., 2005).

Most children below the age of 1 year do not require specialist wheelchairs. Some benefit from specialist seating. In a child under the age of one year, neither specialist wheelchairs nor adaptations to the home are required but early planning for these is important and the child may benefit from specialist seating. Table 22.5 and 22.6 show the measures that may be used to evaluate and classify body structure and function and activity.

Comorbidities
As the lesions that cause CP often affect other brain functions, comorbidities are frequent and need to be actively identified and managed. This requires a multidisciplinary approach (see Table 22.7).

Table 22.5 Classification systems used in the evaluation of the cerebral palsy

Instrument	What is addressed?	ICF dimension	Target age	Clinical value	Literature
Gross Motor Function Classification System (GMFCS)	Classification of motor abilities, oriented to mobility, corresponding to age	Activity	<2, 2–4, 4–6, 6–12, 12–18 years	+++	www.canchild.ca/ Palisano et al. (1997, 2000, 2006, 2008), Russell et al. (2003)
Manual Ability Classification System (MACS)	Classification of manual abilities for children with CP, oriented to activities of daily living	Activity	4–18 years	+++	www.macs.nu Eliasson et al. (2006)
Communication Function Classification System	Classification of communication abilities for individuals with CP. Oriented towards everyday communication performance	Activity Participation	2–18 years	+++	http://faculty.uca. edu/mjchidecker/ CFCS/index.html

+, helpful; ++, very helpful; +++, excellent

Table 22.6 Instruments for evaluation of cerebral palsy

Instrument	What is addressed?	ICF dimension	Target age	Psychometric criteria	Clinical value	Literature
Goal Attainment Scaling (GAS)	Standardized therapy goal setting (in five levels) and determination, which level has been reached	According to individual therapy goal: function, activity, participation	All ages	++	++	Maloney (1993), Maloney et al. (1978), Cusick et al. (2006), Palisano (1993)
Range of Motion (ROM)	Passive assessment of joint mobility with neutral-0-method (goniometry)	Body function/structure	All ages	++	+	McDowell et al. (2000); Allington et al. (2002); Fosang et al. (2003)
Modified Tardieu Scale	'Fast' assessment of joint mobility Differentiates dynamic from fixed limitation of muscles	Body function/structure	All ages	+ Upper extremity ++ Lower extremity	+++	Fosang et al. (2003); Scholtes et al. (2006); Boyd and Graham (1999); Mackey et al. (2003)
Modified Ashworth Scale	Evaluation of the degree of spasticity	Body function/structure	All ages	++ For knee flexors and elbow + For all other muscles	++	Fosang et al. (2003); Bohannon and Smith (1987); Clopton et al. (2005); Scholtes et al. (2006)
Video documentation	Standardized documentation of baseline and follow-up examinations to evaluate therapy progress	Activity	All ages	++	+++	Mackey et al. (2003); Maathius et al. (2005)

Table 22.6 *Continued*

Instrument	What is addressed?	ICF dimension	Target age	Psychometric criteria	Clinical value	Literature
Canadian Occupational Performance Measure (COPM)	Measurers changes of self-evaluated function and performance during a period of time	Function activity participation	From about 8 years (need for self evaluation)	+++	++	www.caot.ca/copm Cusick et al. (2006); Carswell et al. (2004)
Gross Motor Function Measure (GMFM; 88, or 66)	Evaluation of quantitative changes of motor functions within defined time periods; 66 is a shortened version of 88	Activity	0.5–16 years	+++	+++	Russell et al. (2003)
Assisting Hand Assessment (AHA)	Evaluation of bimanual skills of children with unilateral CP	Activity	1.5–15 years	+++	+++	Eliasson et al. (2006)
Pediatric Evaluation of Disability Inventory (PEDI)	Standardized questionnaire for parents to assess the amount of functional deficits of everyday activities	Activity and participation	0.5–7.5 years	+++	+++	www.bu.edu/hdr/ products/pedi

Table 22.7 A multidisciplinary approach to comorbidity management

System	Specialists	Problems	Possible actions
Visual	Ophthalmologist, orthoptist	Strabismus, refractive errors, retinopathies, optic nerve hypoplasia, visual field defects, cortical visual agnosia	Spectacles, patching, strabismus surgery
Hearing	Otolaryngologist, audiometry	Conductive defects Sensorineural hearing loss	Hearing aids
Communication	Speech and language therapist	Bulbar dysfunction, central language disorders	Alternative and augmentative communication methods
Feeding	Speech and language therapist, dietitian, nurse, paediatrician	Bulbar or pseudobulbar palsy, gastro-oesopageal reflux (after first year)	Monitor growth, nasogastric tube or gastrostomy feeding, antireflux medication
Epilepsy	Paediatrician	Seizures	Electroencephalography, antiepileptic medication
Intellectual	Paediatrician, psychologist	Learning difficulties	Early intervention, early nursery placement
Behaviour	Paediatrician, psychologist	Sleep problems, frequent crying	Behavioural techniques, assessment for pain
Family	Paediatrician, social services	Bereavement, education, multiple hospital visits, financial resources	Social support, financial support, respite provision

Some myths and related facts

- Specificity of treatment: there are, in fact, no data showing that one type of physiotherapy intervention is superior to another.

- The more the better: trials of intense versus normal physiotherapy intervention have shown temporary short-term improvement, but have not, in fact, shown any difference in longer-term outcome.

- It is necessary to do everything in order not to miss anything.

- If the outcome is not the desired one, the treatment was wrong or not intense enough or the method was wrong. These are, in fact, usually not the reasons.

- Stem cell treatment: there is, in fact, no indication for any kind of therapy involving stem cell injections or implantations.

Summary

CP is the most common cause of spastic movement disorders in children. Although the cerebral lesion in CP is caused by a single event, CP has to be understood as a developmental disorder described over time as an individual develops. Throughout the last 20 years, intensive research in the field of CP has overcome different ideological 'schools' of (physio-)therapies and complementary medications. Using the above mentioned tools we now have evidence-based information to give the parents and caregivers a *prediction* of motor development by classifying CP with regard to (a) type, (b) severity and (c) etiology. It is the right of every family to be in possession of such information and is a prerequisite for family centered programmes.

Early classification of CP within the first year(s) of life provides the best starting point for a *preventive* strategy to reduce the risk of secondary complications (e.g. hip luxation). This has been shown to be of benefit in large cohort studies during the last two decades. Nevertheless, the clinical profile of each child with CP remains unique and requires a personalised approach to maximize his or her potential functioning. The goal of multidisciplinary treatment is, however, not only to improve functional abilities but also to increase the participation of each child with CP. This has to be the goal for all of our interventions.

References

AACPDM. The definition and classification of cerebral palsy. *Developmental Medicine and Child Neurology*, 2007, 49(s109):1–44.

Allington NJ, Leroy N, Doneux C. Ankle joint range of motion measurements in spastic cerebral palsy children: intraobserver and interobserver reliability and reproducibility of goniometry and visual estimation. *Journal of Pediatric Orthopaedics Part B*, 2002, 11(3):236–239.

Bohannon RW, Smith MB. Interrater reliability of a modified Ashworth scale of muscle spasticity. *Physical Therapy*, 1987, 67(2):206–207.

Boyd RN, Graham HK. Objective measurement of clinical findings in the use of botulinum toxin type A for the management of children with cerebral palsy. *European Journal of Neurology*, 1999, 6, suppl. 4:23–35.

Cans C et al. Recommendations from the SCPE collaborative group for defining and classifying cerebral palsy. *Developmental Medicine and Child Neurology Supplement*, 2007, 109:35–38.

Carswell A et al. The Canadian Occupational Performance Measure: a research and clinical literature review. *Canadian Journal of Occupational Therapy*, 2004, 71(4):210–222.

Clopton N et al. Interrater and intrarater reliability of the Modified Ashworth Scale in children with hypertonia. *Pediatric Physical Therapy*, 2005, 17(4):268–274.

Cusick A et al. A comparison of goal attainment scaling and the Canadian Occupational Performance Measure for paediatric rehabilitation research. *Pediatric Rehabilitation*, 2006, 9(2):149–157.

Eliasson AC et al. The Manual Ability Classification System (MACS) for children with cerebral palsy: scale development and evidence of validity and reliability. *Developmental Medicine and Child Neurology*, 2006, 48(7):549–554.

Fosang AL et al. Measures of muscle and joint performance in the lower limb of children with cerebral palsy. *Developmental Medicine and Child Neurology*, 2003, 45(10):664–670.

Hagglund G et al. Prevention of dislocation of the hip in children with cerebral palsy. The first ten years of a population-based prevention programme. *Journal of Bone and Joint Surgery*, 2005, 87(1):95–101.

Heinen F et al. The updated European Consensus 2009 on the use of Botulinum toxin for children with cerebral palsy. *European Journal of Paediatric Neurology*, 2010, 14(1):45–66.

Hidecker MJ et al. Developing and validating the Communication Function Classification System for individuals with cerebral palsy. *Developmental Medicine and Child Neurology*, 2011, 53(8):704–710.

Krageloh-Mann I, Horber V. The role of magnetic resonance imaging in elucidating the pathogenesis of cerebral palsy: a systematic review. *Developmental Medicine and Child Neurology*, 2007, 49(2):144–151.

Mackey AH et al. Reliability and validity of the Observational Gait Scale in children with spastic diplegia. *Developmental Medicine and Child Neurology*, 2003, 45(1):4–11.

Maloney FP. Goal attainment scaling. *Physical Therapy*, 1993, 73(2):123.

Maloney FP et al. Use of the Goal Attainment Scale in the treatment and ongoing evaluation of neurologically handicapped children. *American Journal of Occupational Therapy*, 1978, 32(8):505–510.

McDowell BC et al. The variability of goniometric measurements in ambulatory children with spastic cerebral palsy. *Gait Posture*, 2000, 12(2):114–121.

Palisano RJ. Validity of goal attainment scaling in infants with motor delays. *Physical Therapy*, 1993, 73(10):651–658.

Palisano RJ. A collaborative model of service delivery for children with movement disorders: a framework for evidence-based decision making. *Physical Therapy*, 2006, 86(9):1295–1305.

Palisano R et al. Development and reliability of a system to classify gross motor function in children with cerebral palsy. *Developmental Medicine and Child Neurology*, 1997, 39(4):214–223.

Palisano RJ et al. Validation of a model of gross motor function for children with cerebral palsy. *Physical Therapy*, 2000, 80(10):974–985.

Palisano RJ et al. Content validity of the expanded and revised Gross Motor Function Classification System. *Developmental Medicine and Child Neurology*, 2008, 50(10):744–750.

Russell DJ, Leung KM, Rosenbaum PL. Accessibility and perceived clinical utility of the GMFM-66: evaluating therapists' judgements of a computer-based scoring program. *Physical & Occupational Therapy in Pediatrics*, 2003, 23(2):45–58.

Sanger TD et al. Classification and definition of disorders causing hypertonia in childhood. *Pediatrics*, 2003, 111(1):e89–e97.

Scholtes VA et al. Clinical assessment of spasticity in children with cerebral palsy: a critical review of available instruments. *Developmental Medicine and Child Neurology*, 2006, 48(1):64–73.

Sullivan PB (Ed). *Feeding and nutrition in children with neurodevelopmental disability*. Mac Keith Press, 2009.

Resources

Australian Hip Surveillance Programme: www.ausacpdm.org.au/activities/hip-surveillance

DeMatteo C et al. *QUEST: Quality of Upper Extremity Skills Test*. Hamilton, ON: McMaster University, Neurodevelopmental Clinical Research Unit, 1992.

Gross Motor Function Classification System (GMFCS): www.canchild.ca/en/

Gross Motor Function Measure (GMFM): www.canchild.ca/en/measures/gmfm.asp

Maathuis KG et al. Gait in children with cerebral palsy: observer reliability of Physician Rating Scale and Edinburgh Visual Gait Analysis Interval Testing scale. *Journal of Pediatric Orthopedics*, 2005, 25(3):268–272.

Supplementary data in Heinen F., et al. 2010: The updated European Consensus 2009 on the use of Botulinum toxin for children with cerebral palsy. *European Journal of Paediatric Neurology*, 2010, 14(1): 45–66; Treatment modalities – Gross Motor Function, a perspective beyond the first year of life.

Surveillance of Cerebral Palsy in Europe (SCPE): www-rheop.ujf-grenoble.fr/scpe2/site_scpe/index.php.

Chapter 23

Central nervous system disorders of movement other than cerebral palsy

Peter Baxter and Florian Heinen

Key messages
- There are many different paroxysmal or persistent movement disorders in the first year of life.
- Most can be diagnosed on clinical grounds.
- Phenomenology discriminates ataxia, athetosis, chorea, dystonia, myoclonus, stereotypies and tremor. Ballismus, parkinsonism and tics are rare in this age group.
- Remember that these motor disorders are most obvious in the mature brain, but in younger people they are less easily distinguished.
- Normal infants can also show mild forms of 'physiological' ataxia and athetosis which are age-related.

Common errors
- Mistaking the normal variation in motor development for disease.
- Mistaking normal motor asymmetry during development for disease.
- Mistaking a paroxysmal movement disorder for epilepsy (or vice versa).
- Assuming that all chronic motor abnormalities are a form of cerebral palsy.
- Inappropriate investigations for benign conditions.
- Inappropriate treatment for normal conditions.

When to worry
- When head control does not develop.
- When sitting without support is delayed beyond 9 months corrected age.
- When new motor findings appear or old ones worsen.

Definitions
See also Sanger et al. (2003, 2006).

Ataxia (literally 'without order')
Inability to generate a normal or expected voluntary movement trajectory that cannot be attributed to weakness or an involuntary muscle activity around the affected joints. Ataxia can result from impairment of the spatial pattern of muscle activity or from impairment of the timing of the activity, or both. It can be specified as dysmetria (undershoot or overshoot), dyssynergia (decomposition of multi-joint movements) and dysdiadochokinesis (impaired rhythmicity of rapid alternating movements; not applicable within the first year of life).

Athetosis (literally 'without fixed position')
Slow, writhing, continous, involuntary movements. This is part of the spectrum of dyskinetic movements disorders (choreo-athetotic versus dystonic). It also occurs in one (sub)type of cerebral palsy (see Chapter 22).

Chorea (literally 'dance like')
Involuntary, continual, irregular hyperkinetic disorder in which movements or parts of movement occur with variable rate, direction and distribution (all body parts may be involved); typically unpredictable and random.

Ballismus
Involuntary, high-amplitude, flinging movements typically occurring proximally. Brief or continual. It may be an extreme form of chorea. If, as usually happens, one side of the body is affected, the term hemiballismus is used.

Dystonia
Dystonia is an involuntary alteration in the pattern of muscle activation during voluntary movement or maintenance of posture. It is thus a syndrome of sustained muscle contractions, frequently causing twisting and repetitive movements, or abnormal posture. Typically both agonists and antagonists co-contract. Dystonia can be action- or posture-induced. Dystonic spasms can resemble tonic seizures and can be painful. Status dystonicus is a medical emergency.

Myoclonus
Quick, shock-like movements of one or more muscles. The term is usually applied to describe positive myoclonus: sudden, quick, involuntary muscle jerks caused by muscle contraction. Negative myoclonus refers to sudden, brief interruption of contraction in active (postural) muscles.

Parkinsonism
Presence of two or more of the cardinal features: tremor at rest, bradykinesia, rigidity and postural instability.

Startles
Brief, generalized motor responses similar to myoclonus. Startle syndrome is a disease entity.

Stereotypies
Involuntary, patterned, coordinated, repetitive, nonreflexive movements that occur in the same fashion with each repetition, often rhythmic.

Tics
Involuntary, sudden, rapid, abrupt, repetitive, nonrhythmic, simple or complex movements or vocalizations. Tics are classified into two categories (motor and phonic) and do not usually occur in the first year of life.

Tremor
Oscillating rhythmic movements about a fixed point, axis or plane that occur when antagonist muscles contract alternately. Usually this involves oscillation around a joint and produces a visible movement. Pathological tremor is also rare in the first years of life.

Introduction and clinical approach

Many different paroxysmal and non-paroxysmal movement disorders can occur in neonates and older infants (see Table 23.1). In most diagnosis relies on clinical

Table 23.1 Movement disorders in the first 2 years of life

Movement disorders	Paroxysmal	Non–paroxysmal
Neonatal	Jitteriness Doggy paddle/bicycling Benign neonatal sleep myoclonus Transient dystonia of prematurity	Floppy baby (hypotonia) Dystonias Stiff-baby syndromes Chorea
Infancy	Shuddering attacks Paroxysmal torticollis Benign paroxysmal upgaze Sandifer syndrome Benign tonic upgaze of infancy Spasmus nutans Opsoclonus-myoclonus Head banging (jactatio capitis) Stereotypies Gratification phenomena (Tics) Benign spasms	Head tilt Dystonia – generalized Lower-limb hypertonia Ataxia Tremor

recognition (for which paroxysmal disorders videos can be particularly useful) rather than investigations. The most important differential diagnoses are, for paroxysmal disorders, from epilepsy (see Chapters 13 and 16), and for persistent disorders, from cerebral palsy (see Chapter 22).

Paroxysmal movement disorders in neonates: clinical approach

Paroxysmal movement disorders can easily be mistaken for neonatal seizures (see Chapter 13). In certain conditions such as pyridoxine dependency, both seizures and non-epileptic movement disorders can occur in the same infant. The differential relies on clinical assessment and electroencephalographic (EEG) recording, both ictal and inter-ictal.

Jitteriness is a common, non-specific feature which can occur in hungry infants but can also be a sign of hypocalcaemia, hypoglycaemia, drug-withdrawal syndromes or a range of acute neonatal encephalopathies. It can be distinguished from epileptic seizures by being interrupted by sleep, by a change of body posture or by restraint of the affected limbs. An exaggerated startle response can be associated. Preterm infants in non-REM sleep can also show excess startles.

Age at onset: first week of life.
Age at resolution: typically before 6 months.
Treatment: underlying cause if appropriate; otherwise information/reassurance.

Bicycling movements of the arms and doggy-paddling movements of the legs, with or without tonic axial hyperextension (back arching), are non-specific signs of acute or chronic encephalopathies due to any cause.

Age at onset: any age.
Treatment: underlying cause; positioning.

Benign neonatal sleep myoclonus is frequently mistaken for epileptic seizures (see Chapter 17). The main distinguishing feature is that episodes only occur while asleep. Typically they are not stereotyped so on one occasion only one limb may be involved while on others several show the typical jerking movements. The infant is otherwise neurologically normal. In cases of clinical doubt a normal EEG record during an episode can be helpful. The outcome is also normal.

Age at onset: less than 1 month.
Age at resolution: latest 6 months.
Treatment: information/reassurance; no treatment is needed.

Persistent movement disorders in neonates: clinical approach

Hypotonia (floppy infant) is a feature of many central motor and other disorders (see Chapter 20 for more details).

Dystonia manifesting as back arching and head retroversion, associated with obligate asymmetric tonic neck reflex and at least transient relaxation with neck flexion, is most commonly associated with severe chronic neurological impairment due to prenatal or perinatal brain damage (e.g. asphyxia, hyerbilirubinaemia). Back arching and head retroversion can also be a symptom of raised intracranial pressure from any cause, including hydrocephalus.

Transient dystonia of prematurity can occur in preterm infants and consists of increased leg extensor tone and asymmetric axial tone with head lag when pulled to sit but not when held prone, sometimes associated with fisting and exaggerated tendon jerks.

Age at onset: few weeks.
Age at resolution: 12 months in most; a minority continue with more definite signs of cerebral palsy.
Treatment: reassurance.

Stiff-baby syndrome is a rare conditions most commonly caused by hyperekplexia, due to a mutation in the glycine receptor gene or the glycine transporter gene. Clinically the diagnosis of hyperekplexia (or startle disease) is suggested by a non-habituating exaggerated startle response to repetitive nose taps. The condition is lifelong but symptoms usually change with age, with hypertonia becoming less prominent by 1 year of age and the appearance of excess sleep myoclonus, 'freezing' to fright, and sometimes epilepsy. In neonates and young infants severe life-threatening episodes with apnoea can be aborted promptly by neck flexion. Prophylaxis with benzodiazepines, valproate or phenobarbital can prevent attacks (see Chapter 17). The differential diagnosis of stiff baby syndrome includes congenital disorders of neurotransmitter metabolism (often associated with oculogyric crisis) and congenital absence of the pyramidal tracts.

Infants with severe bronchopulmonary dysplasia can develop a movement disorder with choreiform movements of the limbs, face and tongue and a general restlessness, which settles when asleep. The etiology is unclear.

Age at onset: third postnatal month; can persist or slowly resolve over 12–18 months.
Treatment: clonazepam can help especially if tongue involvement affects feeding.

Paroxysmal disorders in infancy: clinical approach (see also Chapter 17)
Benign infantile shuddering attacks are best diagnosed by video footage. The child is otherwise healthy with normal development. There may be an association with essential tremor later in life.

Age at onset: infancy, early childhood.
Treatment: information/reassurance

Benign paroxysmal torticollis consists of episodes of head tilt lasting several hours or days, associated with vomiting, abnormal eye movements and, in older children, ataxia. The child is healthy between attacks. Sandifer syndrome (see below) should be excluded. Some cases are linked to mutations in the *CACNA1A* gene. Some also develop migraine in later childhood.

Age at onset: first year of life.
Age at resolution: by 8 years.
Treatment: information/reassurance

Sandifer syndrome often consists of asymmetric dystonic posturing, usually involving the neck with turning and torticollis, followed by distress, which last a few minutes. Occasionally more of the body is involved with back and limb extension. Some episodes occur after meals. They are due to gastro-oesophageal reflux and/or a hiatus hernia.

Age at onset: early infancy.
Age at resolution: early childhood or after treatment.
Treatment: drug therapy of reflux; often surgical fundoplication is needed.

Action dystonia can occur in some chronic dystonias including dopa-responsive disorders, but usually only in older children. Paroxysmal and exertional dystonia can be a feature of GLUT1 deficiency, diagnosed by low glucose levels in the cerebrospinal fluid and treated by a ketogenic diet. Paroxysmal chorea can occur in Allan–Herndon–Dudley disorder (MCT8 deficiency), an X-linked thyroid transporter disorder seen in males and suggested by raised blood T3 levels.

Episodes of benign paroxysmal tonic upgaze of infancy can be associated with unusual head postures and ataxia. The infant is otherwise normal with normal neurodevelopmental findings between episodes.

Age at onset: first year of life.
Age at resolution: 1–4 years.
Treatment: some may respond to l-dopa.

Spasmus nutans consists of the triad of head abnormal head posture, repetitive head nodding (at around 3 Hz), most apparent during visual fixation on near or distant objects and a shimmering nystagmus (at around 11 Hz). The nystagmus is assymetrical and may be monocular. Rarely, this may be mimicked by tumours in the visual pathway or region of the third ventricle but visual impairment is usually also present in such cases. Computed tomography (CT) or magnetic resonance imaging (MRI) may therefore be necessary. Head tilt (without the other components of the triad) may be a presentation of a posterior fossa tumour.

Age at onset: 3–12 months.
Age at resolution: within a few months, but subtle nystagmus may persist for years.
Treatment: none

Episodic or persistent chaotic but conjugate eye jerking is an important feature of the opsoclonus-myoclonus (also known as the opsiclonus-myoclonus-ataxia, Kinsbourne or dancing eye syndrome) syndrome typically together with severe distress/dysphoria/misery that may appear as 'rage attacks'. The majority of cases are associated with occult neuroblastoma, so need specialist investigation.

Age at onset: usually after the first year of life.
Treatment: symptomatic: immunomodulatory agents (e.g. steroid pulses); causative (neuroblastoma, as above).

Head banging while awake is seen in a number of healthy infants when bored or frustrated. It is not usually severe enough to cause any injury or bruising. The equivalent while asleep, jactatio capitis, is a well-recognized parasomnia. Usually the child is otherwise well and wakes completely rested but their parents may not be, as the sound has kept them awake! It may persist for years.

Age at onset: first year of life.
Age at resolution: any, but jactatio capitis can persist.
Treatment: reassurance; protective padding against surfaces, such as a mattress against the wall.

Gratification phenomena are voluntary events when a child will sit or lie, often with their legs crossed, and adopt repetitive postures or movements. Some authorities postulate a link to infantile masturbation. During episodes the child remains aware and the activity can be interrupted but will start again afterwards. Frequently the feet can adopt an inturned supinated dystonic posture.

Age at onset: 3–12 months.
Age at resolution: any.
Treatment: reassurance.

Infantile stereotypies can appear very similar and consist of repetitive semi-voluntary movements. Some occur in specific situations, such as while watching a washing machine spin. There can be an association with autism.

Tic disorders rarely occur in this age group.

Persistent movement disorders in infants: clinical features
Chronic head tilt can be due to torticollis (e.g. benign sternomastoid tumour, hypothesis: residuum of haematoma within the sternocleidoid muscle), posterior fossa abnormalities including cerebellar tumours, and abnormalities of the atlanto-axial joint. If palpation of the contralateral sternomastoid reveals a tumour and there is restricted extension, treatment is by regular gentle stretching. Otherwise sonography of the muscles, neuroimaging focusing on posterior fossa structures and X-ray or CT of the cervical spine are required, with surgical referral for any abnormal findings.

Chronic dystonia involving the trunk and limbs can occur in Lesch–Nyhan disease, ataxia telangiectasia, glutaric aciduria, Aicardi–Goutieres syndrome and mitochondrial cytopathies. All of these can be mistaken for cerebral palsy.

Treatment: mostly symptomatic; in Lesch–Nyhan: allopurinol, dopa; in glutaric aciduria: diet, riboflavin, carnitine.

Hypertonia of the lower limbs raises the possibility of a spinal cord lesion due either to a neural tube defect or a congenital spinal tumour. If the MRI of the brain is normal it is important to assess the spine. Similar findings can be due to dopa-responsive dystonias; biotinidase deficiency; hereditary spastic paraparesis (Strumpell–Lorrain disease) due to a variety of genes; purine nucleoside phosphorylase (PNP) deficiency; arginase deficiency; and L1 syndrome.

Treatment: dopa (dopa-responsive conditions); biotin (biotinidase deficiency); otherwise supportive; symptomatic (e.g. for hypertonia); genetic counselling.

Progressive spasticity, dystonia or ataxia all can suggest a leukodystrophy, such as Pelizaeus–Merzbacher disease and its variants, or Krabbe disease (Chapter 24). Additional features include nystagmus, optic atrophy, stridor and seizures. If this group of disorders is suspected MRI is an essential first step. In Pelizaeus–Merzbacher leukodystrophy, symptoms begin in infancy with hypotonia, nystagmus and sometimes chorea, followed by hypertonia and ataxia. The more severe connatal form causes early stridor and seizures as well. In infantile Krabbe leukodystrophy symptoms begin at a few months of age with marked irritability, feeding difficulties, vomiting and developmental slowing. Progressive hypertonia, epileptic seizures, deafness and blindness follow, with death by 2 years.

Treatment: supportive; symptomatic (e.g. for hypertonia); genetic counselling.

Ataxia is rarely diagnosed in early infancy, partly because young children are intrinsically ataxic when their coordination is compared to older children and partly because early disorders of the cerebellum more usually present with hypotonia and early developmental impairment. However, acute ataxia can be caused by infectious or inflammatory cerebellitis, intoxication and other rarer causes. Chronic ataxia can be a feature of hexosaminidase A and B deficiency or mitochondrial disorders. GLUT1 deficiency can also present in this way.

Treatment: usually symptomatic; for GLUT1 deficiency: ketogenic or Atkins diet.

Tremor can be difficult to distinguish from chorea. Prolonged chorea can follow encephalitis, especially when due to herpes simplex, usually associated with recurrence of the encephalopathy. The exact mechanism is uncertain. Previously it was believed to be due to persistence of the herpes virus infection leading to recommendations of very prolonged aciclovir treatment but it is now recognized that this may have another explanation such as an autoimmune cause. Choreo-athetosis is also associated with glutaric aciduria type 1 and Lesch–Nyhan syndrome. Benign hereditary chorea, can present in infancy with delayed walking and improves slowly with age.

Summary

With a wide range of possible disorders it is difficult to propose a common diagnostic approach. However, always considering a differential diagnosis, even in 'known cases' of 'cerebral palsy' or 'epilepsy', will avoid misdiagnosis. In addition, if the motor condition does not follow an expected course but, for example, shows progression, re-evaluation of the diagnosis is essential.

References

Sanger TD et al. and Task Force on Childhood Motor Disorders. Classification and definition of disorders causing hypertonia in childhood. *Pediatrics*, 2003, 111:e89–e97.

Sanger TD et al. Definition and classification of negative motor signs in childhood. *Pediatrics*, 2006, 118:2159–2167.

Resources

King MD, Stephenson JBP. *A handbook of neurological investigations in children*. London, Mac Keith Press, 2009.

Singer HS, Mink JW, Gilbert DL, Jancovic J. *Movement disorders in childhood*. Philadelphia, Saunders Elsevier, 2010.

Chapter 24
Progressive loss of skills

Meral Topcu, Dilek Yalnızoglu and Richard Newton

Key messages
- Progressive loss of skills in a child with normal or near normal development may be the initial sign of a progressive neurometabolic/neurogenetic disorder.
- Always consider biotinidase deficiency in an infant with seizures, particularly if there is coarse or sparse hair or a skin rash. It is treatable.

Common errors
- Children with progressive neurological diseases may be incorrectly diagnosed as cases of cerebral palsy or epileptic encephalopathy.

When to worry
- Faltering of developmental progress and loss of previously gained skills are crucial problems in neurological evaluation of the young child.
- Onset of seizures, progressive deceleration or acceleration of head growth, hearing loss, visual impairment, hypotonia, dystonia or spasticity are considered red flags.

Introduction

A child, whether following a pattern typical of the general population or an early pattern suggesting developmental impairment, will follow a predictable trajectory of motor and cognitive developmental progress. If the developmental milestones are falling away from the expected trajectory, this raises the question of whether the child has a progressive disease. If the child develops normally and then loses the previously gained mental and/or motor skills, the clinical picture is likely to reflect a progressive disease process. Poorly controlled epilepsy may also cause this clinical picture and mimic a progressive disease.

Clinical approach

The *history* should include history of current symptoms and of any exposure to infectious and toxic agents, previous medical history including prenatal, perinatal and postnatal risk factors and a family history (including parental consanguinity or other affected family members). A personal or family history of febrile or afebrile seizures should be sought. A detailed developmental history, and current level of functioning should be documented. If the family history is uninformative, acquired or sporadic genetic disorders should be considered.

Physical examination should be undertaken with awareness of the possible relevance of abormalities of respiration, dysmorphic features or signs of a storage disorder including cranial or other skeletal abnormalities, organomegaly, retinopathy or heart murmurs; hair (coarse in Menke disease, sparse in biotinidase deficiency) and skin (rashes or signs of a neurocutaneous syndrome) should be examined. The occipitofrontal head circumference is always an important observation to record and plot on a centile chart. Disorders of eye movements may provide clues to a wide variety of disorders. The clinical picture of neurometabolic disorders may, however, be non-specific and with early onset it can be particularly difficult to be sure that the disorder is truly progressive.

Laboratory evaluation (see Chapter 9) in any child with early developmental impairment, with or without suspected regression, should include a complete blood count with differential count, glucose, calcium, phosphate, urea and creatinine, thyroid function tests, amino acids, organic acids, a mucopoly- and oligosaccharide screen and chromosomal karyotype. Comparative genomic hybridization (CGH), which measures DNA copy number differences between a test and reference genome, is now adding to the diagnostic yield but is not available in all settings.

Further investigation of regression (see also Chapters 7–9) should be tailored to fit the clinical picture, as summarized in later sections of this chapter. Capillary pH, plasma and cerebrospinal fluid (CSF) lactate and mitochondrial DNA deletions should be considered if mitochondrial cytopathies seem possible; transferrin isoelectric focusing (abnormal in congenital disorders of glycosylation) should be considered for the combination of early developmental impairment with either unusual subcutaneous fat distribution or cerebellar hypoplasia on cranial imaging; white-cell enzymes for the lysosomal storage disorders; dihydroxyacetone-phosphate acyltransferase (DHAP-AT), phytanic acid and very-long-chain fatty acids (VLCFAs) for peroxisomal disorders; copper for Menke disease. If the picture includes acute encephalopathy, include glucose, ammonia, acid-base status and organic acids (see Chapter 14). For intractable epilepsy include plasma urate concentration, sulphite dipstick test on a *fresh* urine sample to exclude molybdenum cofactor deficiency.

Neuroimaging studies (see Chapter 7) have revolutionized our approach to neurological disorders with a progressive course and, in particular, the leukodystrophies including two disorders of infancy that present with a slowly progressive megalencephaly combined with irritability, spasticity (sometimes preceded by hypotonia), epileptic seizures and bulbar problems: Alexander disease and Canavan disease (or aspartocyclase deficiency).

Electroencephalography (Chapter 8) and, when available, visually evoked potentials, electroretinogram, nerve conduction studies and electromyogram can greatly narrow the differential diagnosis or help to confirm clinical suspicion when their use is tailored to the clinical presentation.

As children mature and you observe the clinical signs or developmental profile, the emergence of an epilepsy or dystonia may allow investigation to become more focused and specific. Targeted testing may then be performed based on individual patient evaluation and the results of previous tests, including CSF analysis and tissue samples as appropriate. For a guide on clinical presentation and approach to specific investigations on neurodegenerative conditions presenting in infancy, see Table 24.1.

Early regression with prominent seizures

Several conditions present with progressive myoclonic epilepsies in which multiple seizure types, including myoclonic seizures, co-occur with abnormal neurological signs and progressive, although sometimes slow, deterioration. Possible underlying diagnoses include *early infantile neuronal ceroid lipofuscinosis* (NCL) (Table 24.1), *Tay–Sachs or Sandhoff disease* (Table 24.1), *tetrahydrobiopterin (BH4) deficiency* and *progressive neuronal degeneration of childhood* (PNDC). In tetrahydrobiopterin deficiency the epileptic encephalopathy may be associated with extrapyramidal features including hypotonia, dystonia and oculogyric crises. Diagnosis is by CSF biogenic amine and pterin profile, along with a phenylalanine challenge. Treatment is with L-DOPA, and biotin, possibly with phenylalanine dietary restriction. PNDC, also known as Alpers disease or Huttenlocher syndrome, may have onset of clinical problems prior to age 12 months but may not declare itself until the second year. After weeks or months of refractory seizures, epilepsia partialis continuans or other forms of status epilepticus, there is progressive loss of developmental skills. Deranged liver function is suggestive, but may be apparent only late in the illness. In those children in whom a specific underlying defect has been confirmed, nearly all have been mitochondrial cytopathies due to

Table 24.1 The clinical presentation and approach to specific investigations in neurodegenerative conditions presenting in infancy

Condition	Presentation	Clinical course	Neurophysiology	Neurometabolic and genetic investigations
Early infantile neuronal ceroid lipofuscinosis (CLN1, Santavouri–Haltia)	Towards the end of the first year, developmental arrest; infrequent seizures; evolving blindness; movement disorder; microcephaly	Irritability, hypotonia, dystonic spasms	Attenuation then loss of ERG with abnormal VEPs; characteristic EEG response to slow-flicker	Histopathology: skin biopsy shows neuronal granular inclusions on electron microscopy Biochemistry: palmitoyl-protein thioesterase (PPT) assay
Krabbe leukodystrophy (common infantile form)	In the first months of life: severe irritability, dystonia, spasticity with excess of extensor tone; developmental impairment	Regression progresses, especially with febrile illnesses; distressing dystonia, decerebration by 1 year, loss of reflexes, decreased visual awareness	Slow peripheral nerve-conduction velocities	Histopathology: needle-like inclusion bodies in macrophages; demyelination on nerve biopsy; foamy histiocytes Biochemistry: raised CSF protein; WCE analysis: low levels of galactocerebrosidase, beta-galactosidase
Tay-Sachs disease (classic infantile GM2 gangliosidosis)	4–6 months, motor weakness, visual failure; excessive startle to sound; macular degeneration and cherry red spot in some	Rapidly progressive hypotonia, seizures by 6 months (frequent myoclonus), blind by 1 year, death in 4 years Macrocephaly from year 2	EEG initially unremarkable, becomes very abnormal; VEPs abolished by 18 months; ERG normal	Neuroimaging: white-matter abnormalities Biochemistry: low levels of hexosaminidase A

Table 24.1 Continued

Condition	Presentation	Clinical course	Neurophysiology	Neurometabolic and genetic investigations
Pelizaeus–Merzbacher disease	Dysmyelinating disorder of white matter Classical and connatal (more severe) forms are distinguished by rate of progression, with considerable phenotypic overlap	Early infancy: pendular nystagmus, spastic paraparesis and movement disorder (usually dystonia) Stridor in severe forms May be mistaken for cerebral palsy as clinical progression is often slow or very slow		Neuroimaging: hypomyelination of cerebral white matter Genetics: (X-linked); mutation in the *PLP* gene (75%)
Metachromatic leukodystrophy (late infantile; sulphatide lipidosis)	18 months; regression, flaccid limb paresis with depression or loss of reflexes (peripheral neuropathy)	Within 3–6 months hypertonia, optic atrophy, decerebration and decorticate posturing; death by 8–10 years	Slow nerve conduction; abnormal VEPs and SSEPs	Neuroimaging: MRI shows symmetrical demyelination (typically frontal and occipital horns) Histcpathology: metachromatic sulphatides in nerves WCE: low levels of arylsulphatase A; raised CSF protein

Infantile neuroaxonal dystrophy (INAD*; Seitelberger disease)	Hypotonic infant with decreased limb reflexes	Evolution of progressive spasticity and dystonia; opisthotonic posturing; optic atrophy; death by 5 years	EMG shows anterior horn cell disease and denervation (nerve conduction studies normal) BAEPs, SSEPs and VEPs progressively worsen; normal ERG	Autosomal recessive: PLA2G6 molecular genetic testing Histopathology: axonal spheroids on axillary skin biopsy MRI shows diffuse cerebellar hyperintensity and atrophy ± iron deposition in basal ganglia
HIV-associated progressive encephalopathy	A developmental plateau appears with later neurological and general cognitive regression.	There is evolution of corticospinal tract signs, hypokinesis and evolving dysphagia with feeding difficulties		Raised CSF protein (60%) and IgG (80%); usually no cells (mononuclear cells in 25%); HIV antibodies detected MRI: hyperintense lesions are noted in the periventricular white matter and centrum semiovale on T2-weighted images These lesions are often patchy in the early stages becoming more diffuse with disease progression.

*INAD is now regarded as a form of neurodegeneration with brain iron accumulation (NBIA). BAEP, brainstem, auditory evoked potential; EEG, electroencephalography; EMG, electromyography; ERG, electroretinography; MRI, magnetic resonance imaging; SSEP, somatosensory evoked potential; VEP, visual evoked potential; WCE, white cell enzymes.

mutations in the catalytic subunit necessary for the replication of mitochondrial DNA, called DNA polymerase gamma (*POLG1*), located on chromosome 15.

Inherited disorders of metabolism presenting as progressive disorders

Nonketotic hyperglycinaemia (see Chapter 13) classically presents in the neonatal period with seizures, hiccoughs and burst suppression on electroencephalography (EEG).

Glutaric aciduria type 1 typically presents between 6 and 18 months with an acute encephalopathy and paroxysmal episodes often interpreted as seizures but which are actually involuntary movements. The bouts are often precipitated by mild intercurrent illness. It is a cause of subdural effusions with associated macrocephaly. The condition may be stabilized by special diet.

Late-onset urea cycle disorders typically predominantly present with recurrent encephalopathy associated with hyperammonaemia (see Chapter 14). Take note of any family history of unexplained death in male siblings.

Multiple carboxylase deficiency typically has dermatological features (rash, which may be subtle, and/or alopecia appearing around 3 months of age) as well as seizures and severe developmental impairment.

Neurotransmitter metabolism defects, including disorders of biogenic amine metabolism in which there is failure of synthesis of dopamine, serotonin, norepinephrine, epinephrine or the cofactor tetrahydrobiopterin. Each has a characteristic CSF neurotransmitter profile. They may present with epileptic encephalopathy or myoclonic epilepsy; intestinal dysmotility or feeding difficulties; early developmental impairment; microcephaly, central hypotonia, peripheral hypertonia. Principles of treatment include the replacement of neurotransmitters, in particular a trial of L-DOPA or the administration of a cofactor or precursor such as biotin, pyridoxine or folinic acid.

Other disorders which may mimic neurodegeneration

The *cerebral palsies* are static conditions but their course is not unchanging; they may mimic progressive disorders. Cerebral palsy is also the most common misdiagnosis in the child with progressive loss of skills without epilepsy. See also Chapters 22 and 23. Other possible mimics of degenerative disorders include conditions that may become evident after a period of apparently normal development. Their onset may lead to a slowing or even plateauing of motor, cognitive or social development, often associated with the emergence of seizures, motor signs and involuntary movements. Nonetheless their course may be stabilized and become static, particularly if appropriate treatment is offered.

Mitochondrial disorders: Leigh syndrome is clinically heterogeneous, but the onset is often in infancy with brainstem involvement (clinically apparent as loss of saccadic eye movement and sighing or sobbing respiration) plus a motor disorder (pyramidal and/

or extrapyramidal). Stepwise deterioration, sometimes precipitated by intercurrent illness, is characteristic; occasionally a long period of stability can lead to misdiagnosis of cerebral palsy that is corrected when the disease leads to further regression. Neuroimaging shows involvement of the brainstem and basal ganglia. As specific laboratory confirmation of diagnosis becomes available in a higher proportion of cases (e.g. in cases of mutations in POLG1; see section covering progressive myoclonic epilepsies, above), it is clear that the range of mitochondrial disorders in infancy is wide and may not correspond to an obvious textbook disease category and should be considered in progressive unexplained neurological disorders, especially poliodystrophies (i.e. those affecting grey matter).

Acute necrotizing encephalopathy (ANE) is an even rarer, dominantly inherited, condition (see Chapter 14). Like Leigh syndrome, ANE has acute deteriorations with intercurrent illness and radiology that is superficially similar to Leigh syndrome. Involvement of the external capsule and brainstem is seen in ANE but atypical for Leigh syndrome. Either may be misdiagnosed as an acute acquired encephalopathy. The importance of ANE lies in identifying pre-symptomatic first-degree relatives who can benefit from immunization and prophylactic antibiotics to reduce the risk of acute deterioration.

Rett syndrome affects female infants only (see Chapter 20). After appearing to be initially normal, there is regression of functional hand movement between ages of 6 and 18 months along with sleep disturbance and agitation, and acquired microcephaly. There follows the evolution of severe cognitive impairment, stereotyped hand movements, progressive deterioration of gait, scoliosis, seizures and non-epileptic 'vacant spells'. Respiratory rhythm disturbances including hyperventilation and respiratory pauses usually evolve after infancy. Identified genetic mutations include the methyl-CpG-binding protein 2 (*MECP2*) gene (85%) and, less commonly, cyclin-dependent kinase-like 5 (*CDKL5*).

Rare static disorders with severe epilepsy and developmental impairment

3-Phosphoglycerate dehydrogenase deficiency presents with microcephaly, severe early developmental impairment, intractable epilepsy and a severely abnormal EEG. Magnetic resonance imaging shows a reduction in white matter.

Guanidinoacetate methyltransferase (GAMT) *deficiency* presents with intractable epilepsy, early developmental impairment and an extrapyramidal movement disorder. Suspect this condition where there is a low plasma creatinine although this finding may sometimes be a non-pathological reflection of reduced muscle mass in a small infant. Additional laboratory evidence for this condition comes from the demonstration of low urine creatinine/calcium and creatinine/protein ratios. Brain MRS shows an absent creatine peak. The condition may improve with creatine administration.

Progressive encephalopathy, peripheral oedema, hypsarrhythmia and optic atrophy (PEHO) is a recessive condition with hypsarrhythmia and optic atrophy. Magnetic resonance imaging shows atrophy of the temporal lobes and atrophy of the cerebellar folia.

Management of neurodegenerative conditions

Palliation
There are some issues common to all; palliative interventions may be non-specific or disease-specific. They should include an explanation to parents of the condition involved, in terms they can understand (see Chapter 21).

Common attendant problems and treatment include the following:

- feeding difficulties (often requiring nasogastric feeds as the condition progresses; gastrostomy may or may not be appropriate);
- sleeplessness (use of melatonin or sedation);
- distressing irritability (morphine can help);
- seizure control which can be very difficult. Benzodiazepines are good for myoclonus and clonazepam may also help control distressing dystonia. When the standard approach does not help, consider using phenobarbitone in high doses; and
- spasticity and dystonia. Benzodiazepines can relieve and are a good choice when epilepsy is also a feature.

Community support networks or a *hospice movement* can be called on to help support the family and the family should be encouraged to express their wishes on whether they would prefer the death of the child to take place at home, in hospital or in a hospice. The emphasis should always be on a good palliative approach for the child, and easing distress which, in turn will ease distress for the family as a whole.

Prenatal screening is possible for several disorders such as lysosomal storage diseases and peroxisomal disorder wherever there is a neurometabolic or neurogenetic marker. Where parents wish to pursue this the result offers important information and choices. Pre-test counselling is an important part of this process.

Interventions that modify the underlying disease process
These again may be non-specific or disease-specific. Detailed consideration is beyond the scope of this book but general principles are:

- reducing the metabolic load on the affected pathway (e.g. dietary manipulation);
- correcting product deficiency (e.g. biotin in biotinidase deficiency);
- decreasing metabolite toxicity (e.g. sodium benzoate and sodium phenylbutyrate in hyperammonaemia; L-carnitine in organic acidaemias; substrate reduction therapy used with some success in animal models of Tay–Sachs disease);
- stimulating residual enzymes, with cofactors;
- pharmacological enzyme replacement (e.g. glucocerebrosidase for Gaucher type III). This and other enzymes are targeted for uptake by the mannose-6-phosphate receptor system present on the surface of nearly all cells, which facilitates their

entry. The blood/brain barrier still offers the greatest hindrance to progress with many enzymes; and

- transplantation/gene therapy. Cell-mediated therapy brings significant improvement in central nervous system pathology in the lysosomal storage diseases largely through release of enzymes by transplanted cells for uptake by deficient cells. This can be enhanced through gene overexpression and the use of receptor-mediated uptake systems. Direct implantation of cells and the use of bone marrow transplant to deliver microglial/brain macrophage precursors to the central nervous system have resulted in improvement in animal models. Neural progenitor cells coupled with enzyme overexpression show promise and but do not yet have any place in clinical practice.

Resources

Aicardi J. *Diseases of the nervous system in childhood*. London, Mac Keith Press, 2009.

King MD, Stephenson JBP. *A handbook of neurological investigations in children*. London, Mac Keith Press, 2009.

Appendix 1: Growth charts

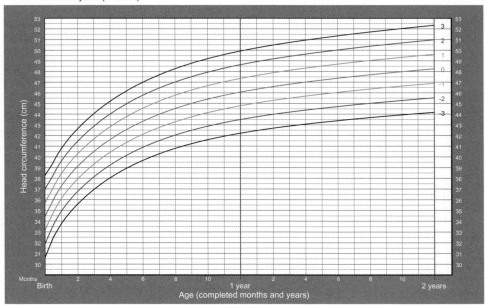

Head circumference-for-age BOYS
Birth to 2 years (z-scores)

World Health
Organization

Head circumference (cm)

53
52
51
50
49
48
47
46
45
44
43
42
41
40
39
38
37
36
35
34
33
32
31
30

3
2
1
0
-1
-2
-3

Months
Birth   2   4   6   8   10   1 year   2   4   6   8   10   2 years
Age (completed months and years)

WHO Child Growth Standards

340

Head circumference-for-age GIRLS
Birth to 2 years (z-scores)

World Health Organization

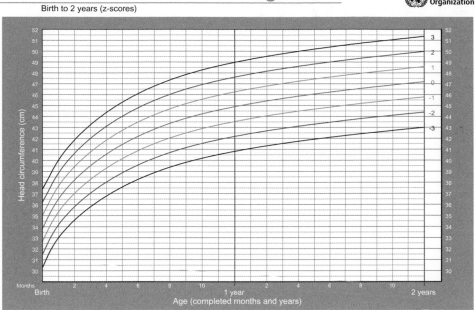

WHO Child Growth Standards

Length-for-age BOYS
Birth to 2 years (z-scores)

World Health Organization

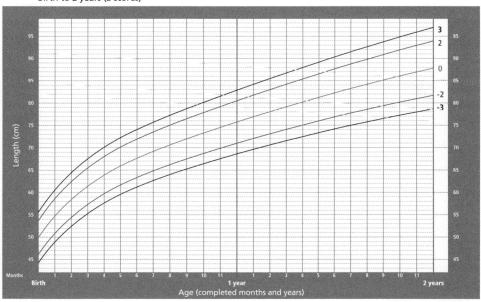

WHO Child Growth Standards

Length-for-age GIRLS
Birth to 2 years (z-scores)

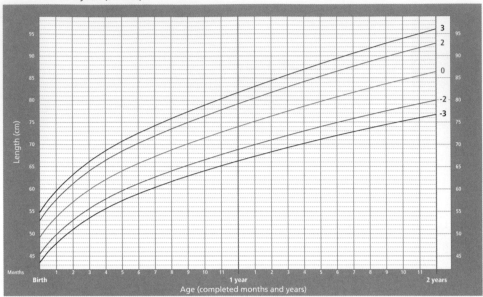

WHO Child Growth Standards

Weight-for-age BOYS
Birth to 2 years (z-scores)

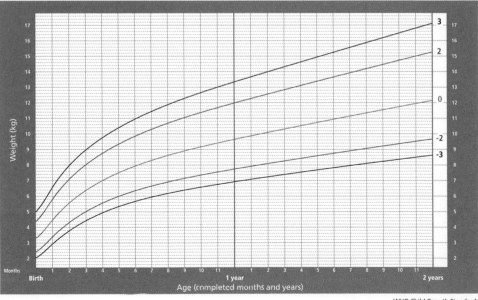

WHO Child Growth Standards

Weight-for-age GIRLS
Birth to 2 years (z-scores)

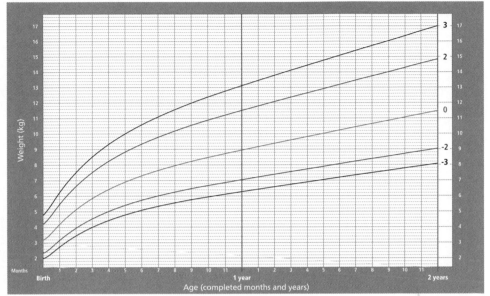

WHO Child Growth Standards

Index

Index

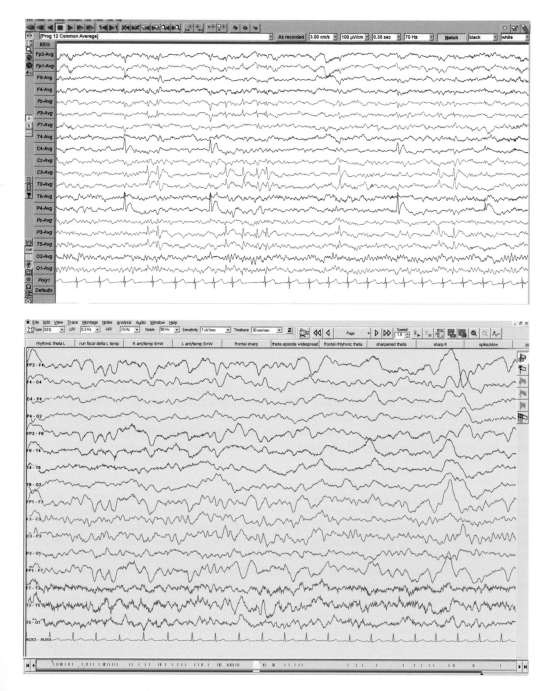

Plate 1 (Figure 14.5, see page 201) Electroencephalography. Top: bilateral independent discharges, occurring in typical doublets (and a quadruplet) on the left, typical of benign Rolandic epilepsy, in a child presenting with a persistent, but ultimately reversible, hemiparesis. Bottom: unilateral slowing on electroencephalography in a child with familial hemiplegic migraine and a calcium-channel gene mutation.

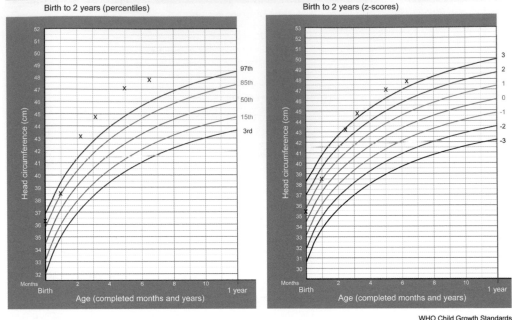

Birth to 2 years (percentiles)

Birth to 2 years (z-scores)

Head circumference (cm)

Age (completed months and years)

WHO Child Growth Standards

Plate 2 (Figure 18.3, see page 258) Trajectory of head growth from birth in a well male infant whose father and paternal grandfather had OFCs of 60.0 and 62.0 cm. At the time of the most recent measurement he was sitting alone, passing objects from hand to hand and babbling communicatively. The two charts are based on identical data plotted against (a) centiles and (b) z scores. This shows how perception of the need to take action might be influenced by the specifics of chart construction.

Plate 3 (Figure 22.1a, b, see pages 309, 310) The first figure plots motor performance on y axis against age in years on x-axis. The five curves shown correspond to the five levels (I–V) of the GMFCS (Russell et al., 2003; Palisano et al., 2008). A careful history and repeated clinical assessments provide the basis for estimating the likely trajectory and brain imaging within the first two years will provide additional information. The graph provides parents, caregivers and the multidisciplinary team with a vehicle for discussion of management options for the individual child and a means of visualizing the projected future course of the child's motor development. The basal green curve represents therapist input to which orthoses/aids (bright green), oral medication (yellow), botulinum toxin (orange), intrathecal baclofen (red) and orthopaedic surgery (blue) can be added as necessary. The thickness of the lines A to D indicates an approximation to the percentage (0–25%, 25–50%, 50–75%, 75–100% respectively) of patients having the need for each type of therapy with a broken line indicating an intermittent requirement. The second figure gives the indications, principles and summary of limitations of the different treatment options indicated by the different coloured lines in the first Figure, illustrated by examples. Indications for selective dorsal rhizotomy are not shown. For each treatment, the potential for benefit has to be weighed against the limitations.

These figures can be downloaded from Heinen et al., 2010, supplementary data, *European Journal of Paediatric Neurology.*

CP GRAPH TREATMENT MODALITIES-GROSS MOTOR FUNCTION

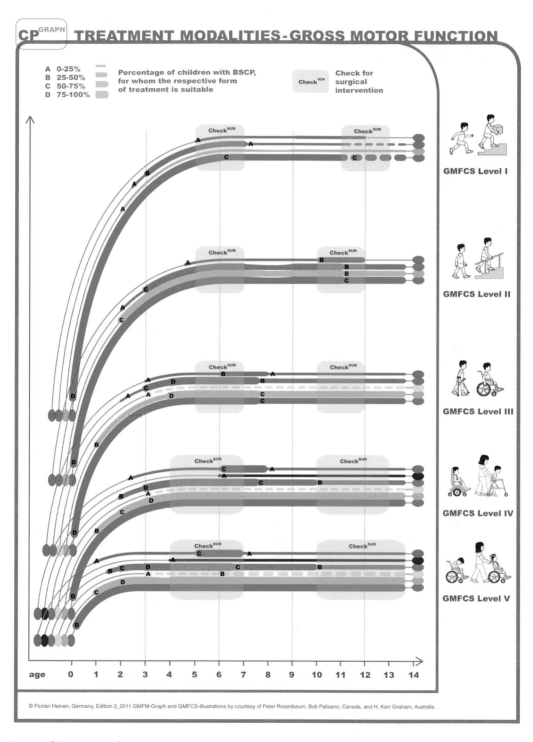

A 0-25%
B 25-50%
C 50-75%
D 75-100%

Percentage of children with BSCP, for whom the respective form of treatment is suitable

Check^SUR — Check for surgical intervention

GMFCS Level I
GMFCS Level II
GMFCS Level III
GMFCS Level IV
GMFCS Level V

age 0 1 2 3 4 5 6 7 8 9 10 11 12 13 14

Plate 3 (Figure 22.1a)

INDICATION, PRINCIPLE & LIMITATION

Orthopaedic surgery

- Treatment indication: Established for each level of severity. Surgical intervention: The higher the GMFCS level, the earlier it should be considered.
- Aim: Correction of spasticity-induced structural misalignments involving one or more joints (multilevel) to prevent secondary bone deformities. In the case of irreversible bone deformities: Reconstruction for functional improvement or to facilitate care and ameliorate secondary injuries.
- Principle: The experienced paediatric orthopaedic surgeon is the key-member of the decision making team.
- Limitations/controversies: Irreversibility, morbidity, repeat surgery, lack of evidence.

Intrathecal baclofen

- Treatment indication: Starting with higher GMFCS-Levels (III) - IV, - V.
- Aim: Reduction of spasticity to enhance quality of life - extent of side effects and complications depend on the experience of the centre. Functional improvement: Improved ability to sit up, increased mobility, orthosis tolerance. Improved quality of life: Simplified care, pain relief, improved sleep, lower sedative doses, weight gain. Prophylaxis: Contractures, hip (sub-) luxations, scoliosis.
- Principle: Agonist of the inhibiting neurotransmitter GABA-B: Modulation at spinal circuits. Intrathecal administration with programmable drug pump via a spinal catheter enables effective treatment using 100 to 1000 times lower doses than with oral administration.
- Limitations/controversies: Technical complications, infection. Possible negative influence on scoliosis.

Botulinum Toxin

- Treatment indication: Established for each level of severity.
- Aim: Correction of dynamic spastic misalignments over one or more joints (multilevel).
- Principle: Local inhibition of acetylcholine release as messenger for the motor end plates and muscle spindles, and hence reduction in tone of injected muscle (dose-dependent). Reduction in muscle strength of approx. 20%. Duration of effect approx. 3-6 months (or more). Adherence of 1/2 to2/3 of patients, treatment will be renewed 1 (-3) times a year.
- Examples: GMFCS I-III: Functional indication: Reduction in muscular hypertonia, and hence prevention of imbalance between flexors and extensors given (still) passively correctable or repositionable deformities in the legs or arms. Structural indication: Delay in development of contractures, improved orthosis tolerance. GMFCS IV-V: Functional indication: Rarely, possibly improved operation of accessories. Structural indication: Reduced pain, simplified care, improved orthosis tolerance. Reduced salivation.
- Limitations/controversies: Focal treatment for non-focal disease, potential for distant action and systemic action of substance, only acts in active dynamic muscle. Action in muscle and its control circuits only partially understood. Ongoing discussion on labeling, please see[1] for update information.

Oral medication

- Treatment indication: Rare, time-constrained treatment option for higher levels of severity starting with GMFCS IV (rarely III), e.g., benzodiazepine, oral baclofen (if intrathecal baclofen treatment is contraindicated), etc.
- Aim: Tone reduction, e.g., to relieve pain, facilitate positioning and care, bridge treatment in acute situations.
- Principle: Reduction in spasticity/GABAergic action.
- Limitations/controversies: Cognitive side effects/sedation, development of tolerance.

Orthoses/aids

- Treatment indication: depending on more national standards, interdisciplinary, continuous cooperation with experienced paediatric orthopaedic surgeons and (paediatric) orthotists.
- Aim: improvements in function and participation, prevention and/or reduction in muscle contraction (contracture formation and bone deformities) to minimize surgery.
- Principle: Extremities: Functional improvement and maintenance via maximum utilization of functional reserves. Trunk: Propping up through stabilization and trunk support.
- Limitations/controversies: Lack of evidence, Compliance and adherence, no international standards, variability of concepts even on national level between treatment centers.

Functional therapies

- Treatment indication: Concomitant treatment by a qualified therapist.
- Aim: Assist motor development, handling instruction, to avoid development of joint misalignments caused by spasticity.
- Principle: Problem-related focus of treatment depending on the severity of the disease: Define objective, repeat targeted, functional exercises, document changes. Muscle activation immediately after botulinum toxin treatment and subsequent strengthening of paretic, non-injected musculature. Conversion of change in muscular equilibrium (between agonists and antagonists) in everyday life toward functional objectives/participation. Treatment breaks (to avoid compliance loss) as reward for achievement of treatment objective.
- Limitations/controversies: lack of evidence, concept is only partly based on scientific foundation, bias to tradition and ideologies.

1: European Medicines Agency (EMEA: www.wmwa.europe.eu), The German Federal Institute for Drugs and Medical Devices (BfArM: http://www.bfarm.de), Swiss Agency for Therapeutic Products (Swissmedic: www.swissmedic.ch), Food and Drug Administration (FDA: www.fda.gov).

Plate 3 (Figure 22.1b)

Related titles from Mac Keith Press www.mackeith.co.uk

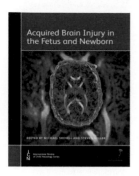

Acquired Brain Injury in the Fetus and Newborn
Michael Shevell and Steven Miller (Eds)

International Review of Child Neurology Series
2012 ▪ 320pp ▪ hardback ▪ 978-1-907655-02-9
£125.00 / €155.00 / $195.00

Given the tremendous advances in the last five years in the
understanding of acquired neonatal brain injury and in the care of
affected newborn infants, this book provides a timely review for the
practising neurologist, neonatologist and paediatrician.
The editors take a pragmatic approach, focusing on specific populations
encountered regularly by the clinician. The contributors, all
internationally recognized clinician scientists, provide the clinician
reader with a state-of-the art review in their area of expertise.

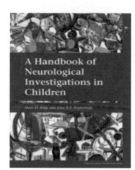

A Handbook of Neurological Investigations in Children
Mary D. King and John B. P. Stephenson

A practical guide from Mac Keith Press
2009 ▪ 400pp ▪ paperback ▪ 978-1-898683-69-8
£39.95 / €48.00 / $73.95

The management and treatment of neurological disorders in children
depend on establishing the diagnosis, which usually requires
investigation, but the number of possible investigations is now very
large indeed. This book sets out the investigations that are really needed
to establish the cause of neurological disorders. Its problem-oriented
approach starts with the patient's presentation, not the diagnosis, with
more than 60 case vignettes to illustrate clinical scenarios.

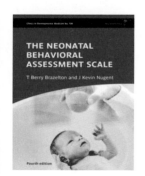

The Neonatal Behavioral Assessment Scale
T. Berry Brazelton and J. Kevin Nugent

Clinics in Developmental Medicine No. 190
2011 ▪ 200pp ▪ hardback ▪ 978-1-907655-03-6
£50.00 / €60.00 / $63.95

The Neonatal Behavioral Assessment Scale (NBAS) is the most
comprehensive examination of newborn behaviour available today and
has been used in clinical and research settings around the world for
more than 35 years. The scale assesses the newborn infant's behavioral
repertoire with 28 behavioral items and also includes an assessment of
the infant's neurological status on 20 items. The NBAS items cover the
following domains of neonatal functioning: autonomic regulation; motor
organization; state organization and regulation and attention/social
interaction.